Harold W. Preiskel
Precision Attachments in Prosthodontics:
The Applications of Intracoronal and Extracoronal Attachments
Volume 1

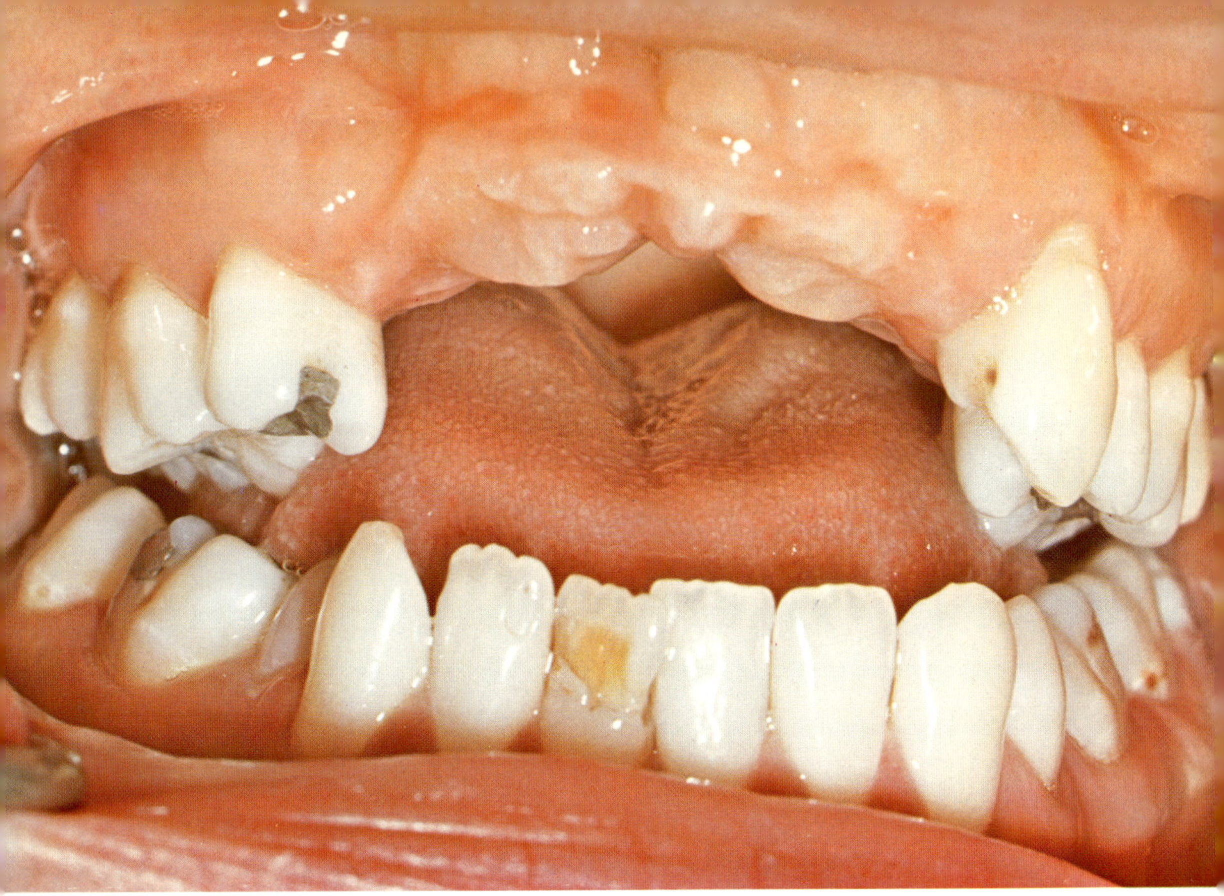

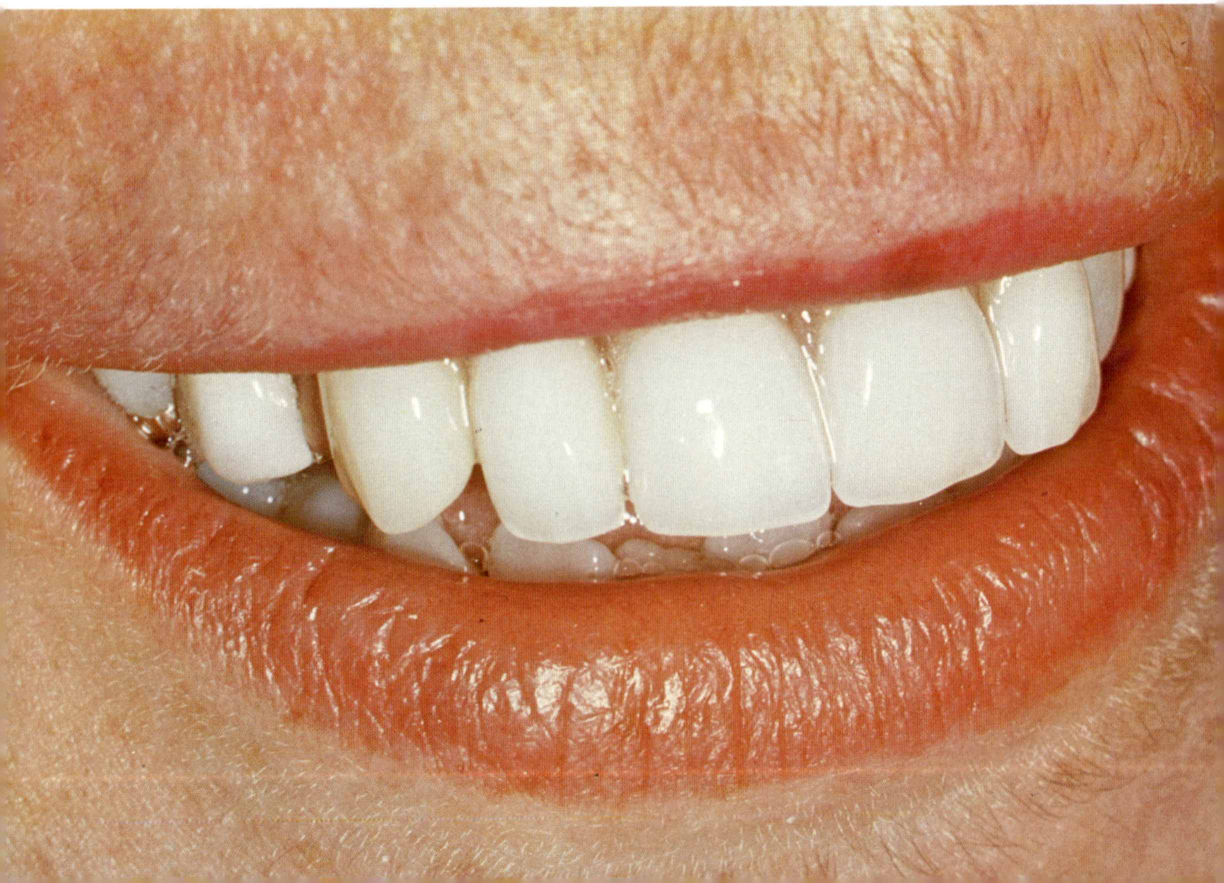

Precision Attachments in Prosthodontics: The Applications of Intracoronal and Extracoronal Attachments

Volume 1

Harold W. Preiskel

M.D.S. (London), M.Sc. (Ohio), F.D.S. R.C.S. (England)
Consultant
Department of Prosthetic Dentistry
The United Medical and Dental Schools
of Guy's and St. Thomas's Hospitals
Guy's Tower, London SE1 9RT

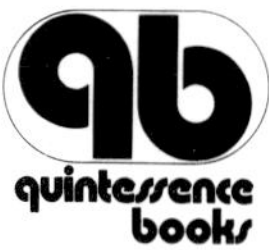

Quintessence Publishing Co., Inc.
Chicago, London, Berlin, Rio de Janeiro and Tokyo   1984

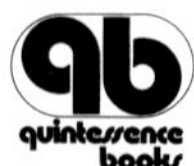

Composition and Printing: Kupijai & Prochnow, Berlin
Binding: Lüderitz & Bauer-GmbH, Berlin
Printed in Germany

ISBN 0-86715-119-6

Contents

3. The Occlusal Surfaces 77

4. Distal Extension Prostheses 95

Contents

Introduction

This work is concerned with the role of attachments in restoring the partially dentate mouth. It is directed to the experienced practitioner, specialist and postgraduate student, although I hope it will be of interest to the advanced undergraduate as well.

Our ever-increasing knowledge of the oral environment, together with the technological improvements of the last few years, have meant that, of necessity, the text is of considerable size and for this reason it has been divided into two volumes. This volume, the first, deals with problems that arise when relatively few teeth are lost. Volume 2: 'Overdentures and Telescopic Prostheses' is concerned with replacement of far more extensive loss of dental tissue.

Colleagues from all over the world have helped to produce this book and have shared with me both their ideas and their experience. Step-by-step guidance of clinical techniques have been given whenever possible, but procedures that are covered in standard undergraduate texts have been omitted in order to save unnecessary expansion. Nevertheless, the reader is referred to these works when necessary.

This is a practical book about a practical subject, but I believe it is important to understand the environment in which one is working and what is being achieved by the clinical procedures undertaken. The clinician needs to be aware not only of the oral environment, but to understand the materials and the technical problems involved in the tasks he is considering. Wherever he practices, today's practitioner requires a broad based education, considerable knowledge and the clinical expertise to carry out the therapy that has been deemed necessary. I hope that this work will assist in meeting these goals.

Harold W. Preiskel
1984
25 Upper Wimpole Street
London W.I

Acknowledgement

I have received so much help and encouragement with the production of this book that it is impossible to thank all concerned by name. Colleagues from several continents have shared their knowledge with me, while the following have kindly lent me illustrations: *Neville Bass*, FDS (Figs. 28, 29, 31–38, 41–47), *Harry Gelfant*, DDS (Figs. 186–188), C. Obreschkov (Figs. 164 [a] [b]) and *William R. Scott*, DDS (Figs. 286–288). My particular thanks to those who have continued to share their most precious secrets—information about their failures. This knowledge has been so helpful in improving our methods of treatment. Mr *J. O. Forrest*, Mrs *Patricia Knightley* and the late Dr *D. Preiskel* have spent many hours correcting the manuscripts, while Drs *Kratochvil, Mensor* and *Scott* have all read parts of the text. Dr *Alex Koper* has made an interesting contribution. Most of the attachment manufacturers have checked the proofs concerning their own products. Many of the restorations illustrated have been constructed with the help of Messrs *Bernard* and *Walter Muhlgay, Paul Portanier, Brian Reardon*, the late *Brian Dance* and other skilled dental technicians.

Mrs *Gillian Lee* has drawn most of the new illustrations and I am grateful for the time and care she has taken over the task.

I would also like to express my thanks to Miss *P. Archer* and to all members of the Medical Illustration Dept at Guy's who have so willingly come to my assistance on many occasions. Miss *J. Hodgkin* and the staff of the Dental Photographic Department have cheerfully carried a heavy burden, while Mr *G. Rytina* and his staff have gone well beyond their normal bounds of duty to help with awkward problems. My thanks are also due to Professor *D. J. Neill* for his cooperation.

My team in the practice have given invaluable help in collecting information and material for the book. It is, of course, thanks to their efforts that we were able to treat the patients from whom the illustrations have been obtained.

Mrs *Elsie Crook* has been a constant source of encouragement in the production of the manuscript, organising the illustrations, and cheerfully carrying a monumental burden.

My wife and family have suffered from my preoccupation with my work on this project and I am grateful for their forbearance.

Finally, my thanks to the publishers, Mr H. W. Haase, Mr Neumann, and all the staff at Quintessence for their attention to detail, their patience and cooperation.

Chapter 1

Treatment Planning and Preliminary Therapy

Humourists have suggested that clinicians who do not like communicating with their patients be directed to careers in forensic or veterinary medicine—yet there is some basis for these jokes. The importance of communication with one's patient was stressed by many of the speakers at the International Prosthodontic Symposium (1982) held in London. Today's practitioners are provided with an ever-improving armamentarium of materials, changing techniques and a better understanding of the oral environment. This makes it all the more important to reconcile what is actually feasible with the patient's own expectations. Without an adequate history and a proper examination this will not be possible. Mutual understanding leads to rapport, an essential commodity for any prosthodontic therapy. To continue therapy without rapport is, in the words of Dr *Samuel Johnson*, 'A triumph of hope over experience'.

Misunderstandings over removable prostheses are notoriously common and can often be tracked down to lack of explanation at an early stage of treatment. Maintenance requirements can sound like an excuse if not explained until they become necessary. This important aspect of treatment needs to be stressed before prosthodontic therapy is commenced.

Relief of pain and other emergency procedures must come first. Before deciding upon making a restoration, or even further preliminary therapy, six important questions must be answered.

1. Is the patient healthy?
2. Is a prosthesis necessary?
3. Is the patient suitable for a prosthesis?
4. How large a space is to be restored?
5. By what structures is the prosthesis to be supported?
6. How is the prosthesis to be made?

Answers to these questions cannot be found by a few polite enquiries and a cursory glance inside the mouth. Nor can any type of examination or planning be carried out in this manner. The examination of the patient is one of the most important aspects of treatment by prosthetic restorations, and it is noticeable that the most experienced operators are those who spend the greatest amount of time on this step. It is also sensible to select a stage in the therapy at which treatment can be discontinued if satisfactory progress has not been made.

Is the patient healthy?

The dental practitioner must be concerned with the general well-being of his patient.

Prosthodontic replacement of missing teeth can hardly have anything but a beneficial effect and many of the procedures can be carried out even upon moderately sick patients, should the need arise.

Should any surgical procedure be required it will have to be considered, together with the attendant type of anaesthesia, in relation to the patient's health and any medical treatment he is receiving. Account must also be taken of the emotional strain involved in the treatment.

Patients with heart disease are probably the most frequently at risk. They may require antibiotic protection against bacterial endocarditis, while others may be on anticoagulant or antihypertensive therapy. It is therefore wise to work in cooperation with the patient's physician. Routine blood pressure evaluation is now being advocated for the age group to which many of these patients belong.

Apart from potential hazards to the patient during the treatment, the dentist must be aware of possible dangers to himself and to other patients. Hepatitis B, also known as serum hepatitis, is diagnosed by detection in the blood of Australia antigen, now called hepatitis B antigen. The incubation period is long, between 6 weeks and 6 months, and the antigen may be present in the blood for 6 weeks or more before the onset of symptoms. The antigen is present in saliva in serum positive patients. The problem is that the virus can be transmitted between a patient and the dental surgeon. It is also possible for a dental surgeon, whose blood group is positive, to infect his patient. There is evidence that the incidence of hepatitis is higher in dentists than in a comparable population of lawyers. Furthermore, at least one report has suggested that transmission by the dentist was responsible for an outbreak of viral hepatitis in a community in the USA.

In order to reduce risk to himself, the dentist should be wary of patients with a history of jaundice, multiple blood transfusions and renal dialysis. Patients who may be drug addicts or male homosexuals also appear to have higher carrier rates.

Infection is spread by the virus in the blood of the patient, bloodstained saliva and, possibly, normal saliva. The common route is by inoculation or accidental abrasion of the skin or mucosa. Since the dentist cannot hope to identify incubating cases, it is prudent to take precautions, such as careful examination of the hands and covering these, wearing eye protectors and a mask. Fortunately, a vaccine is now available that seems a sensible prophylactic measure for health care personnel.

Is a prosthesis necessary?

This is a most important, yet one of the more difficult decisions to be made. Both the patient and his oral conditions require consideration.

A detailed history should be taken, paying particular attention to the reasons for the loss of teeth and, if extractions took place in phases over several years, a record should be made of the sequence in which these were carried out. Should the patient be wearing a partial denture a great deal can be learnt from an assessment of the prosthesis and the patient's reaction to it. If this denture must be replaced, it may still have value, in modified form, as a transitional prosthesis.

The examination should start with a general investigation of the mouth, noting the number and distribution of the remaining teeth together with any apparent discrepancy between centric jaw relation and the centric occlusion of the teeth (see Chapter 3). The individual teeth should naturally be checked for caries. Since all partial prostheses derive support from the periodontal structures, it is important that these tissues should be sound and healthy before the prosthesis is made. It is also essential that the prosthesis be designed carefully to cause only the minimal interference with the periodontal structures. An assessment of the periodontal condition should therefore be made, ensuring that the gingivae are pink, firm and stippled with the gingival margins knife-edged. The crevice should not exceed 1 or 2 mm, and probing should not cause bleeding. If there is evidence of periodontal disease, as is commonly the case, this must be treated before any restorative work is carried out. This treatment always includes bringing the patient's plaque control up to a satisfactory standard. The appearance of the soft tissues, including the floor of the mouth, cheeks and tongue, should be noted.

Even at this early stage, lack of denture space or other problems may become apparent.

The patient's cooperation during this course of treatment may be a useful pointer to the way ahead. If necessary, a halt may be called before patient and operator are involved in unnecessary expenditure.

Two important diagnostic aids are necessary to complete the examination—full-mouth radiographs and mounted diagnostic casts. Full-mouth radiographs should show the level of the alveolar bone around the teeth, the width of the periodontal ligament space and periapical structures, and any retained roots or other pathological structures.

Diagnostic casts should include details of the entire denture-bearing area as well as of the natural teeth, for the shape of these areas plays an important part in the design of the restoration.

A centric relation record will be required. Of the common methods used, the horse-shoe-shaped piece of wax is least likely to give acceptable results. A method recommended by *Dawson* (1974) has now been found simple to employ and gives excellent results. There are many alternative methods, the result not the technique being the important factor. Diagnostic casts of each jaw are made and an occlusal rim made on the upper. Where sufficient teeth are standing, the wax is built across the occlusal surfaces of the premolar and molar teeth and out of contact with the areas representing soft tissues and clear of the upper anterior teeth (Fig. 1). One important feature is to cut the wax back so that it is flush with the buccal cusps. (An extremely hard base wax must be employed, such as Moyco Extra Hard Beauty Wax*.) Three thicknesses of wax is the maximum that should be employed. When it has been adapted it will probably be somewhat thinner.

Before placing the rim in the mouth, only the outer sections are softened. The upper

* J. Bird Moyer Co. Philadelphia PA19132, USA.

teeth are dried so that the record will tend to adhere to them, while the wet lower teeth will separate from the record without dislodging it. The operator is then free to manipulate the jaw with both hands. This technique is described in Chapter 3, p. 83. Once the record has been made, it is cooled with air, removed and chilled in ice water. Care should be taken that no penetration of the wax has occurred. Any excess wax that has flowed over the buccal cusps is cut back with a disposable scalpel blade. The record is now tested again in the mouth and, after subsequent chilling, can be used for mounting the diagnostic casts. The record must fit these casts as it fits the mouth, otherwise it will need to be remade and a new jaw relation made. Since this type of centric relation record must be made at an increased vertical relation of occlusion, a facebow record is essential. The centric relation record should be made at a vertical relation just sufficient to prevent contact of the teeth. *Dawson* (1974) has also described a modification of this technique, useful where mobility patterns are demonstrated in posterior teeth or where patients find it difficult to hold their mandibles still. An anterior stop is made with compound or acrylic resin at the desired vertical relation. This anterior stop will help stabilise the mandible while the record material of choice is setting or hardening.

Where a quadrant of teeth is missing, or insufficient remain to allow an entirely tooth-supported rim to be made, a conventional rim will be required, supported by the mucosa in the edentulous regions. The centric relation record is again made with the natural teeth just separated, and a facebow record is again essential.

It is a pity that adjustable articulators are surrounded with an aura of mystery by some practitioners. Others appear to worship the instrument and regard it as the *raison d'etre* for the treatment, rather than as a tool. Sensibly employed, adjustable articulators simplify treatment. Trying to occlude two hand-held casts is a difficult procedure and the result may be hopelessly inaccurate. If casts are to be mounted on an articulator (Figs. 2 to 4), it takes no longer to mount them on an adjustable one than on a plane-line type. An adjustable articulator allows examination of the casts mounted in positions corresponding with centric relation or centric occlusion (Fig. 5) and, in addition, it enables an assessment to be made of lateral and protrusive excursions that would otherwise have to be carried out by guesswork. Examination of the casts on the articulator allows an assessment to be made of the relationship of palatal and lingual cusps. Looking at the buccal aspect alone can be deceptive (Fig. 6 a, b).

Planning the appearance is also simplified, as the infra-orbital marker of the facebow ensures that the occlusal plane of the casts mounted on the articulator is the same as that in the mouth, when the head is level. There is certainly a place for more complex methods of occlusal analysis employing 'hinge-axis' locating facebows and gnathological articulators that allow more comprehensive adjustments, but not for routine use.

The method outlined for mounting diagnostic casts is a compromise. It is simple and quick to use and provides an accuracy that will match the jaw relation records that most operators can obtain. No articulator can be more accurate than the records

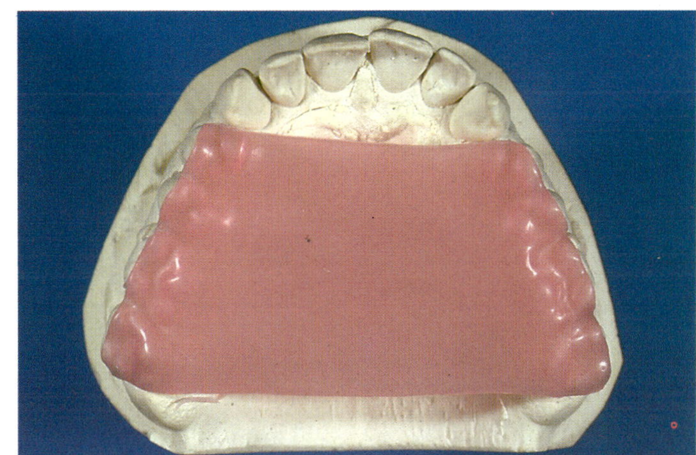

Fig. 1 Where sufficient teeth are standing, the wax rim is built across the occlusal surfaces of the premolar and molar teeth, out of contact with areas representing soft tissues.

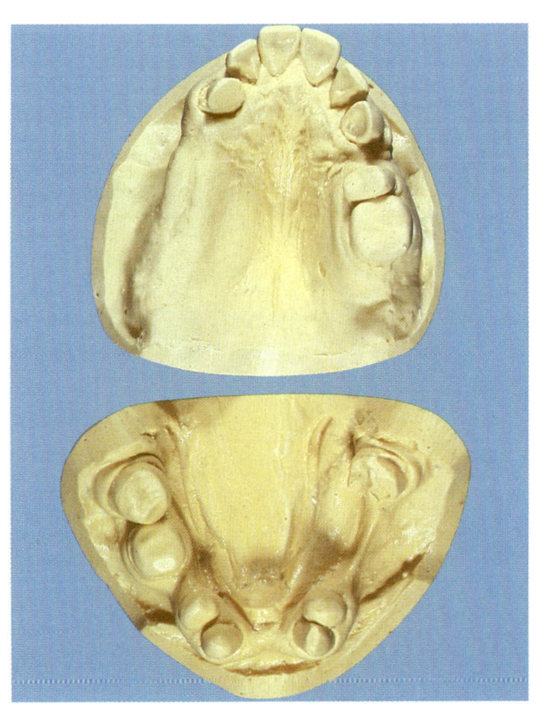

Fig. 2 Upper and lower diagnostic casts. Their value for treatment planning is greatly increased if they are mounted on an adjustable articulator.

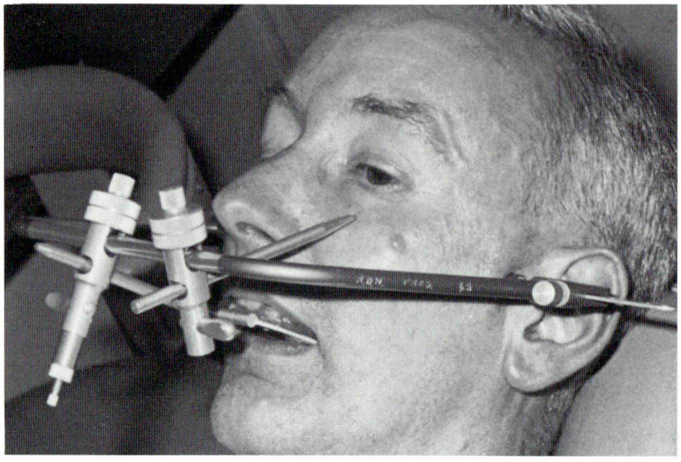

Fig. 3 Dentatus facebow record with the infra-orbital marker in position.

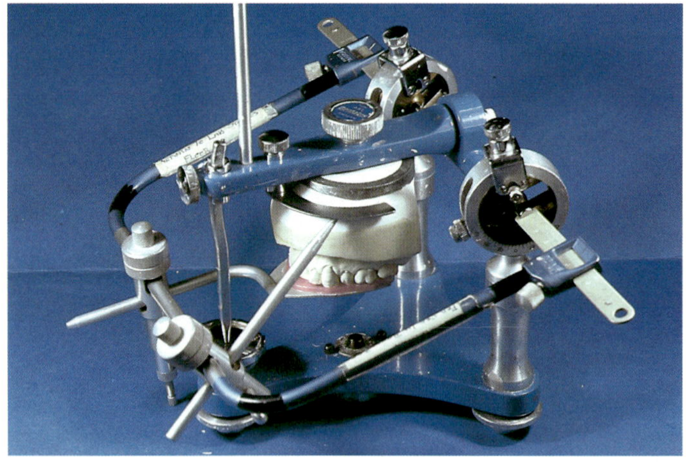

Fig. 4 An upper cast mounted on articulator by means of facebow record.

used in it. However, of the various jaw relations made, by far the most important is that of centric relation.

Why make a prosthesis?

A prosthesis may be required to restore appearance and speech, to improve chewing, or to spread occlusal load over a wider area. It may also be used to correct the occlusion of natural teeth. Constructing a restoration may prevent migration of teeth adjacent to a space, or overeruption of the opposing teeth. A restoration may also help prevent the development of abnormal speech habits or jaw postures.

On the other hand, construction of a prosthesis is time-consuming, it may require tooth preparation and will probably involve coverage of some of the gingival margins and mucosa. Wearing a prosthesis makes good plaque control

Fig. 5 The casts mounted on the articulator. A thorough examination of the occlusion can now be made, and the difficulties of restorative procedures assessed.

Fig. 6(a) Examination of the occlusion and articulation from the buccal aspect alone can be deceptive.

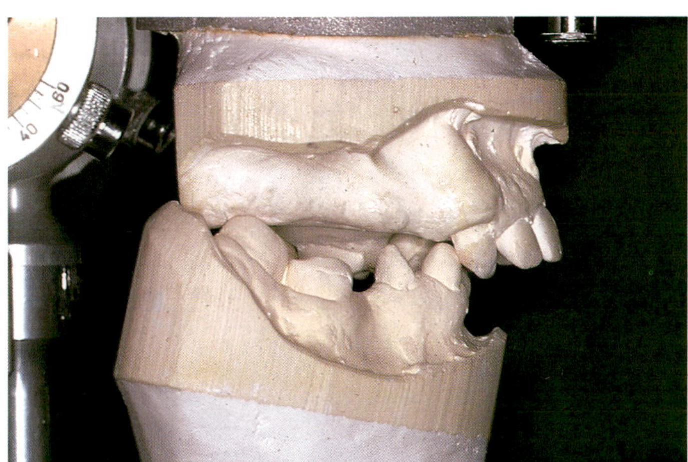

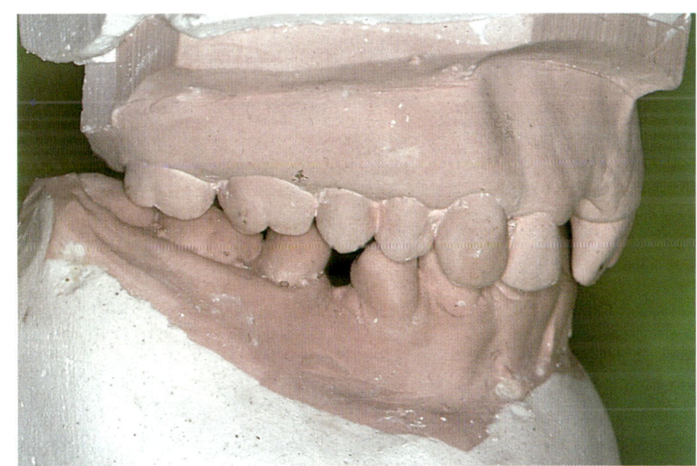

Figure 6 a

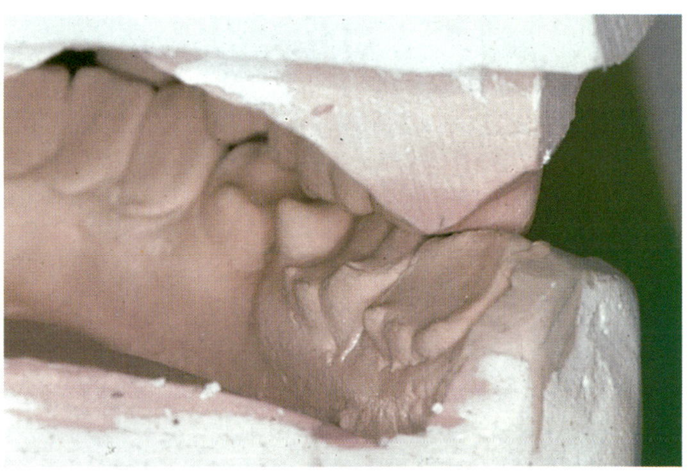

Figure 6 b

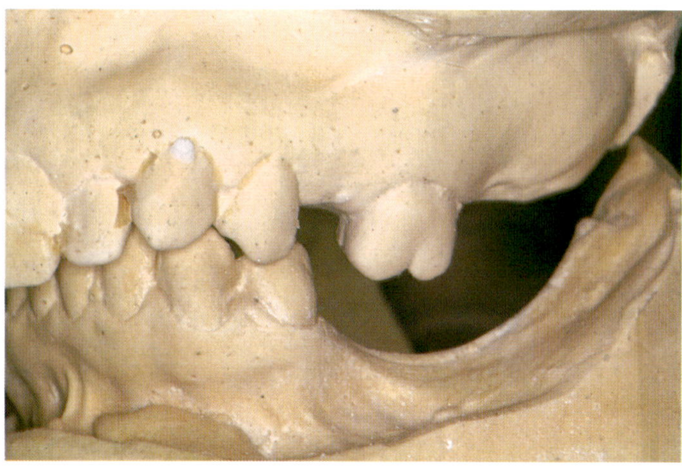

Fig. 7   Examination of the opposing occlusal surfaces is essential to enable reshaping to be planned.

imperative, while the prosthesis itself will require periodic inspection. The only firm rule to guide the operator in his decision is to ensure that he is in possession of all the facts.

How large a space is to be restored?

The span of the restoration is the key to the treatment plan. It determines the work the prosthesis will do, as well as the loads to which the prosthesis and the structures supporting it will be subjected. Articulated diagnostic casts are necessary when making this decision, and their value is enhanced if lateral and protrusive records have been made. It is important to realise that with most articulators these records are only accurate at the particular positions in which the records have been made. Intermediate positions are an approximation. Wear facets on the remaining teeth are a useful guide to the

magnitude and direction of forces that may be applied to the prosthesis. After careful analysis of the diagnostic casts, it is surprising how often a decision is made not to construct a restoration. If a prosthesis is justified, the opposing occlusal surfaces should be examined and a note made of any reshaping required (Fig. 7).

Overeruption of opposing teeth can usually be corrected by grinding, which should be planned at this stage. The occlusal surfaces of the adjusted teeth must not be widened by these procedures and it may be necessary to place restorations on these teeth. The time to make the decision is at the beginning of the treatment.

Typical spaces to be restored are anterior or posterior gaps bounded by natural teeth, or spaces with no distal abutment. If the prosthesis chosen requires prefabricated attachments, these should be selected and measured against the teeth on the diagnostic casts before any tooth preparation is carried out. It is easy to misjudge the space (especially vertical space)

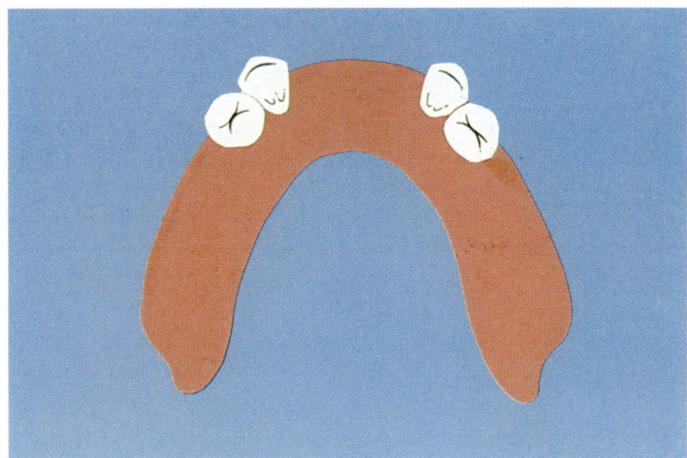

Fig. 8 A typical situation favouring a combined lower anterior fixed prosthesis and a removable bilateral distal extension denture.

required for an attachment, and it is important to discover any error as early as possible so that either the treatment plan can be changed or another attachment substituted.

Frequently, several gaps are found in one jaw. They may be restored with one prosthesis, such as a partial denture, one or more fixed prostheses, or a combination of fixed and removable restorations. Such a combination may be used where there is an anterior gap and bilateral posterior distal spaces (Fig. 8).

A partial denture restoring all these gaps would have a tendency to rotate about the abutment teeth (Fig. 9). A better approach is to construct a fixed prosthesis for the anterior teeth (Fig. 10). The posterior spaces can then be restored with a bilateral distal extension partial denture that can be clasp-retained (Fig. 11 a), or attachment-retained (Fig. 11 b).

Combined restorations of this nature frequently result in problems with the articulation, particularly when opposed to a complete denture. The development of a balanced articulation is important if the stability of the complete denture is to be ensured. It is tempting to complete the construction of the fixed restoration first before considering the dentures. However, it may then be quite impossible to produce the arrangement of the teeth and compensating curves required for a balanced articulation. The fixed restoration determines the vertical relation of occlusion, the occlusal plane, and the position of the anterior teeth. A trial insertion is necessary to determine the position of all the teeth before the denture framework is made.

By what structures is the prosthesis to be supported?

Once the decision has been made to restore a space, the manner in which the prosthesis will be supported against

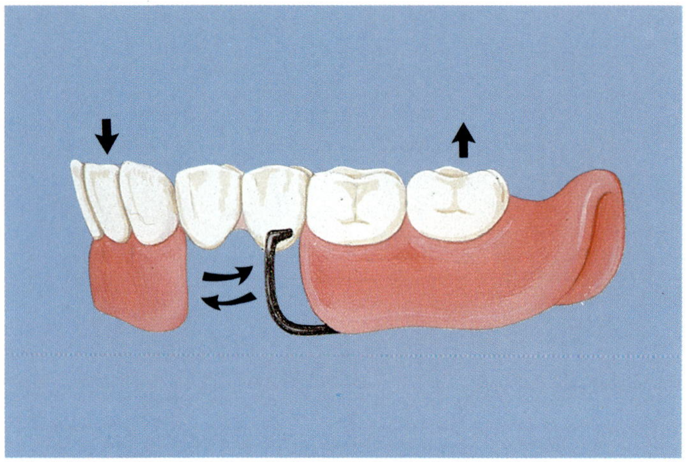

Fig. 9 A partial denture restoring all these gaps has a tendency to rotate about the abutment teeth.

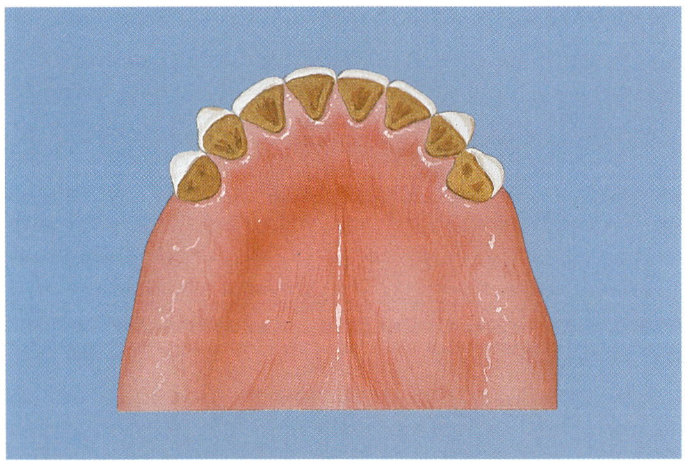

Fig. 10 A fixed prosthesis restoring the anterior space splints both groups of abutments.

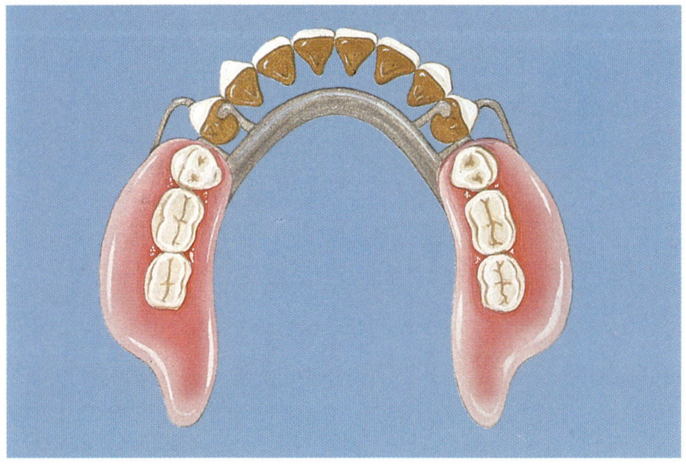

Fig. 11 (a) The distal extension clasp-retained removable partial denture made in conjunction with an anterior fixed prosthesis.

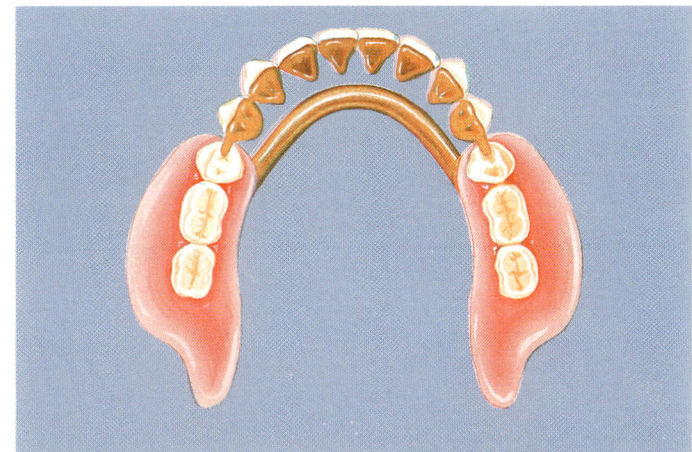

Fig. 11(b) An attachment-retained denture made in conjunction with the anterior restoration.

Fig. 12 (a) (b) A fixed prosthesis is normally the restoration of choice for replacing missing anterior teeth.

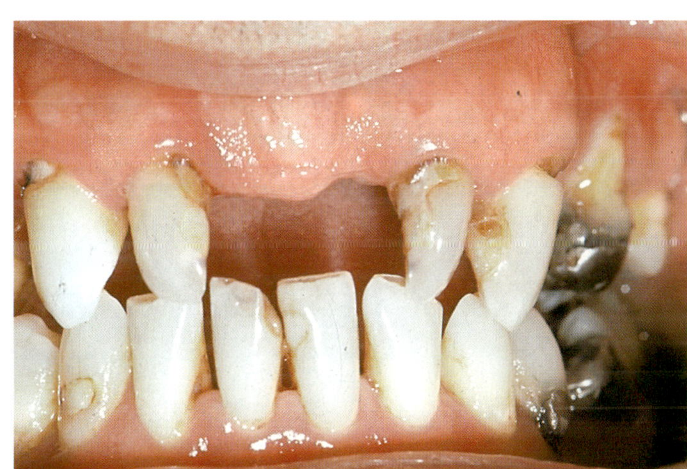

Figure 12 a

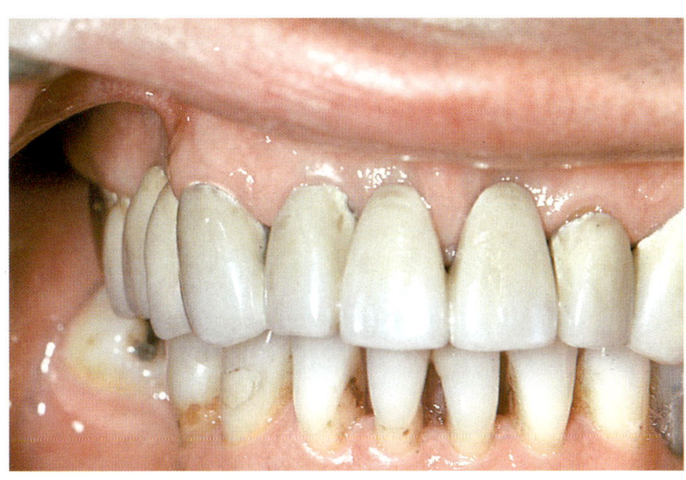

Figure 12 b

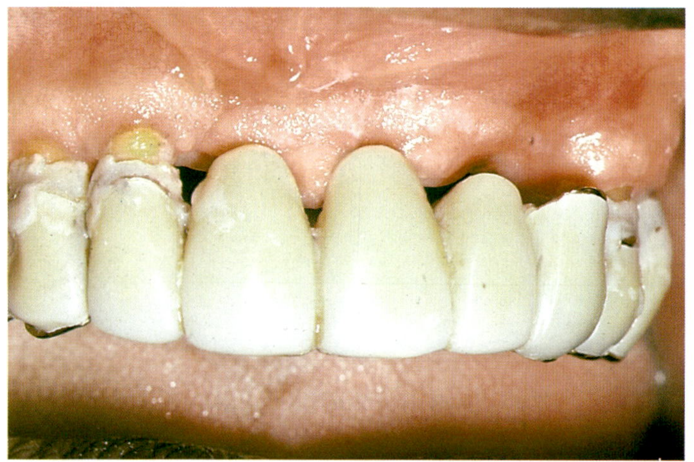

Fig. 13 Note bone loss in canine region following root removal from this fixed prosthesis. This loss will dictate a removable replacement prosthesis if the canine eminence is to be restored.

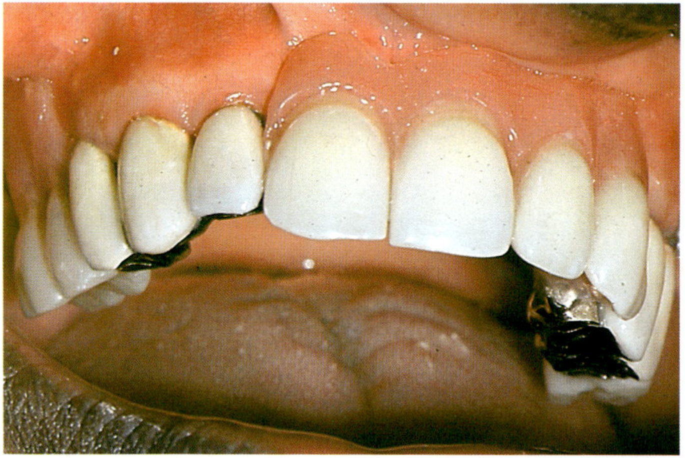

Fig. 14 (a) Edentulous span restored with a removable prosthesis.

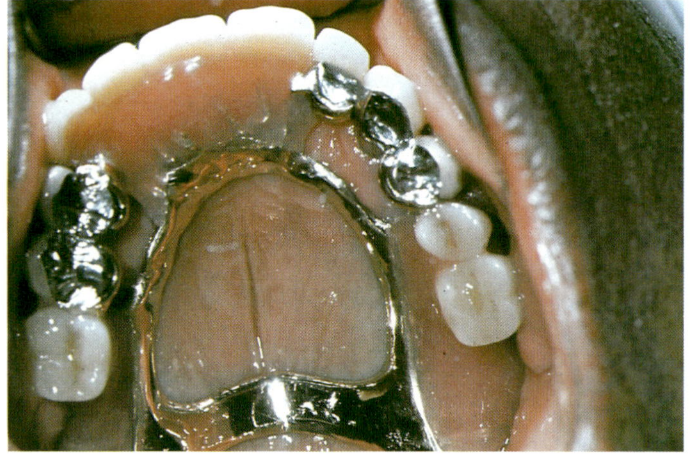

Fig. 14 (b) Occlusal view to show lip support.

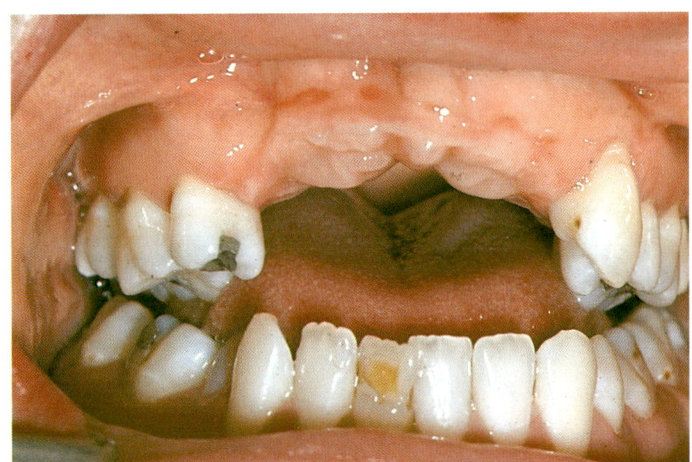

Fig. 15 Replacing extensive bone loss and long edentulous spans requires the use of a removable prosthesis. The denture base will provide mucosal support and allows correct placement of the anterior teeth.

vertical and horizontal forces must be planned.

If the restoration can be tooth-supported, the fixed prosthesis should be considered. The fixed prosthesis is normally the restoration of choice for missing anterior teeth (Fig. 12 a, b), or for small bounded spaces elsewhere.

Contraindications for fixed prostheses

Fixed restorations are neat, usually good-looking and preferred by most patients. Nevertheless their applications cannot be universal.

Aesthetics

Vertical loss of edentulous ridge structure can result in the need to make pontic teeth almost twice the length of the abutment crowns. This is particularly unsightly in the anterior region (Fig. 13). The problem is overcome once artificial mucosa is incorporated, but plaque control considerations normally dictate a removable restoration. Artificial mucosa is also important where there has been bone loss labio-palatally in the maxilla. A common mistake is to place the pontic teeth directly over the crest of the edentulous ridge, despite the fact that they are now grossly palatal to the teeth they replace. The result is the destruction of labial support. In order to provide the necessary lip support, the artificial teeth must, in these instances, be placed labial to the crest of the ridge. A removable prosthesis gives excellent results in these circumstances (Fig. 14 a, b). It is true that detachable labial flanges can be made on occasions, but only at the expense of considerable complication and space. Preprosthetic surgery involving ridge augmentation techniques have shown promise in overcoming problems of this type (*Siebert* 1981), but 5-year results are not presently available.

Removable restorations allow considerable versatility with the arrangement of artificial teeth. Spaces and other irregular-

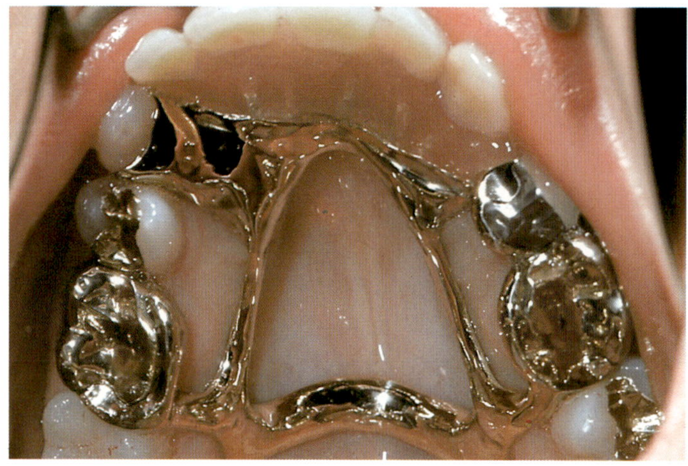

Fig. 16   Restoration in place following mucogingival surgery.

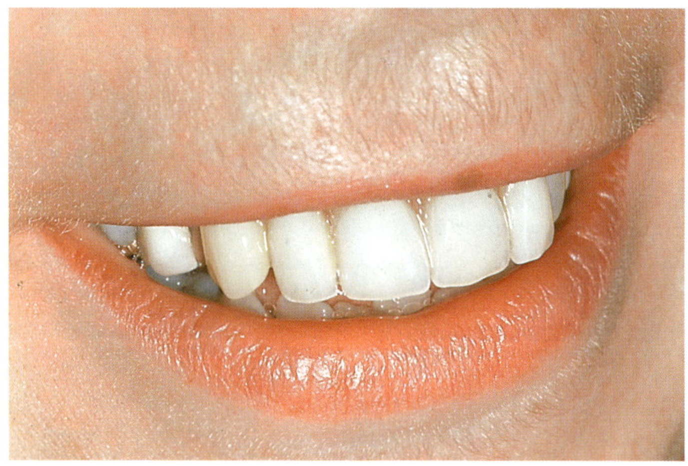

Fig. 17   Note labial support, particularly to margin of lip. Artificial mucosa is essential to allow correct positioning of anterior teeth.

ities of placement are easily incorporated.

Support

If the extent of the restoration is too great for the abutment teeth, additional support will be required from the mucosa (Fig. 15). This effectively precludes making a fixed prosthesis.

Cost and complexity

Removable prostheses can be simple, and transitional restorations of this type can be rapidly produced. However, bearing in mind the problems of the denture abutment interface, some removable prostheses are far from straightforward. For restoring multiple spaces in one jaw the partial denture has obvious advantages. Furthermore, correct lip support and tooth placement are simplified (Figs. 16 and 17). Where splinting across the edentulous

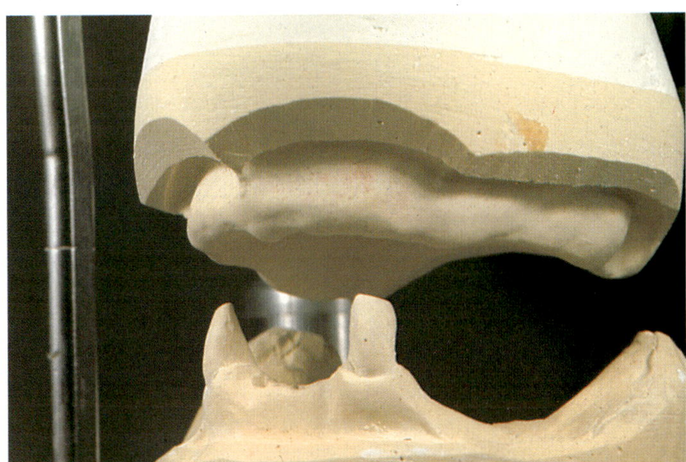

Fig. 18 Vertical space available is the key to planning overdentures.

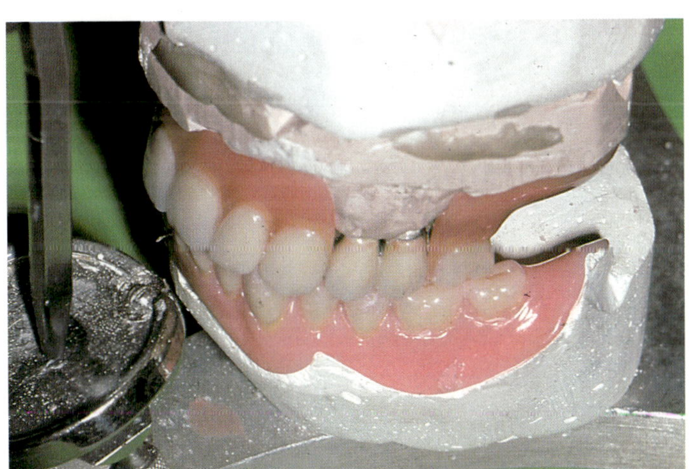

Fig. 19 A lower overdenture opposed to an upper partial prosthesis will require a balanced articulation.

space is required, bar attachments may be employed to connect the abutments either side. Decisions relating to the design, however, can only be made with the aid of mounted diagnostic casts. Where just a few teeth or roots remain, the assessment of vertical space is especially important as the planning of the restoration depends upon the room available (Fig. 18).

A removable partial prosthesis may be tooth-borne, tooth and mucosal-borne, or mucosal-borne. The principles involved are simple. Loads falling on the prosthesis must be reduced to a minimum; any loads that do fall on it should be spread as widely as possible. Reduction of occlusal load is achieved by keeping the artificial occlusal surfaces small, by reshaping the opposing occlusal surfaces if necessary, and by ensuring there is even contact with the opposing dentition (Fig. 19). The occlusal requirements of various types of prostheses are discussed in Chapter 3.

Loads falling on the prosthesis should be

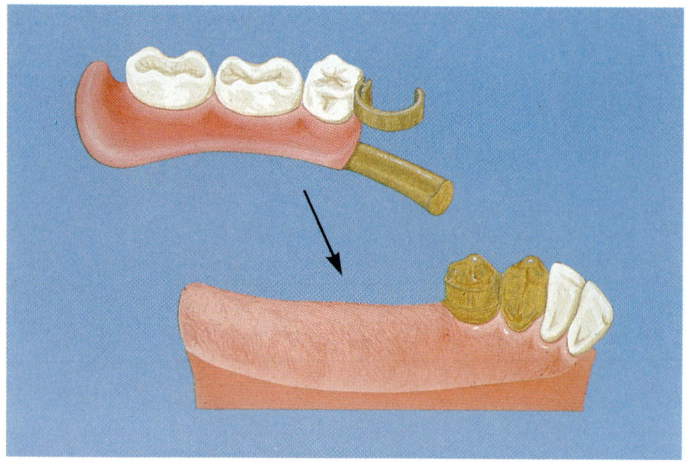

Fig. 20 A bilateral distal extension denture should normally be given a path of insertion that approaches from the distal aspects of the abutments.

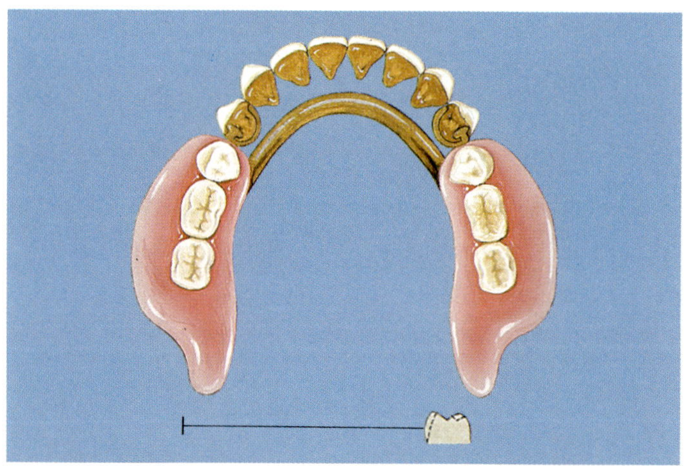

Fig. 21 A major connector, such as a rigid lingual bar, allows lateral displacing forces to be shared by the teeth and mucosa of both sides of the jaw.

spread over as many natural teeth as possible, and maximum support from the mucosa obtained by wide mucosal coverage, where necessary. However carefully the restoration is made, some additional load is likely to be placed on the abutment teeth and their prognosis must be evaluated with care.

Distal extension and complete overlay dentures raise the problem of load distribution between teeth and mucosa. Once it is understood that a correctly designed and constructed prosthesis has only the slightest tendency to move around the abutment teeth in function, the way is clear to understand the controversy over 'stress-breaking'. Prefabricated attachments allowing movement between the two components have many uses; however, it is generally their shape and size rather than the 'stress-breaking' properties claimed for them that allow their use where a more rigid unit would be contraindicated. A 'stress-breaker' may be used as a

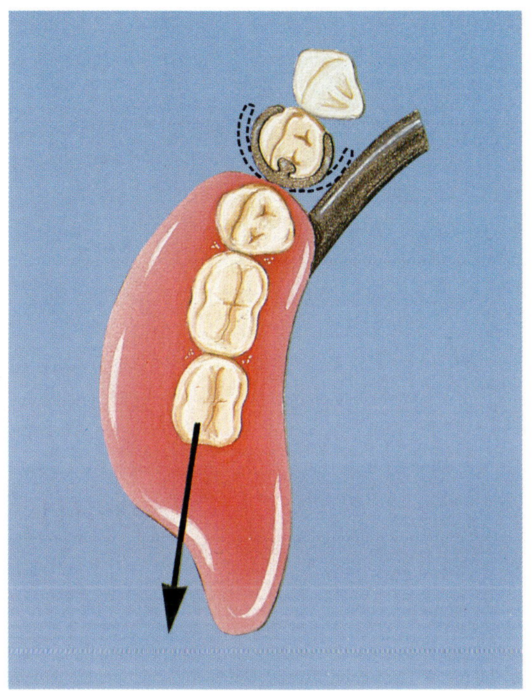

Fig. 22 A posterior displacing force tends to 'open up' this type of clasp arm. A mesial occlusal rest is usually to be preferred.

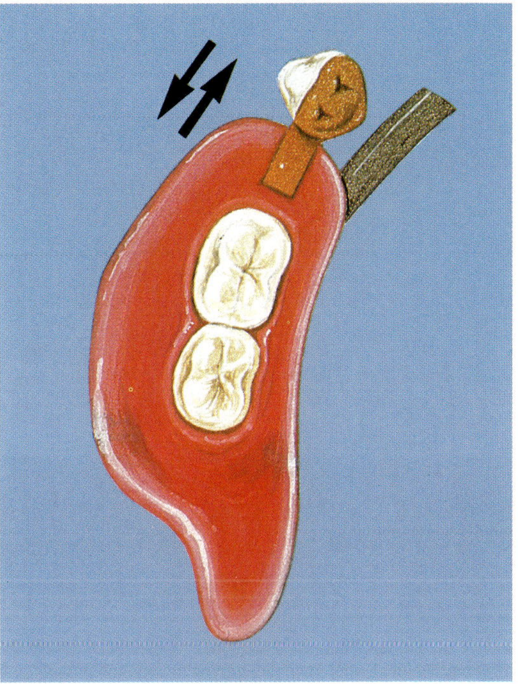

Fig. 23 A distally placed attachment must be able to withstand these forces.

safety valve, but never as a means of anchoring an unstable denture to a rigid abutment. Perceptible movements of a prosthesis in function are potentially harmful to the abutment teeth, to the underlying mucosa, and to the edentulous ridge. The aim must always be to design and construct an inherently stable denture and to pay attention first to the prosthodontic principles involved before considering technical details of the various attachments.

How is the prosthesis to be made?

1. The path of insertion

With the aid of a surveying instrument, the casts should be inspected to determine the most favourable path of insertion for the prosthesis. When prefabricated attachments are used, the path of insertion is critical, so it is important to ensure there are no mucosal undercuts relative to this path. It is usually necessary to give a lower distal extension denture a path of insertion that approaches from the distal aspect in order to extend the lingual flanges into the retromylohyoid fossae (Fig. 20): removable anterior restorations commonly require a path of insertion inclined to approach from the labial aspect.

2. Retention and stability

Once in place, a prosthesis has to resist displacing forces along its path of insertion. Anterior, posterior and lateral displacing forces, acting individually or in combinations, tend to rock and rotate the prosthesis out of position.

Direct retention can be considered to be the force resisting removal of the prosthesis along its path of insertion. The resistance of a clasp arm to deformation, friction between the denture components and the natural teeth, or friction between the sections of an attachment, may all provide direct retention. Mucosal coverage by the denture base also provides direct retention. The forces of adhesion, cohesion and surface tension acting between the denture base, saliva and mucosa, cause a pressure reduction under the denture base when the base is slightly displaced. Further denture movement is thereby resisted.

Resistance to lateral displacing forces is provided by rigid bracing components of the prosthesis, and by mucosal support. If a bilateral prosthesis is constructed, lateral displacing forces can be shared between the teeth and the mucosa of both sides, while a force tending to dislodge one side is resisted by the retainer on the opposite side. These retainers act with a mechanical advantage corresponding to the width of the dental arch (Fig. 21). A bilateral prosthesis is, therefore, inherently more stable than a unilateral restoration.

Anterior and posterior displacing forces are normally resisted by the natural teeth. However, the anterior removable prosthesis frequently needs additional support from the mucosa. When clasp retainers are employed for distal extension prostheses, posterior displacing forces must be resisted by rigid components of the metal framework. It is insufficient to rely on mucosal coverage and the clasp arm, for the flexible retaining arm is likely to flex under distal displacing forces (Fig. 22). An attachment in this position must be designed to resist these displacing forces (Fig. 23).

It is more difficult to provide resistance to forces tending to rock and rotate the prosthesis out of place, yet this is commonly the manner in which a patient tends to dislodge a prosthesis.

Resistance to these displacing forces is provided by the forces of retention, and the mechanical efficiency with which these retaining forces act is determined by the stability of the prosthesis. The more precise the path of insertion of a prosthesis the better it will resist displacing forces tending to rock it out of place. A denture with several widely spaced retainers is likely to prove more stable than one in which the retainers are close together.

A distal extension prosthesis has a tendency for the posterior section of the denture base to lift away from the mucosa when sticky foods are chewed. Some types of clasp-retained dentures do not prevent this movement, as the denture pivots around the tip of the clasp arm (Fig. 24). This tendency to rotate around the clasp can be prevented by incorporating a structure known as an 'indirect retainer'. An indirect retainer is a rigid component of the

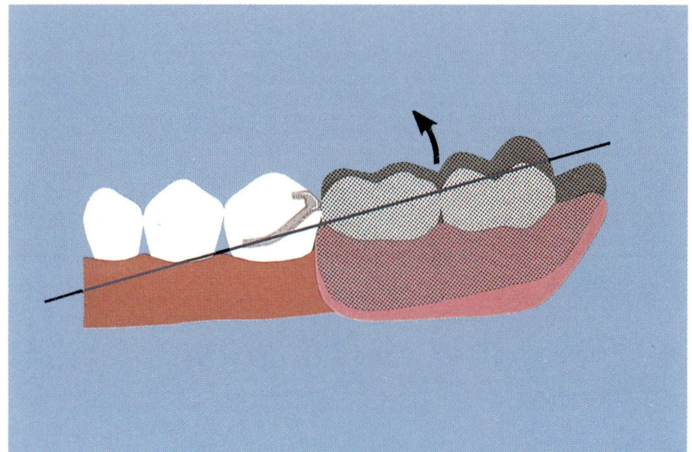

Fig. 24 When sticky foods are chewed the denture tends to rotate around the tip of the retainer.

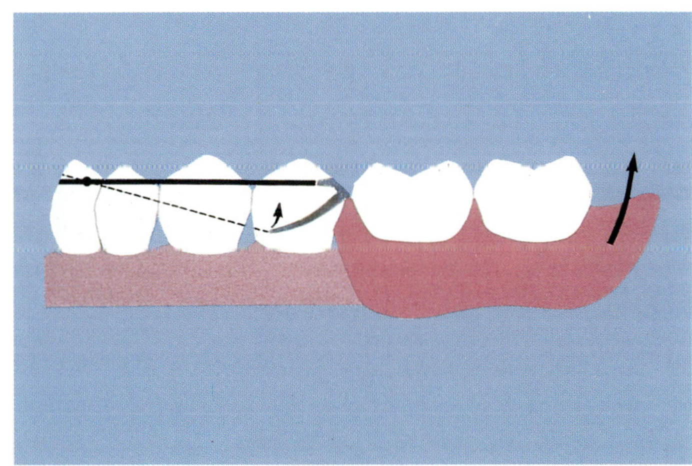

Fig. 25 An indirect retainer becomes the point around which the denture tends to rotate. The tip of the clasp is now in an undercut relative to this movement which it can therefore prevent.

denture and becomes the point around which the denture tends to rotate. As a result, the tip of the clasp arm is now in an undercut relative to this movement, which it can therefore prevent (Fig. 25). The greater the distance between the indirect retainer and the clasps, the more efficient is its action. Guide planes augment the stabilising effects of indirect retainers. However, where there are only six anterior teeth remaining in a somewhat square arch, it may be impossible to provide enough indirect retention to make the denture stable (Fig. 26).

Prostheses with prefabricated attachments have precise paths of insertion and so the need for indirect retention is reduced. Many extracoronal units specifically incorporate a device to prevent tipping of the base. It is, however, essential to select sturdy attachments, and splinted abutments are usually necessary.

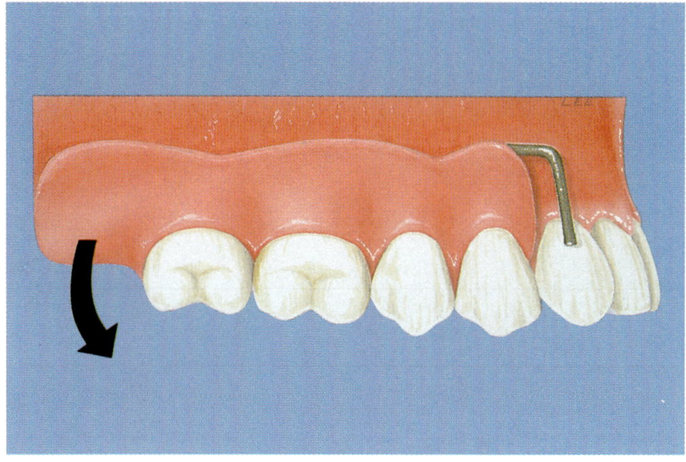

Fig. 26   With only six anterior teeth remaining in a square-shaped arch, it may be impossible to provide enough indirect retention to make the denture stable.

If attachments are to be employed, the amount of vertical and buccolingual space available needs to be examined with care. This is best carried out with the aid of mounted diagnostic casts (Fig. 27*). A minimum of 4 mm vertical space is usually required for prefabricated attachments. Where less space is available, miniature attachments are available or could be constructed. In most instances, crown lengthening procedures are the method of choice as they not only simplify subsequent plaque control but also improve the retention of the crown and the design of the restoration.

When prefabricated attachments are used, the retention between the abutment crowns and the tooth preparations should be planned as well; it is pointless having a retentive denture if the abutment crowns are dislodged when it is removed. Abutment preparations should, therefore, be restricted to full coverage, unless a three-quarter coverage restoration is indicated and can be made with adequate retention and strength.

3. The major connector

The major connector is the chassis of a bilateral prosthesis to which all other components are joined. Since it connects the bases on each side, the major connector acts as a load distributor and makes a large contribution to the stability of the prosthesis. Significant flexibility within the framework will detract from its ability to carry out these tasks. Equally apparent is the fact that the connector should cover the least possible area of gingivae, and that its overall bulk be as small as possible. The high modulus of elasticity of chrome cobalt alloys compared with yellow golds has advantage in this respect, but the design of the connector must be considered with care. Some major connectors, such as

* E. M. Gauge, Bell International Inc., 1320 Marston Road, Burlingame, CA.90401, U.S.A.

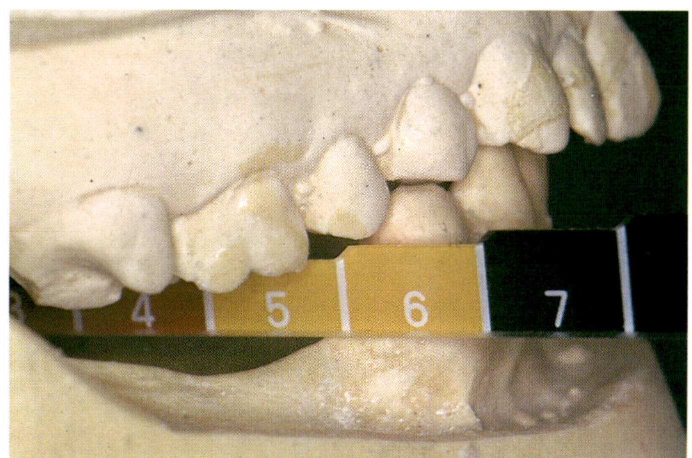

Fig. 27 Vertical space available for attachments can be measured on the diagnostic casts by means of a gauge. Buccolingual room should be assessed as well.

palatal plates, may themselves transmit occlusal loads to the mucosa, in which case the weight of the structure may become important.

Attachments introduce additional complications that can only be overcome with proper understanding of the clasp retainer.

The principles of major connector design vary little between clasp-retained and attachment retained dentures. For a detailed consideration the reader is referred to a standard text on partial denture construction (e.g. *Neill* and *Walters*, 1983). Suggested reading is provided at the end of this chapter and those succeeding it.

4. Compatibility of denture base components

At one time thought was given only to the relative surface hardness of materials. The adaptation between the two surfaces and the coefficient of friction between them was largely ignored. Many intracoronal attachments require to be soldered to the major connector, a procedure that is simplified when the components are of similar metals. Furthermore, the adaptation of lingual bracing arms, or semi-precision devices is easier to obtain. Unfortunately the limited stiffness of precious metal alloys and the corresponding increase in bulk is a significant drawback, to say nothing of weight and cost of the metal. Intracoronal attachments can be soldered to chrome cobalt alloys, albeit with some technical complication. It is also possible to adapt chrome-cobalt lingual bracing arms, or semi-precision components, to gold abutments. None of these complications occur when attachments are buried in the acrylic resin of the denture base. Many extracoronal units are employed in this manner.

Nowadays, chrome-cobalt alloys are normally the material of choice for major connectors. Their use is essential where there is a wide arch or where significant palatal coverage is required.

5. Adaptation of the framework to the abutments

Recent improvements with investment material, matched with new alloys of chrome-cobalt have gone a long way to improve the accuracy of castings. While gold alloys are far easier to employ when anything other than a simple lingual arm is contemplated, the difference in hardness between a gold crown and a chrome-cobalt denture is a factor that is normally over-rated. Problems, when they occur, usually result from inaccuracy of adaptation.

6. Indirect retention

Since many attachments incorporate effective tilt preventing components, the major connector design can be simplified accordingly. Since all the components of a removable prosthesis are joined to the major connector, its importance cannot be over emphasised. Apart from function, consideration should be given to patient tolerance and appearance. Mounted diagnostic casts are invaluable when making this decision.

Preliminary treatment

The health of the periodontal structures is one of the most important influences on the success or failure of the entire treatment. Thorough scaling and plaque control are essential for nearly every patient. There is much to be said for accepting patients on a probationary basis until their plaque control practice is adequate and their mouths are healthy. No tooth preparation should be started until the periodontal structures are sound. Muco-gingival surgery may be necessary to eliminate pocketing and to restore an adequate zone of attached gingivae. Short clinical crowns may require to be lengthened and small irregularities of the denture-bearing mucosa removed. Any necessary root canal therapy should be carried out as part of the preliminary therapy, rather than as emergency endodontics, when preparing the abutment crowns.

Preparation of the tissues covering the edentulous area is overlooked all too frequently. An impression made over inflamed tissues can only produce a restoration that maintains the structures in this state. Mildly abused tissues may recover if the denture causing the problem is left out for about 3 days. More extensive problems will require the use of tissue conditioners. Where complications of this nature are associated with problems of jaw postures, the existing partial denture may be converted into a transitional denture by means of base extension and correction of the occlusal surfaces.

Nowadays, there is seldom need to accept malaligned or malpositioned teeth as a basis for prosthodontic therapy. While crowns can be used to mask small rotations of the teeth, or to make minor corrections to their alignment, tooth preparation can never be an effective substitute for tooth position. *Ross* (1974) has described minor tooth movements without appliances.

Orthodontic therapy can drastically change the problems of prosthodontics (Figs. 28 and 29), producing results impossible to achieve in any other way. The diastema between central incisors is difficult to obliterate by oversized crowns if the restoration is to remain good-looking.

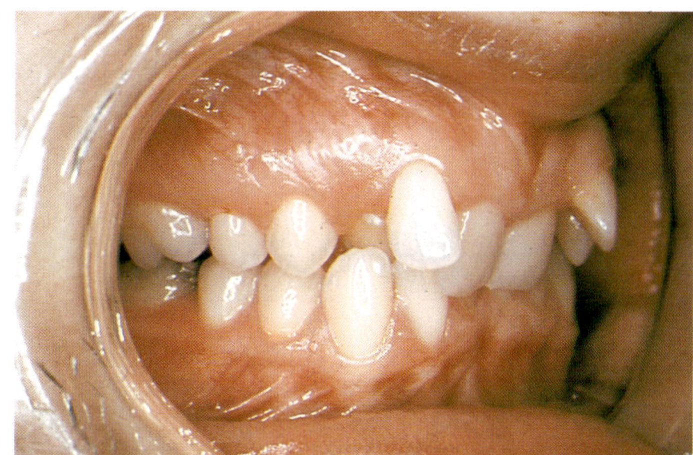

Fig. 28 Unsightly appearance from a deranged occlusion.

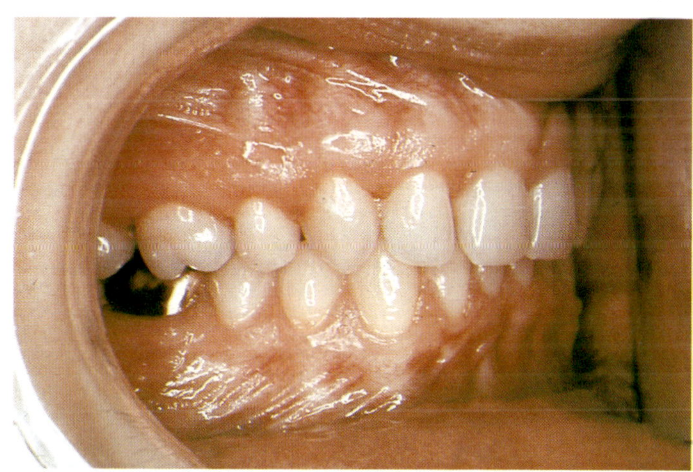

Fig. 29 Result achieved by a judicious extraction and preliminary orthodontic therapy.

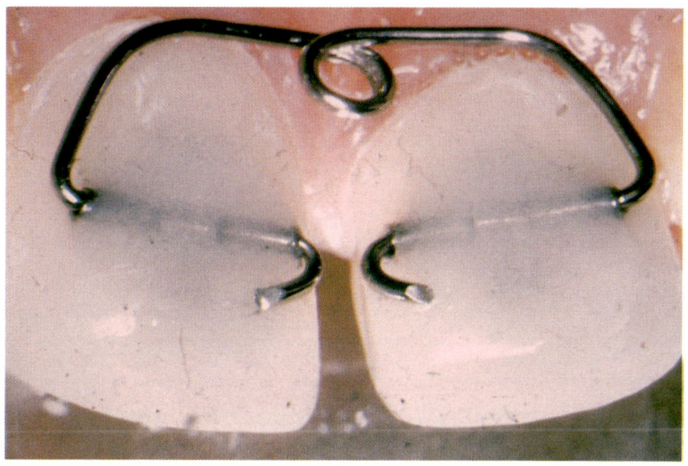

Fig. 30 Simple orthodontic treatment may be used to appose some spaced incisors.

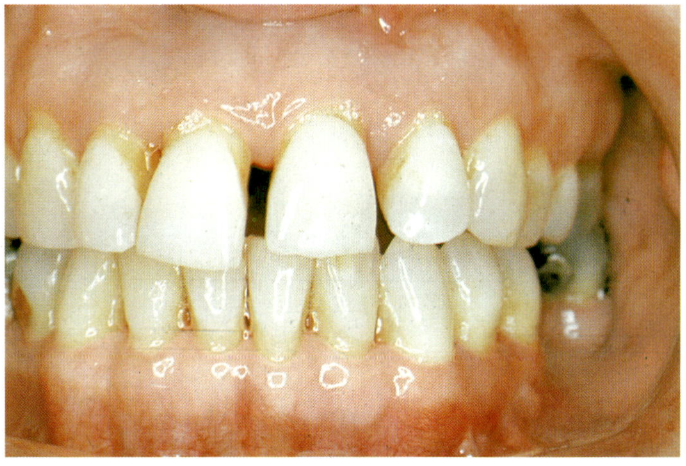

Fig. 31 Adult with spaced incisors before orthodontic treatment.

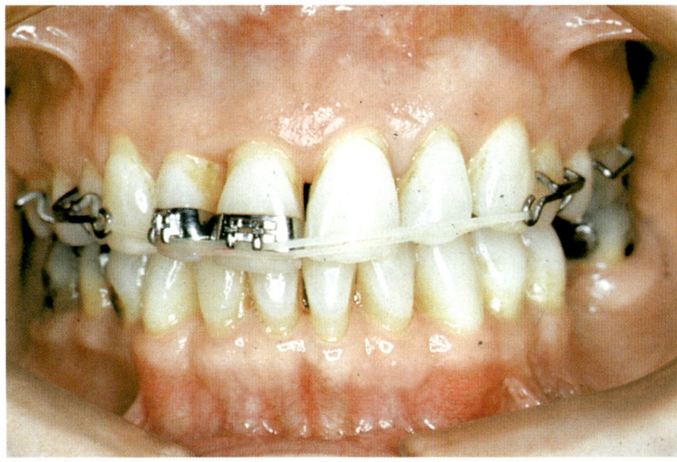

Fig. 32 Patient during the course of active treatment.

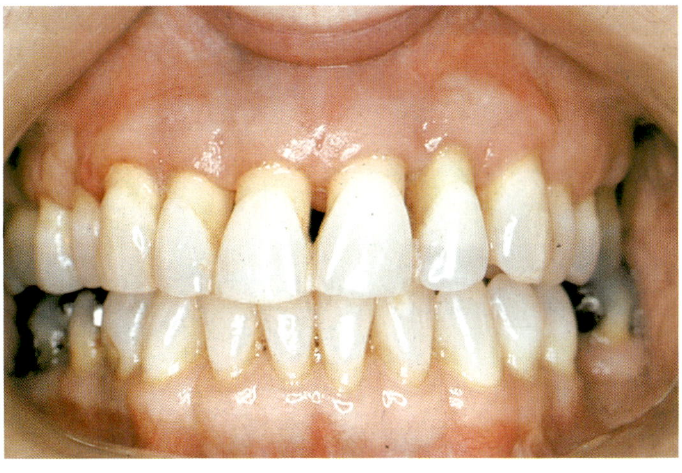

Fig. 33 Same patient after 6 weeks of treatment and with a provisional splint.

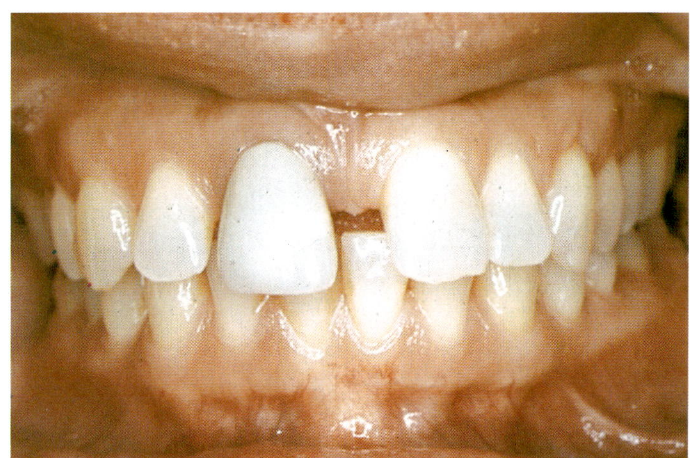

Fig. 34　Another example before orthodontic therapy.

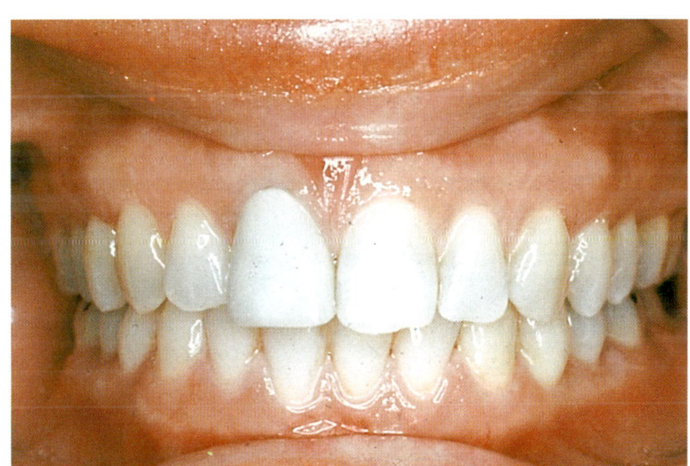

Fig. 35　After orthodontic therapy.

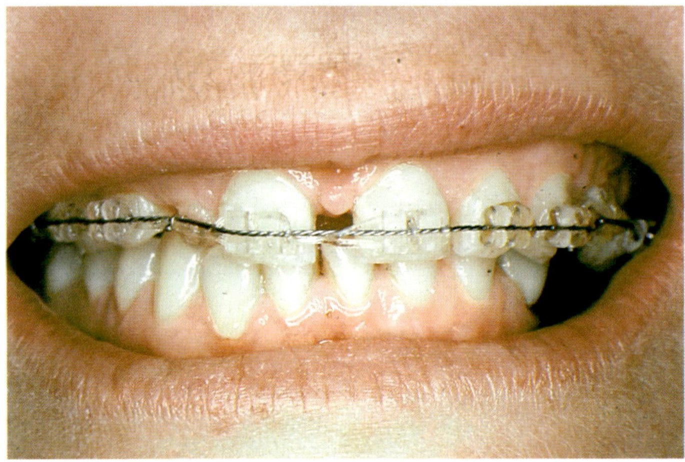

Fig. 36 Retraction and realignment of anterior teeth.

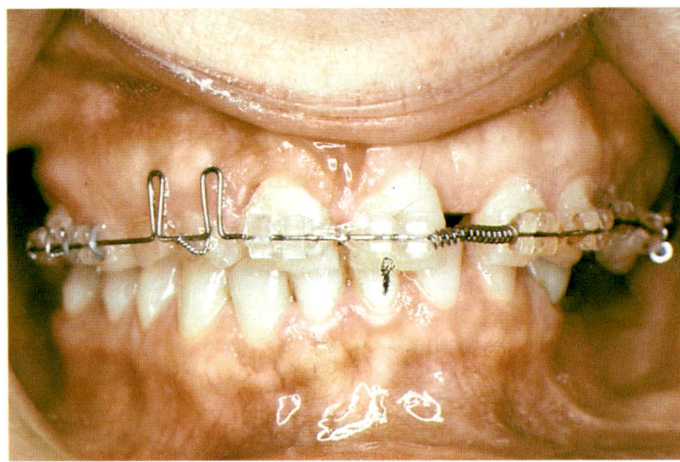

Fig. 37 Subsequent distal movement of the upper left lateral incisor to provide space for a pontic.

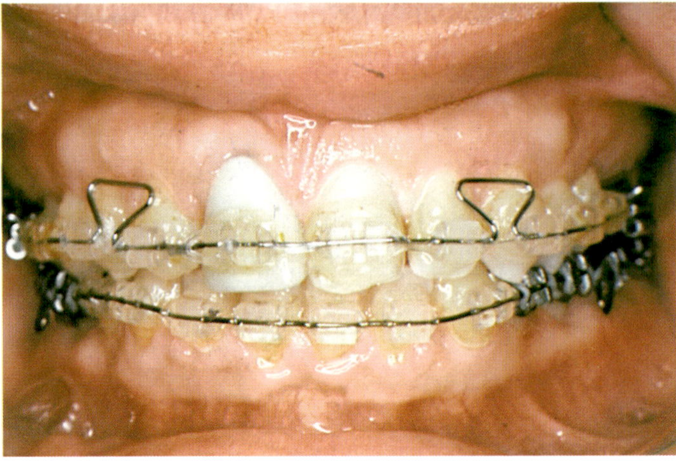

Fig. 38 Moving apart closely opposed roots to provide proximal space between the crowns.

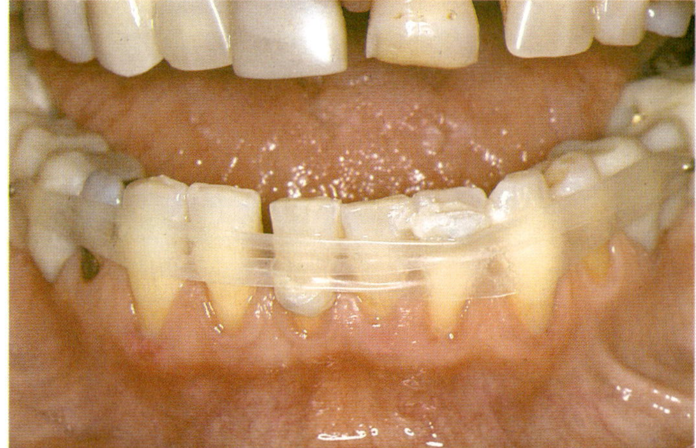

Fig. 39 When loss of posterior occlusal support has caused the incisors to spread out, the occlusal table can be built up with acrylic resin temporary bridges. These restorations form a base for retraction of the incisors.

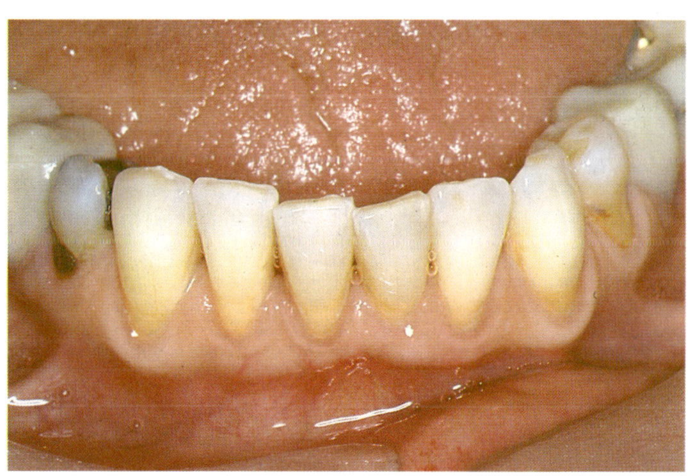

Fig. 40 The same patient one month later.

Simple appliances can be employed in some instances. Retraction of incisors, quite apart from placing them in a more stable position, will remove unwanted spaces, improve angulation, periodontal health and facilitate subsequent restorative dentistry (Figs. 30 to 33).

Apart from the problems of the orthodontic therapy, considerable care in planning is essential to prevent awkward spaces that cannot be restored in a pleasing manner (Figs. 34 and 35).

Another point to consider is the root relationships of adjoining teeth. If these roots are close together it will be impossible to provide adequate proximal space between the crowns when the teeth are subsequently restored (Figs. 36 to 38).

Where loss of posterior occlusal support has been combined with spreading of the incisors, a simple plan is to restore the posterior occlusion with transitional acrylic resin prostheses made with gold collars around the teeth. Small hooks can be

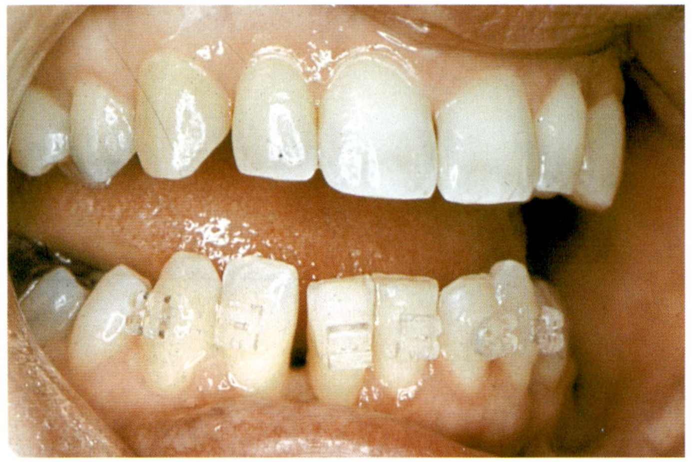

Fig. 41 Brackets applied to labial surfaces.

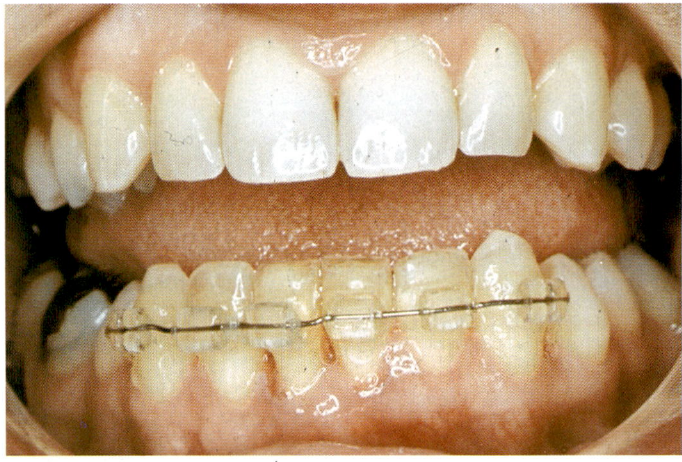

Fig. 42 Active treatment.

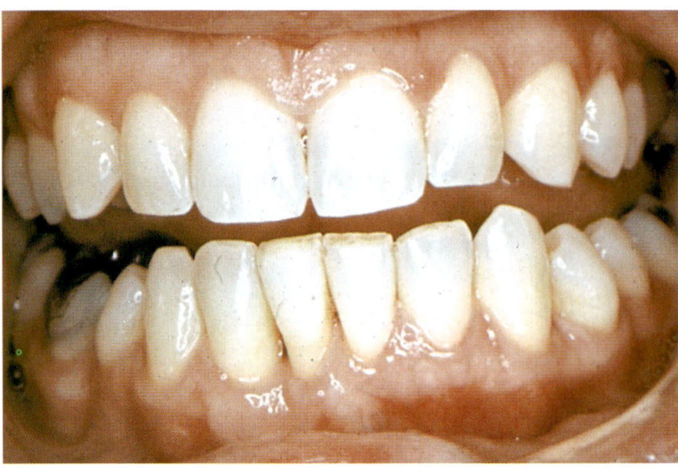

Fig. 43 Completion of orthodontic therapy.

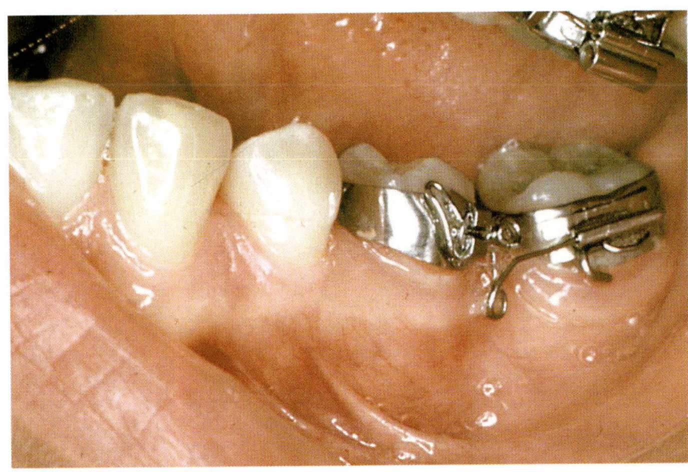

Fig. 44 The realignment of a tilted distal abutment.

inserted in these prostheses and elastic used for retraction. This retraction is really a tipping movement, rather than a bodily movement of the teeth. As a safety measure, a small orthodontic wire ligature covered with acrylic resin can be placed around the neck of one of the teeth to be retracted, and a similar ligature placed near the incisal edge of another tooth. These ligatures will prevent the tubing from sliding onto the gingivae or jumping off the teeth (Figs. 39 and 40).

Simplified techniques now available with orthodontic brackets have made possible a range of therapy that might otherwise have been dismissed as too complex. The modern brackets are far better-looking and can be applied with adhesive to the labial surfaces of the teeth. As a result, combinations of rotations and malangulations can be corrected (Figs. 41 to 43).

Tilted distal abutments are another common complication to prosthodontic therapy. While mechanical answers are available to ease the problems of malalignment, they do not solve the associated periodontal problems. It is far better to restore the tilted abutment to an upright position (Fig. 44). If this is carried out, the preparation of the tooth is simplified, and additional retention for the crown may be obtained. Furthermore, loads will be applied at a more favourable angle, while the changes in angulation of the tooth may well contribute to removal of a mesial infra-osseous pocket.

A modified approach can be employed where there is little space between tilted molars and the more mesial teeth. The apices of the molar tooth are brought forward so that while the tooth is made upright there is no space between it and the adjacent premolar (Figs. 45 to 47).

The examples illustrated are only a few of the possibilities available with adult orthodontics today. Specialist help is recommended and it should be understood that the periodontal condition should be reassessed after orthodontic therapy.

Once a patient has become accustomed to

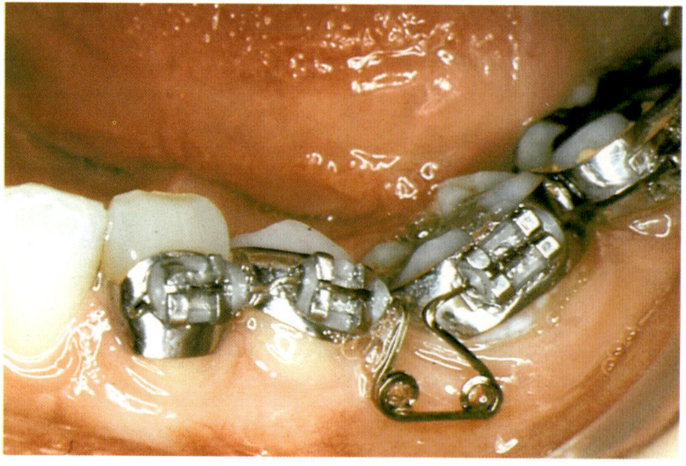

Fig. 45 The apices of a tilted molar being rotated.

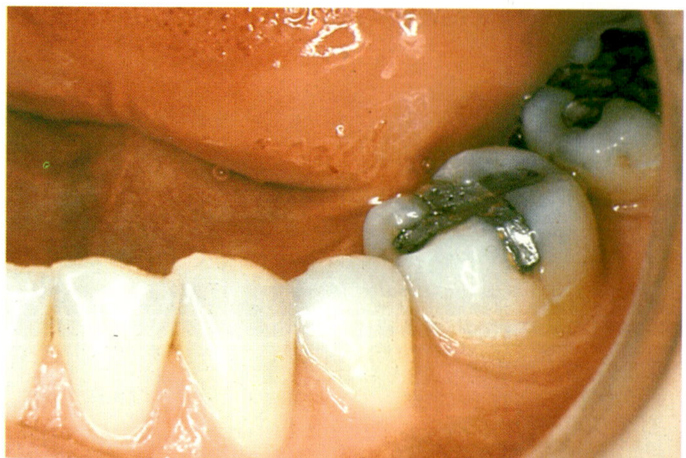

Fig. 46 The molar now in contact with the premolar. A new restoration will be required for the tooth.

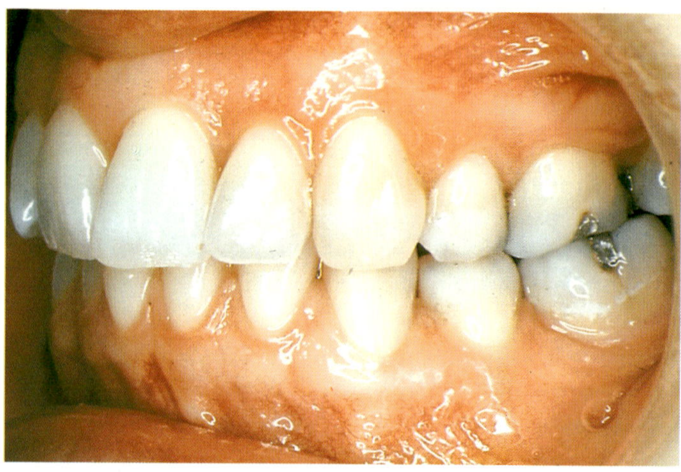

Fig. 47 The occlusion before restorative dentistry.

his restored posterior occlusion, he frequently reverts to centric jaw relation, or a position nearby. If the occlusion of the restoration had been adapted to an acquired protruded mandibular posture, most of the posterior teeth of a removable prosthesis may need to be replaced. A fixed prosthesis, however, may need to be completely reconstructed as the crown preparations may have to be modified.

This type of construction allows accurate adaptation of the gingival margins and wide proximal spaces. For this reason occlusal splints are so useful where the bulk of the remaining dentition remains. Where possible, an upper anterior occluding plane is provided to separate the posterior teeth and break the proprioceptive feedback. This is a rapid and easy method to employ as a mandibular repositioner that facilitates subsequent treatment.

References

Adams D. and Zwink R. (1976)
Treating Australia antigen positive patients. Practical experience. Brit. Dent. J., 141, 341.

Bates J. F., Neill D. J. and Preiskel H. W. (1984)
Proceedings of the International Prosthodontic Symposium: Restoration of the Partially Dentate Mouth. Quintessence Publishing, Berlin.

Benington I. C., Watson I. B., Jenkins W. M. M., and Allan G. R. J. (1979)
Restorative treatment of the cleft palate patient. Brit. Dent. J., 146: 144.

Dawson P. E. (1974)
Evaluation, Diagnosis and Treatment of Occlusal Problems. C. V. Mosby, St. Louis, Mo.

Henderson D. and Steffel V. L. (1981)
McCracken's Removable Partial Prosthodontics. 6th Edn. C. V. Mosby, St. Louis, Mo.

Nagington J. and Varley E. W. B. (1976)
Hepatitis B and the dental surgeon. Brit. dent. J., 141, 337.

Neill D. J. and Walter J. D. (1983)
Partial Denture Prosthetics. 2nd Edn. Blackwell Scientific Publications, London.

Ross I. F. (1974)
Tooth movement and repositioning of the mandible without appliances. J. Prosthet. Dent., 31 : 3 : 290.

Siebert J. (1981)
Personal communication.

Zarb G. A., Bergman B., Clayton J. A. and Jackay H. F (1978)
Prosthodontic Treatment for Partially Edentulous Patients. C. V. Mosby, St. Louis, Mo.

Chapter 2

Periodontal Therapy Before Restorative Dentistry

John Saville Zamet M. Phil., F.D.S., R.C.S.
Consultant in Periodontics
University College Hospital, London

Periodontal disease is responsible for the majority of tooth loss, yet it is seldom treated. This fact must present modern dentistry with one of its greatest challenges. There is conclusive evidence to show that bacteria within dental plaque are responsible for the disease (*Sockransky* 1970), but as yet there is no chemotherapy available that can be used on a permanent basis. The disease has to be controlled by mechanical means such as toothbrushing, woodsticks and floss.

Restorative dentistry may influence the pattern of health and disease in three ways:

1. Inadequate restorations and attachments placed in a healthy mouth may distort the anatomy of the tissues to the extent that good plaque control can no longer be maintained and periodontal breakdown will start to occur.
2. The underlying periodontal problems may have escaped recognition during the examination, diagnosis and treatment planning phase. Indeed it may have been the major reason for tooth loss, for which the patient is now seeking replacement.
3. All well-made restorations should exert a protective function to the surrounding healthy periodontal tissues and allow easy access for plaque control.

The control of disease

Nearly all epidemiological studies have shown a close correlation between dental plaque and periodontal disease. Experimental gingivitis has been induced in healthy subjects by withdrawing oral hygiene over a number of weeks. The disease has then been eliminated by the reinstitution of good plaque control, without the need for any further treatment (*Löe et al* 1965). An analogy can be drawn between periodontal disease and diabetes. Neither disease can be cured, but both are amenable to control—diabetes by means of diet and insulin, periodontal disease by the total elimination of plaque from the teeth every day. In the same way that diabetes can be monitored by the assessment of blood sugar levels, a method has to be found to monitor the plaque control abilities of the patient. One advantage of this method is the development of a baseline of oral hygiene ability before the onset of treatment. This will allow an accurate representation of failure or improve-

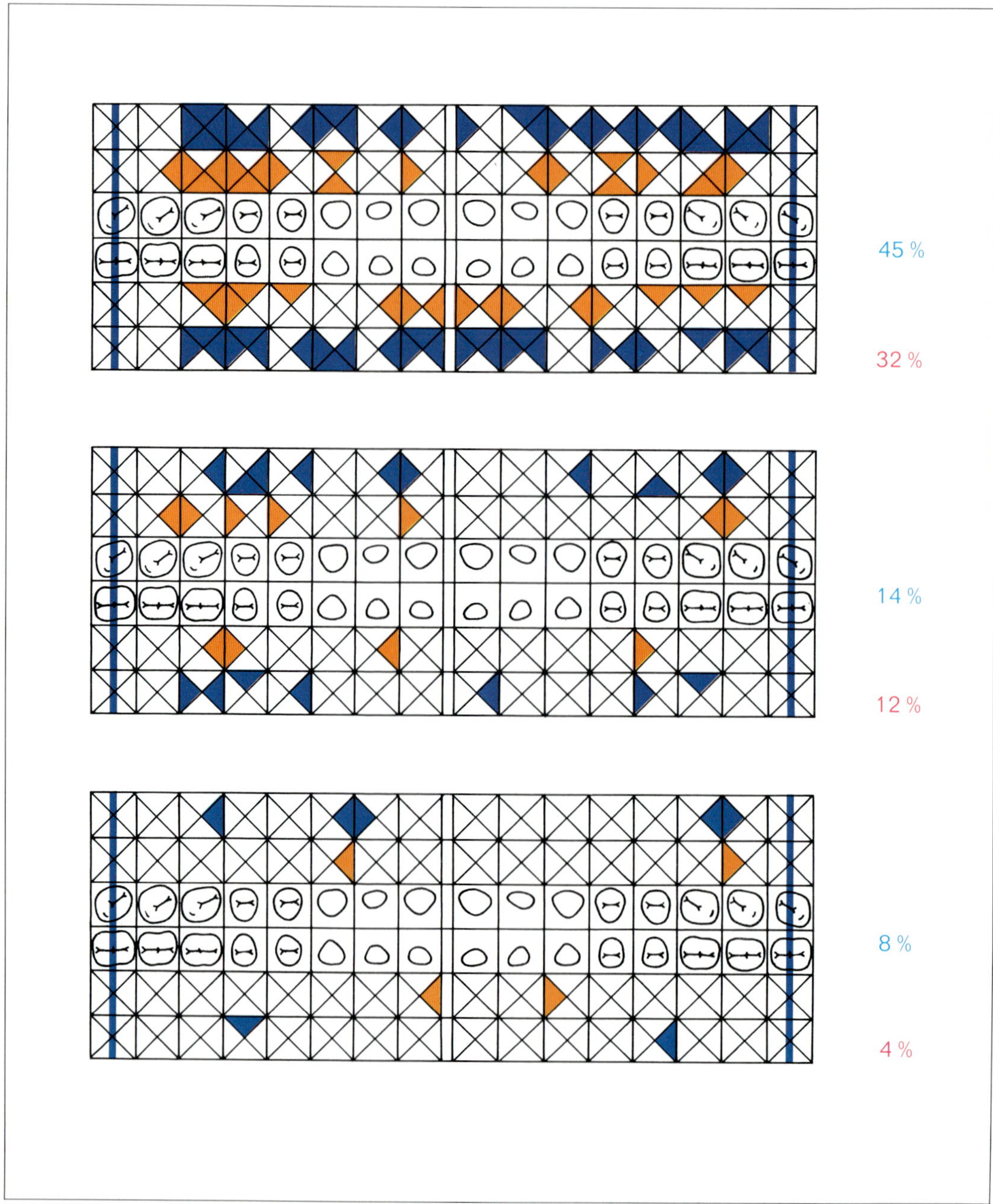

Fig. 48   The plaque index is based on the presence or absence of plaque on four surfaces of each tooth after staining with erythrosin. The surfaces involved are shaded. The bleeding index is established by the presence or absence of oedema, bleeding or redness adjacent to the four surfaces of each tooth. These tooth surfaces involved are shaded in turn.

ment, rather than using the vague description of 'poor' or 'good', which are too general to have meaning for either the patient, hygienist or dentist.

Measurement of plaque and bleeding index scores

Representative diagrams of the maxillary and mandibular dental arches are required (Fig. 48). Each tooth surface is subdivided into four parts, the dotted outlines of the teeth are left unchanged where they are missing and blocked in where the teeth are present.

The plaque index is based on the presence or absence of plaque on four surfaces of each tooth after staining with erythrosin. The surfaces involved are shaded blue. The bleeding index is established by the presence or absence of oedema, bleeding, or redness adjacent to the four surfaces on each tooth. The tooth surfaces involved are again shaded red as required. The percentage of tooth surfaces with plaque or bleeding out of the total number of surfaces present can be measured on a chart (Fig. 49). The number of teeth in the mouth are plotted against the number of tooth surfaces involved and, by following the oblique lines downwards, the percentage of tooth surfaces with either plaque or adjacent gingival bleeding can be obtained.

The advantage of this type of charting is its simplicity compared with the more complex indices that have been used in the past. The patient will also readily appreciate the meaning of a percentage system based on the presence or absence of plaque, or bleeding, and this can be used as an instructional tool during the course of oral hygiene teaching. In addition, the diagrams demonstrate the distribution of plaque or bleeding and again can be compared from visit to visit, highlighting the areas where the patient's plaque control is inadequate or where alternative methods may need to be tried.

A considerable divergence of opinion exists as to whether the plaque control programme should be undertaken as a separate entity or as part of the overall initial preparation of the mouth, which will include scaling and root planing. Some clinicians also recommend that the plaque control programme be undertaken on 5 consecutive days; others advocate longer intervals. It should be emphasised that there is no scientific data to prove that any particular regime is superior to the other. The longterm goal is a permanent change of behaviour. However, in many cases this cannot be expected even from a successful plaque control programme. The problem is that many factors, which are beyond the control of the practising dentist, are decisive in the attitude that the patient has to preventive health and behaviour. Nevertheless, nearly all the studies on oral hygiene show that repeated motivation is likely to give positive results. The dentist will, therefore, have to arrange for an ongoing plaque control programme over the long term.

Anatomical relationships of teeth and restorative dentistry

The normal interdental papilla between teeth which are in contact is never truly pyramidal. Its shape is determined by the

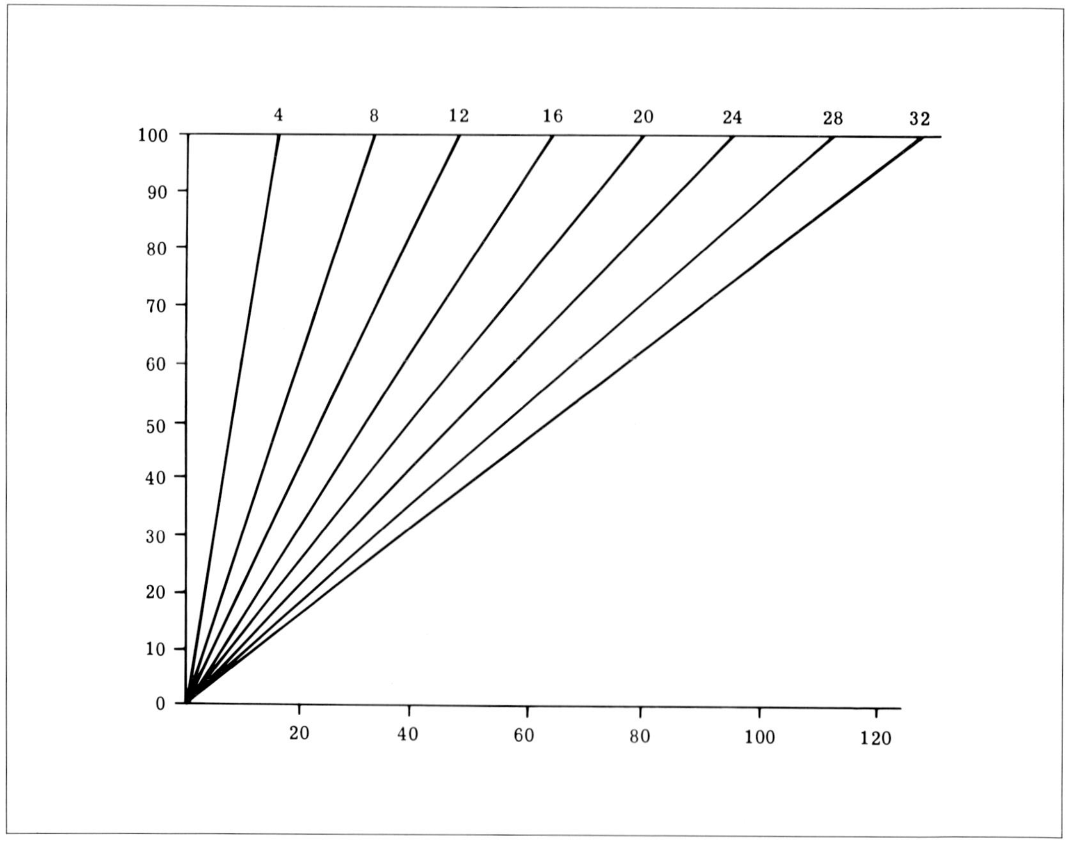

Fig. 49   The number of teeth in the mouth are plotted against the number of tooth surfaces involved and, by following the oblique line downwards, the percentage of tooth surfaces with either plaque or adjacent gingival inflammation can be obtained.

interdental embrasure, which in the healthy mouth should be completely filled by gingival tissue. The crest of this gingiva is knife-edged and directed towards the contact points or areas between approximating teeth. Diagrams of normal interdental gingiva between incisor and molar teeth are shown in Figures 50 and 51. *Cohen* (1959) has described the shape as a 'col'. The shape of the interdental col is like a 'U' between the gingival peaks when teeth are grossly overcrowded (Fig. 52). With the crowns instanding or outstanding from the arch, the contacts between teeth are nearer to the cervical regions of the crown and, occasionally, part of the roots may also be in contact. The space for inaccessible bacterial plaque between the teeth is much larger than between teeth in regular alignment. This 'U' may well be further enlarged if swelling of the buccal and lingual gingival peaks has resulted from bac-

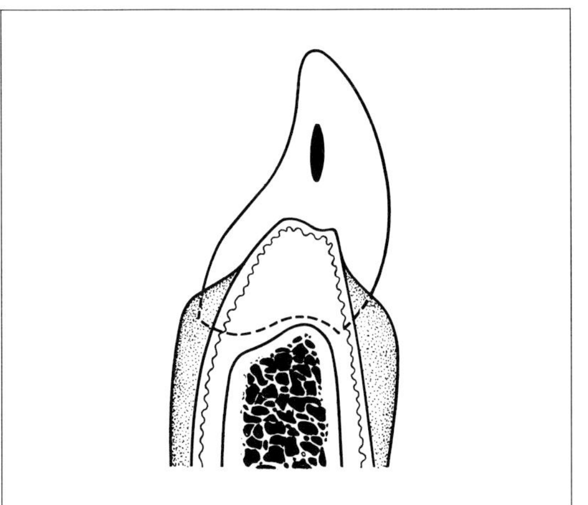

Figure 50

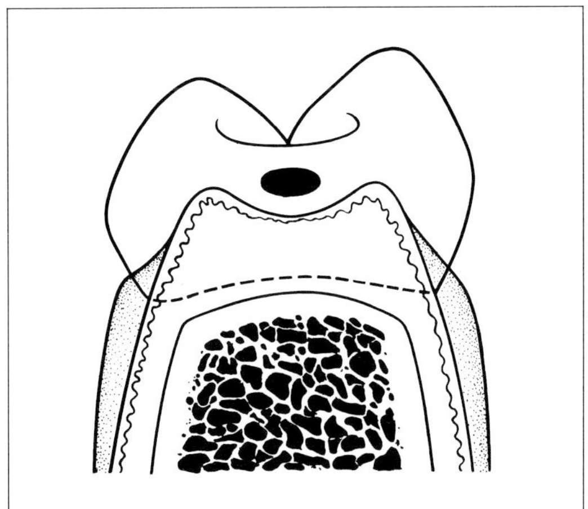

Figure 51

Fig. 50   Diagram of a vertical labiolingual section through the contact points of lower incisors, with clinically normal gingiva. The gingival col is short and dips only slightly between the peaks.

Fig. 51   Diagram of the normal col between premolar or molar teeth. This col is long and dips below the contact zones.

Fig. 52   Diagram of a gingival col between overcrowded lower incisors. This dips deeply between the gingival peaks, providing considerable space between the teeth for undisturbed growth of bacterial plaque.

Figure 52

terial inflammation. Although the problems of overcrowding and malalignment of teeth can be found in any part of the mouth, the classic areas are between the maxillary central and lateral incisor, the distobuccal root of the maxillary first molar and the mesiobuccal root of the maxillary second molar, the mandibular lateral and canine teeth and the mandibular incisor teeth. A difference of opinion exists as to whether tooth irregularity is a major predisposing factor in the development of periodontal disease. There is no disagreement that it poses a severe problem to the construction of effective restorations. Further encroachment on remaining embrasure space inevitably occurs, together with the inflammatory swelling of the buccal and lingual gingival peaks, resulting from the presence of inaccessible plaque between the teeth. This is particularly true of full coverage porcelain to gold restorations,

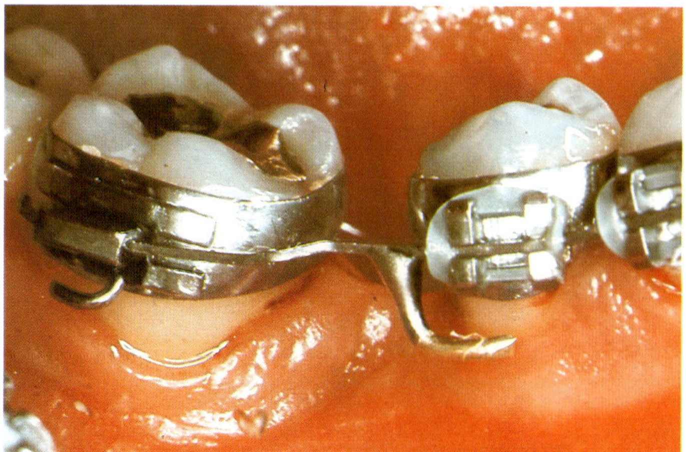

Fig. 53 (a) Second molar tooth is tilted mesially. (b) Intra-oral radiograph shows a vertical bony lesion on its mesial surface.

Figure 53 a

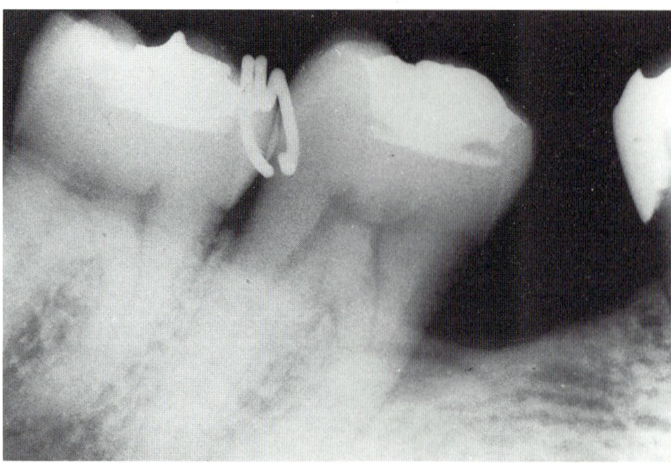

Figure 53 b

where the tendency is to under-prepare the gingival third of the tooth and to over-contour this area of the restoration, in order to retain a sufficient width of porcelain and the correct shade (*Parkinson 1976*).

The early extraction of posterior teeth, especially in the mandible, may eventually result in tilting of one or more of the remaining molar teeth (Fig. 53 a, b and 54 a, b). This presents a problem in treatment planning because on many occasions the mesial surface of the tilted tooth shows an area that is inaccessible to plaque control and inevitably a progressive periodontal lesion, usually infrabony in type, will occur. The construction of a restoration on this tooth will locate the mesial margin in a periodontal pocket; there would also be inadequate vertical space for the use of a precision attachment. The periodontal lesion in such cases is a direct extension of the

Fig. 54 (a) (b) The second molar tooth is uprighted by an orthodontic appliance. The mesial pocket and associated bony defect is eliminated as the bony morphology changes and the area is debrided with intermittent curettage.

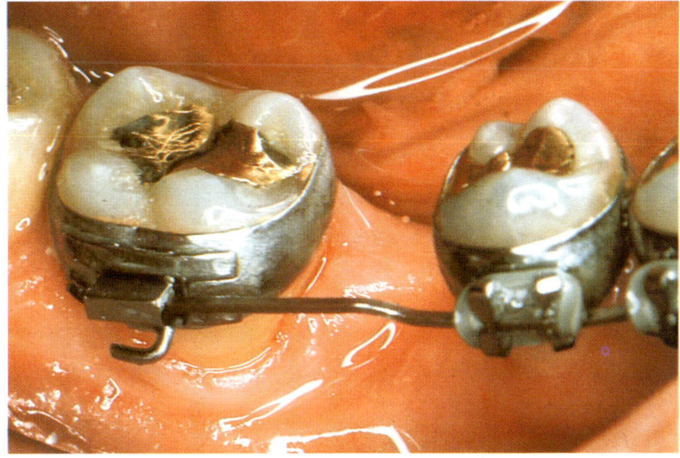

Figure 54 a

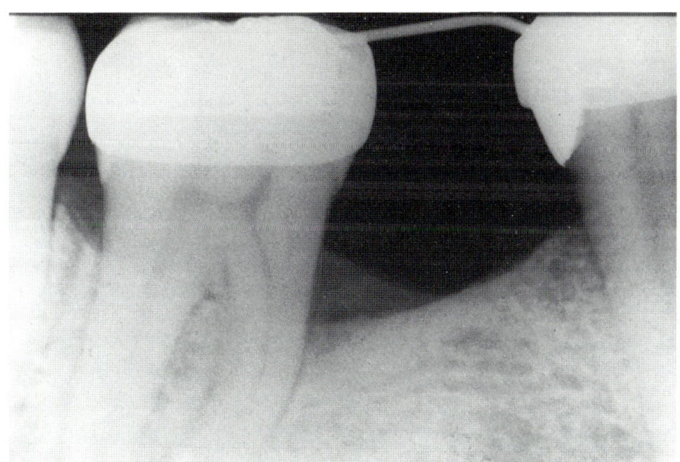

Figure 54 b

tissue morphology that has resulted from the tilted position of the tooth. Pocket elimination procedures will therefore fail because the periodontal structures will return to their original form. The best solution where tilted molar teeth are to be used as abutments, is to upright them by means of minor tooth movement (*Brown* 1973). This has the following advantages:

1. An easier path of insertion.

2. Increased retention, since all the crown is now available for preparation.
3. The margins of the restoration can be made supragingival.
4. The bone and soft tissue morphology change as the tooth is uprighted. This will lead to the elimination of the mesial bony defect and an increased zone of attached gingiva, as the epithelium of the pocket wall becomes evaginated and keratinized.

Effect of restorations on the periodontium

G. V. Black's concept that proximal restorations should always be placed beneath the free gingivae is no longer acceptable. Both animal and human studies have shown that the extension of restorations into the gingival crevice is a contributing factor in causing periodontal breakdown (*Marcum* 1967; *Silness* 1970; *Valderhaug* 1972; *Newcomb* 1974; *Leon* 1975). Scanning electron microscopic studies have shown that the irregularities in the margins of restorations, microporosities and cement margins, all attract sufficient plaque to cause gingival inflammation.

It is often stated in the dental literature that a convexity in the gingival third of the crown is essential for protection of the gingival sulcus area from the impaction of food (*Wheeler* 1962). Evidence against this theory has been advanced by *Yuodelis et al* (1973), who contend that perfectly healthy gingival tissues can be maintained without the protection of crown contours, providing that plaque control is adequate. The commonest mistake is to make bulging rounded crowns (*Eissmann et al* 1971). Such an overcontour interferes with the sealing of the gingival cuff around the neck of the tooth and enhances both supragingival and subgingival plaque accumulation.

The proximal contour of fillings, crowns and pontics should maintain sufficient space for a normal interdental papilla. The tendency is for these restorations to be overcontoured during construction. A long area of contact corono-apically will result in a distortion of the col area, which becomes deeply U-shaped as swelling of the displaced buccal and lingual papillae progresses (Fig. 55). At right angles a wide contact area buccolingually will distort the col area into a wide shallow 'U'-shape, as the buccal and lingual peaks are displaced. This situation will again be exaggerated by inflammation as plaque control becomes increasingly difficult (Fig. 56).

Effect on the periodontium of partial dentures

The concept that a partial denture is a device for losing one's teeth slowly, painfully and expensively, has received support from a number of studies (*Koivumaa* 1956; *Tomlin et al* 1961; *Carlsson et al* 1965; *Derry et al* 1970). The correlation between caries and periodontal injury to the residual dentition, on one hand, and the patient's oral hygiene on the other has been well demonstrated by *Koivumaa et al* (1960). If oral hygiene was unsatisfactory, denture construction contributed to carious lesions in the abutment teeth and gingivitis around them within 1 year, even if metal-based tooth and mucosal-borne partial dentures were designed according to accepted principles.

Fortunately, a more hopeful picture begins to emerge when a concerted effort is made to improve and maintain oral hygiene. *Bergman et al* (1977) found no deterioration to the denture-supporting structures in a 6 year study. Patients had undergone periodontal treatment that included concentrated instruction and motivation in oral hygiene. Subjects were reviewed at yearly intervals when remotivation, scaling and prosthetic adjustments were carried out.

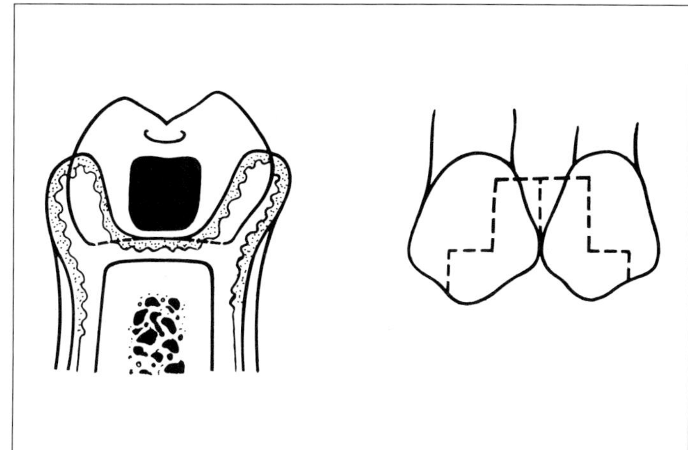

Fig. 55   A long contact area buccolingually distorting the col area into a wide but shallow 'U' shape.

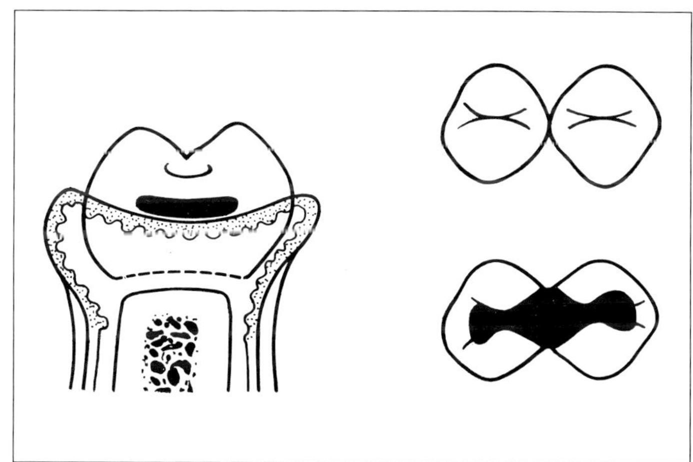

Fig. 56   A wide contact area buccolingually distorting the col area into a wide but shallow 'U' shape.

A rationale for periodontal Surgery around abutment teeth

Where moderate to severe pocket depths are present (4 mm or more), surgical procedures allow for access and visibility so that thorough root planing can be carried out. Depending on the circumstances, gingival tissue during these procedures may be resected, replaced or apically positioned. Osseous surgery may be required where extensive underlying bony deform-ities are present. This would allow the over-lying soft tissues to assume correct form and function. The surgical lengthening of short clinical crowns also has an important role to play in allowing (1) for adequate retention, (2) for the margins of restorations to be supragingival and (3) for adequate embrasure space to be formed. Surgery of this type would also extend to involve saddle areas, tuberosity and retro-molar areas. Although controversial, the establishment of a functional zone of

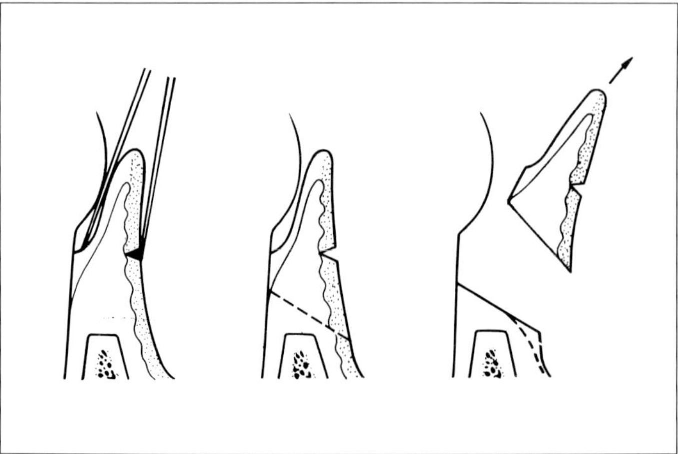

Fig. 57 The gingivectomy incision showing the Krane Caplan pocket marking forceps *in situ*. The incision starts apically to the puncture marks in order to achieve a 45° angle to the long axis of the tooth. The pocket wall is resected and a physiologic contour achieved.

attached gingiva around abutment teeth is still considered desirable for the maintenance of longterm periodontal health.

Gingivectomy

The resection of the pocket wall, using a 45° incision to the long axis of the teeth, provides a useful method for eliminating pocket depth (Fig. 57). This technique should only be used when there is an adequate width of attached gingiva, so that a functional zone of attached tissue will remain post-operatively, and also when there are no underlying bony deformities. The gingivectomy incision can be embellished by gingivoplasty, accentuating the knife edge of the gingival margin and interdental grooving. Gingivectomy is particularly useful in correcting hyperplastic marginal and interdental areas prior to the construction of new restorations; in addition, gingivectomy will expose additional tooth structure where altered passive eruption is resulting in a shortened clinical crown, and it

will also expose carious lesions at the amelo-cemental junction. It should be remembered that as the gingivectomy wound heals, the reforming gingival tissue will tend to cuff out coronally, and allowance will have to be made for the change in level of the gingival tissues if the margins of restorations are to remain supragingival. For the same reason, gingivectomy would be unsuccessful as a means of lengthening crowns in relation to teeth that are unaffected by periodontal disease.

The Modified Widman flap

This method of treating pocket depths lies midway between that of curettage and the full reflective methods of flap surgery. The original technique was described by *Widman* in 1918, but has been modified and used extensively by the Ann Arbor group in Michigan (*Ramfjord* and *Nissle* 1974). The internally bevelled incision follows the scalloped outline of the gingival crest and the entire outer wall of the pocket is retain-

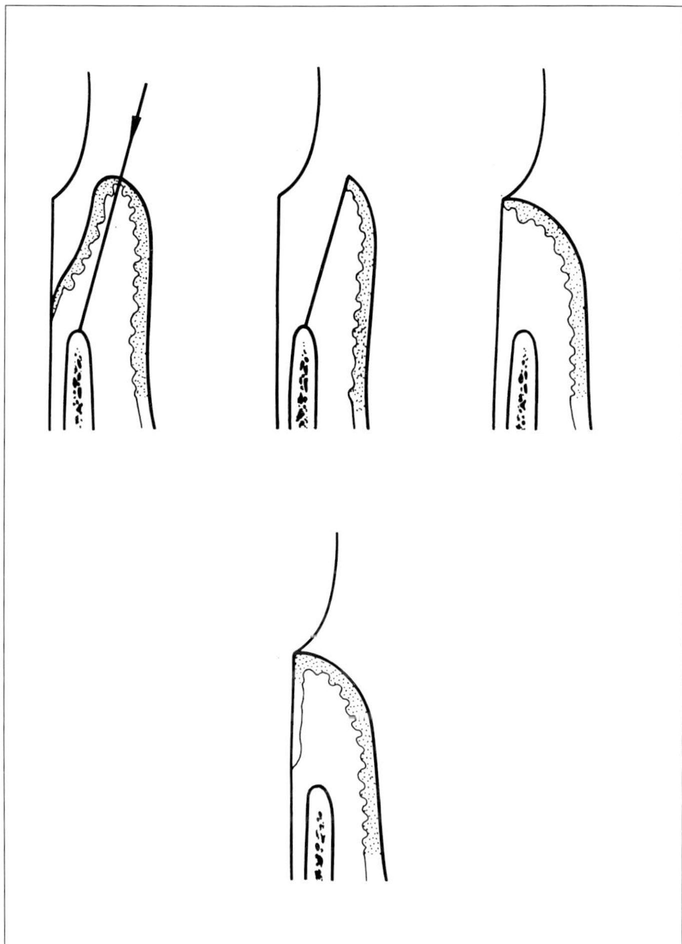

Fig. 58 The modified Widman flap. The internally bevelled incision is made from the gingival margin labially (an exaggerated scollop is made on the palatal side to allow for good tissue approximation interdentally). Flap reflection is conservative and sufficient to allow the resection of the marginal wedge of tissue and debridement of the area. The flap is replaced to its original position and secured with interrupted sutures. Osseous surgery may sometimes be necessary to ramp interdental areas to allow for better approximation of labial and palatal flaps.

ed (Fig. 58). On the palatal side, the internally bevelled incision has an exaggerated scallop and should also allow for some thinning of the palatal mucosa by undermining dissection.

The interdental collar of tissue is carefully incised and curetted away and the root surfaces and adjacent bone debrided. No osseous reshaping is carried out unless the interdental bone is thickened and will not permit accurate flap adaption interdentally.

Maintaining the full height of gingival tissue, labially or buccally, and with the exaggerated scallop and thinned tissue palatally, good approximation of tissue can usually be obtained interdentally without the formation of a soft tissue interdental crater. The flaps are stabilised with interrupted sutures.

The modified *Widman* flap technique is particularly valuable in maxillary anterior parts of the mouth, where aesthetic factors are important. The inductive potential, with the filling-in of vertical bony defects following this technique, has recently been demonstrated in a comparative clinical trial of various methods of pocket elimination by *Rosling et al* (1976). Repair following the modified Widman flap procedure is by means of a long junctional epithelium, not by a new attachment of connective tissue. It has been suggested that this may be a disadvantage with the potential for new pocket formation (*Barrington* 1981). However, a recent study by *Magnusson et al* (1983) suggests that the barrier function of a long junctional epithelium against plaque infection is not inferior to that provided by a dentogingival epithelium of normal length.

The replaced flap and open flap curettage

Where the pocket depths are well within the zone of attached gingiva, but underlying bony deformities are present, usually in maxillary posterior areas, pocket elimination and correction of gingival and osseous contours can be obtained by means of the replaced flap. The crest of the bone is detected by probing through the base of the pocket and the internally bevelled incision is carried out 2 mm coronal to the crest of the bone, both on the buccal and palatal sides (Figs. 59 and 60). Following debridement and osseous reshaping, the tissue flaps are replaced. Pocket depth, of course, will be eliminated by removal of the coronal cuff of gingival tissue.

Open flap curettage, in contrast, is used as a 'clean out' procedure in areas where pocket depths and osseous deformities are severe. The internally bevelled incision is kept close to the gingival margin on the buccal and palatal or lingual sides. The full

thickness flaps are widely reflected beyond the mucogingival junction for access and visibility. Following debridement, the flaps are replaced. However, because the mucogingival junction has been reflected, the buccal and lingual flaps will tend to drop apically. This procedure is useful where bone grafting procedures are to be employed.

The apically positioned flap

Pocket depths may extend close to or beyond the mucogingival junction; either an externally bevelled gingivectomy, or an internally bevelled incision related to the crest of the bone would result in incisions being placed in alveolar mucosa and with little or no gingiva remaining postoperatively. Under these circumstances, the entire gingival wall of the pocket is retained on the labial or buccal side. The internally bevelled incision is carried out around the necks of the involved teeth, keeping the incision close to the gingival margin. It is not related to the underlying bone. The split thickness incision will thin the gingival tissue and ends at the crest of the bone. The flap is then detached from the underlying bone with a periosteal elevator in an apical direction.

The mucogingival junction will be freed and the extent of bone exposure usually depends on the visibility that is required for osseous correction. If further detachment of the flap is required beyond this point to obtain adequate apical positioning, then the dissection can be split thickness, leaving periosteum to protect the underlying bone. The apically positioned flap, therefore, is really a three-part flap: split thickness to thin the flap coronally, full thick-

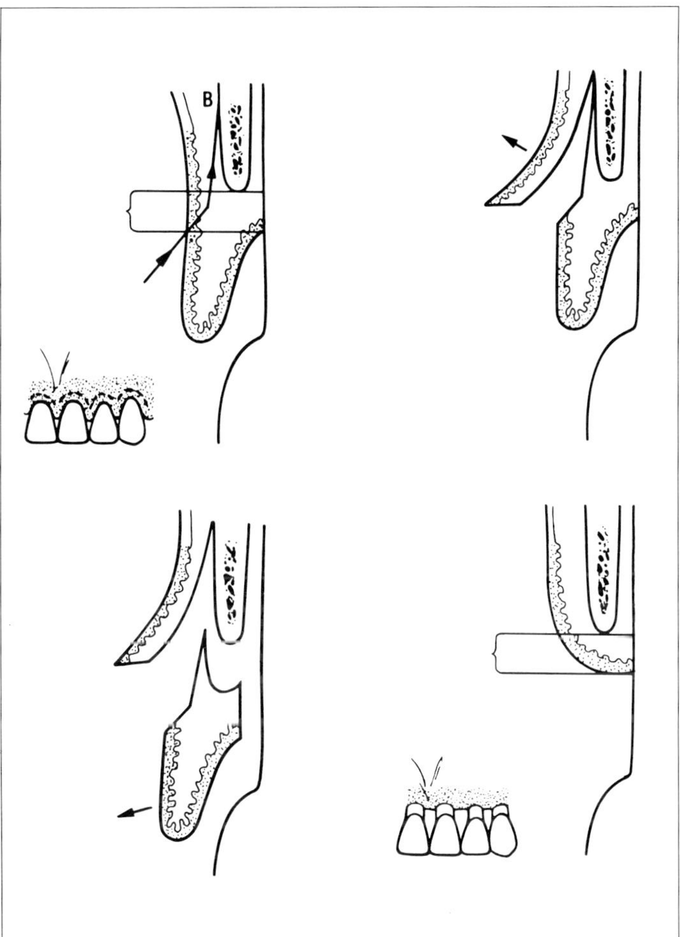

Fig. 59 The replaced flap. Where pocket depths are well within the zones of attached gingiva (usually in the maxilla) the position of the internally bevelled incision on the labial or buccal is made 2 mm coronal to the crest of the bone, that can be sounded by pushing a probe through the base of the pocket. When the marginal cuff is resected, the flap can then be replaced, but the gingival margin is now in its normal anatomical relationship to the underlying bone and pocket depth has been eliminated. Flap reflection is not carried beyond the mucogingival junction so that the tissue is not apically positioned.

ness to expose the underlying bony deformities, and split thickness again to obtain depth for the flap to be positioned apically (Fig. 61). On the palatal side, the reverse bevel incision is carried out 2 mm coronal to the crest of the bone and a similar procedure can often be used lingually in the mandibular molar areas, where the gingival width is greater. Circumferential or continuous sutures are used to suspend the flap around the necks of the teeth. Periosteal sutures improve the reliability of the procedure by preventing a coronal displacement of the flap. The apically positioned flap is the procedure of choice for crown lengthening procedures, osseous resection being carried out if necessary. A marked disadvantage of the procedure is root exposure in anterior parts of the mouth and problems with aesthetics.

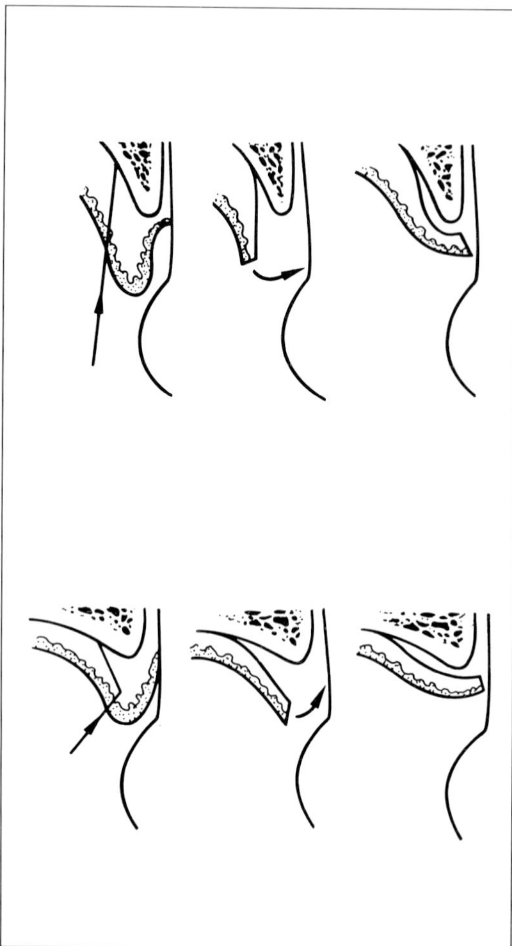

Fig. 60   The internally bevelled incision on the palate. When the gingival tissue is thin and the palatal vault deep, the internally bevelled incision to eliminate pocket depth is made 2 mm coronal to the crest of the bone and angulated to thin the flap at the same time. When the internal wedge of tissue is resected away, the margin of the flap is displaced along the same horizontal plane to fit tightly around the neck of the tooth and to cover the underlying bone. When the palate is shallow and the gingiva thick and detached, the crown of the tooth will restrict the positioning of the scalpel blade. Accordingly an initial incision, some 2 or 3 mm deep, is made using a Bard Parker No. 15 scalpel blade. This incision is then re-entered using a Goldman Fox No. 7 knife, which will allow the secondary incision to be angulated, so thinning the flap. Following the removal of the cervical wedge of tissue, the flap margin is adapted to cover the crest of the bone. It should be noted, however, that the flap margin is displaced through the arc of a circle, in contrast to the steep palate and therefore an increased length of flap will be required for adequate coverage of the crestal bone and close contact with the necks of the teeth.

The importance of a functional zone of attached gingiva

The attached gingiva, under normal conditions, appears as a ribbon of keratinized tissue, firmly bound down to the underlying bone and cementum around the necks of the teeth, and with a marginal cuff of about 2 mm that is detached and forms the gingival sulcus. The function of attached gingiva is to accept the shearing stresses of mastication and to dissipate muscle pull on the marginal tissues. It has been suggested that the dense, closely packed collagen fibre groups found in zones of attached gingiva are better deterrents to the infiltration of inflammation than the loosely arranged fibre apparatus of alveolar mucosa. Support for this contention was given by *Lang* and *Löe* (1972) in their study of attached gingiva. They found that areas with a band of attached gingiva of less than 2 mm had more persistent gingi-

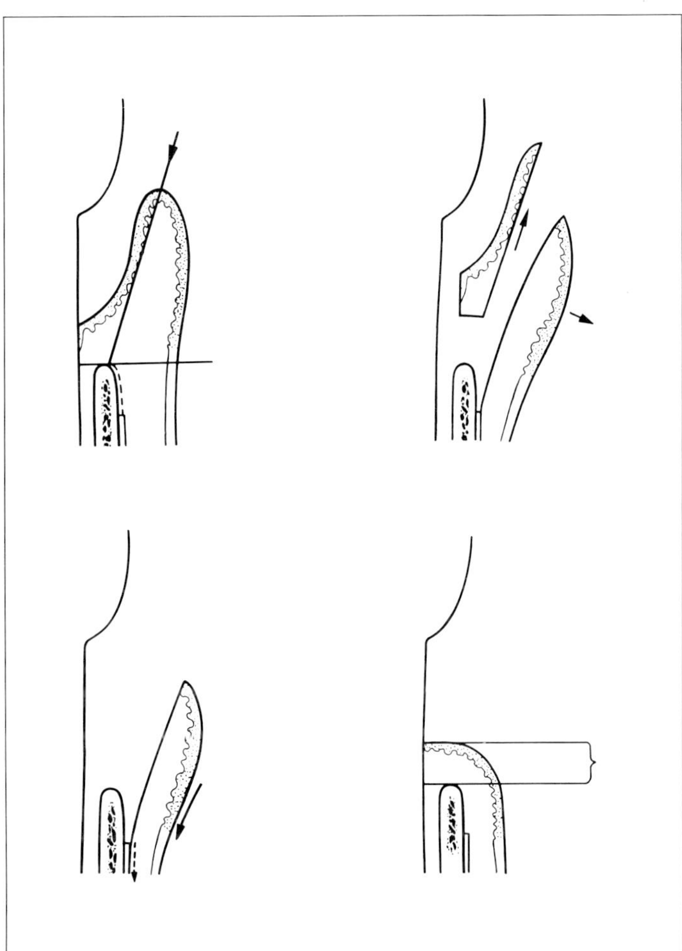

Fig. 61 The apically positioned flap. When pocket depths
extend close to or beyond the
mucogingival junction, the internally bevelled incision is
kept close to the gingival margin. The thinned outer wall of
the pocket is reflected beyond
the mucogingival junction and
apically positioned 2 mm coronal to the crest of the bone.

val inflammation. On the other hand, experiments in humans by *Miyasato et al*
(1977) and *DeTrey* and *Bernimoulin* (1980),
in which no tooth cleaning measures were
exercised for 21 to 25 days, showed that
no significant differences were observed
with respect to development of clinical
signs of inflammation between areas with
presence or absence of attached gingiva.
These findings were further substantiated
by the report of *Wennström* and *Lindhe*
(1983) on beagle dogs. It was concluded by
these workers that a free gingival margin,
which is supported by loosely attached
alveolar mucosa, is not more susceptible
to inflammation than a free gingival margin
which is supported by a wider zone of attached gingiva.

Whether the findings from these experimental models can be related to the clinical
situation in periodontally susceptible patients with extensive restorations, and

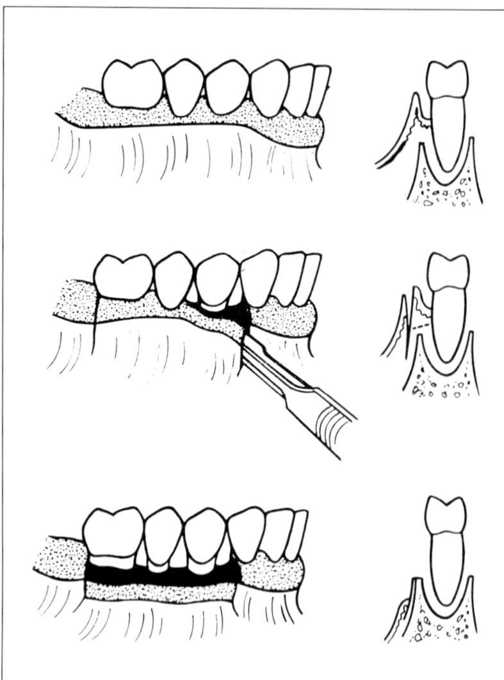

Fig. 62   The split thickness apically positioned flap. Where gingival width needs to be increased and sufficient vestibular depth exists, a split thickness flap is displaced apically to the crest of the bone. New attached gingiva is formed over the exposed periosteum and blends in with the existing gingival tissue to give an increased width of attached gingiva.

perhaps less than perfect plaque control, still has to be established. A minimal zone of attached gingiva may be increased by one of two methods. The split thickness apically displaced flap, or soft tissue grafts.

The split thickness apically displaced flap

This procedure can be used to increase the zone of attached gingiva and eliminate pocket depths that are close to or beyond the mucogingival junction, provided there is an adequate depth to the vestibular fornix. In order to conserve all the existing gingiva, an internally bevelled incision is made close the gingival margin. A vertical releasing incision will often be helpful in providing a plane of dissection for the scal-

pel blade in an apical coronal direction. The marginal cuff is curetted away and the mucoperiosteal flap apically positioned to the desired level and securely stabilised with sutures. During healing, granulation tissue covers the exposed periosteum and matures to form keratinized attached gingiva; depending on the level to which the flap was positioned, an overall gain in gingival width will result (Fig. 62). The split thickness apically displaced flap is used most commonly in the mandibular labial and buccal areas, where gingival width is inherently small. The mandibular lingual area presents a more difficult problem because of the difficulties of split thickness dissection. A full thickness flap is therefore employed, apically positioned, to expose a small area of marginal bone.

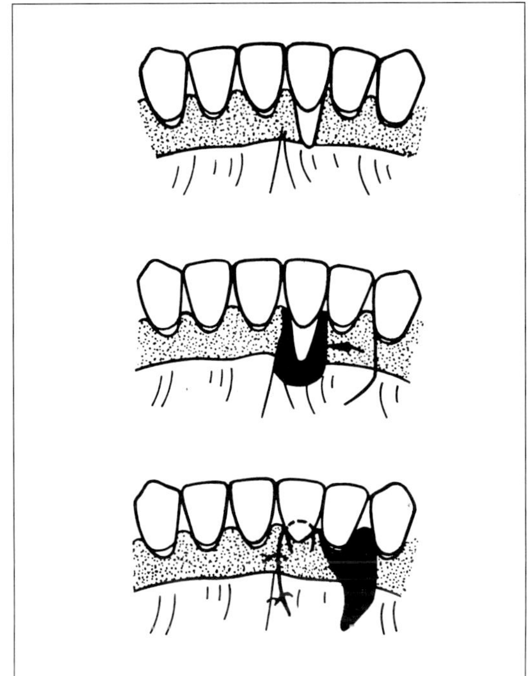

Fig. 63   The laterally positioned flap. This form of repair can be used to treat isolated areas of recession, providing vestibular depth is adequate, sufficient gingival tissue is present laterally and underlying bony dehiscences or fenestrations are not suspected. Opinions vary in the literature as to whether this flap should be full thickness, periosteum over the donor area, but also providing periosteum to cover the exposed root surface, which will be of benefit during healing.

Pedicle grafts

Grupe and *Warren* (1956) were the first to introduce pedicle graft procedures in periodontics and later modifications have been suggested by *Corn* (1964) and *Cohen* and *Ross* (1968). The laterally repositioned flap can be used where there is a lack of attached gingiva on one particular tooth (Fig. 63; 64 a, b, c). It is essential that adequate vestibular depth is present and that donor tissue is of adequate width and quality. Prominent root surfaces on palpation and thin gingival tissue may point to an underlying dehiscence in the donor area and, in such instances, the lateral graft is contraindicated.

A gingivectomy incision is made along the margins of the defect and, where necessary, is extended apically to include frena and muscle attachments that are encroaching on the area. The bevel of the gingivectomy incision on the stable side of the recipient area should be long to provide for a good overlap with the donor flap. The root surface is planed to remove the surface layer of cementum, with its entrapped endotoxin and plaque. Where the root surface is prominent, reduction may be required with a fine diamond stone in an air turbine to bring the root prominence within the boundaries of the alveolus. The donor flap is then dissected, using an internally bevelled incision marginally and a vertical incision 1½ tooth widths lateral to the recipient site. The donor tissue is dissected on a partial thickness basis to ensure adequate periosteal and connective tissue protec-

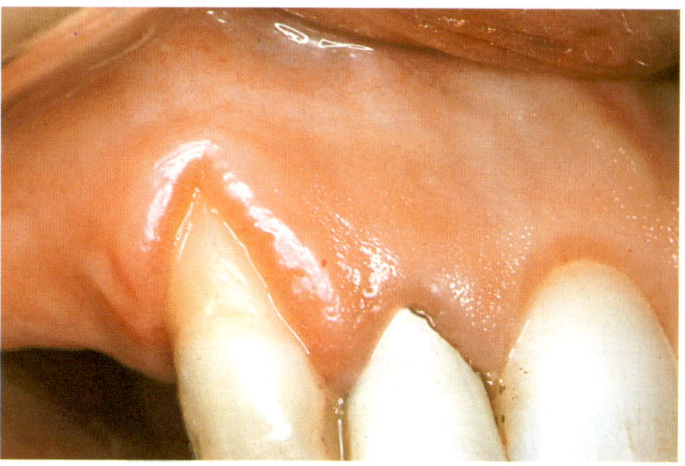

Fig. 64 (a) Lesion prior to surgery. (b) A split thickness laterally repositioned flap to repair recession on the maxillary right canine. A marginal cuff of tissue is left around the neck of the tooth in the donor area to avoid unnecessary recession. In this instance the thin delicate tissue that was present in the saddle area did not represent good donor tissue and the more anterior area was preferred. (c) The postoperative result shows good root coverage prior to restorative dentistry, but a small amount of gingivoplasty would be an advantage to thin the tissues at this stage.

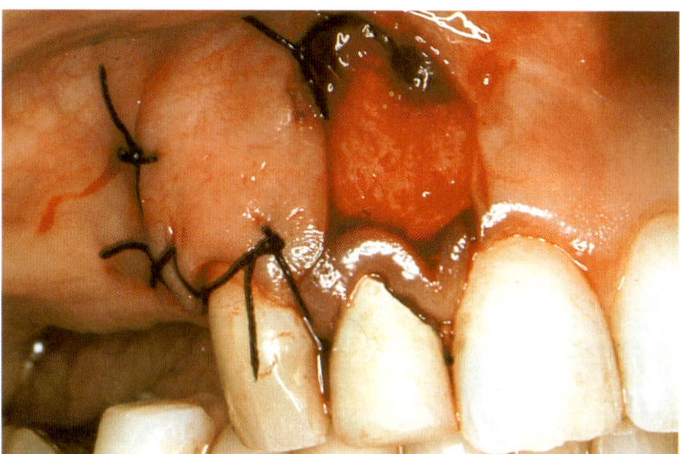

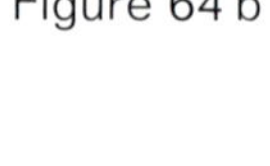

Figure 64 b

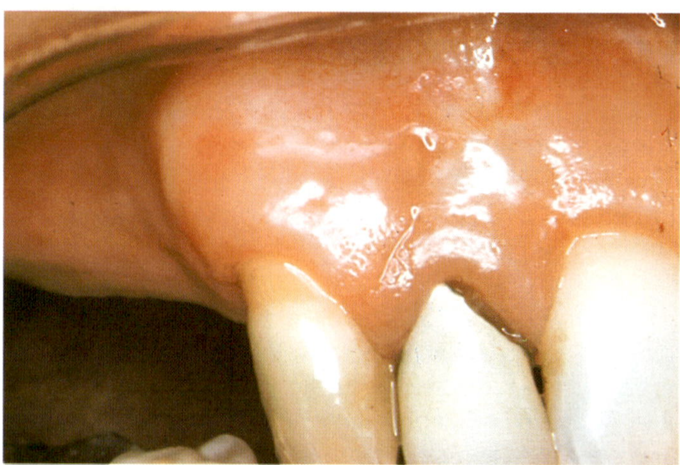

Figure 64 c

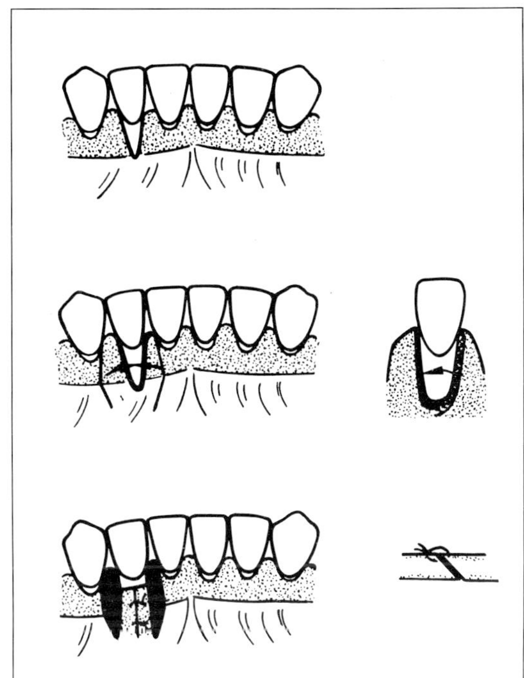

Fig. 65   The double papilla flap allows the use of papillary tissue mesially and distally to the defect and avoids the exposure of marginal bone. The delicate flaps should be full thickness and overlapped to avoid a butt joint.

tion of the exposed area. A cut-back incision in the direction to which the flap is to be repositioned will ensure adequate mobility and lessen tension on the flap in its new position. The flap is then sutured into place with a circumferential suture around the neck of the recipient tooth and interruptal sutures at the area of overlap.

The double papilla flap provides a useful alternative form of treatment for repairing isolated areas of recession (Fig. 65). In this technique the donor tissue is mobilised solely from the adjacent papillae. The ideal situation for its use would be in treating a narrow cleft with insufficient donor tissue to construct a lateral flap, or where the possibility of dehiscence may exist over the root surface in the potential donor area.

The distal papillae is bevelled to expose connective tissue, which will be covered by the overlap of the mesial portion of the flap, thereby avoiding a butt joint. The papillae are then sutured together, a delicate operation, and stabilised with periosteal sutures at their lateral margins. A sling suture is also employed around the neck of the tooth.

The edentulous area pedicle graft was described by *Corn* (1964). This modification of the laterally repositioned flap makes use of keratinized tissue from an edentulous saddle area. With careful dissection and use of a cut-back incision to improve mobility, the mucoperiosteal flap can be positioned both apically and laterally to cover the prepared root surface (Fig. 66; 67 a, b, c).

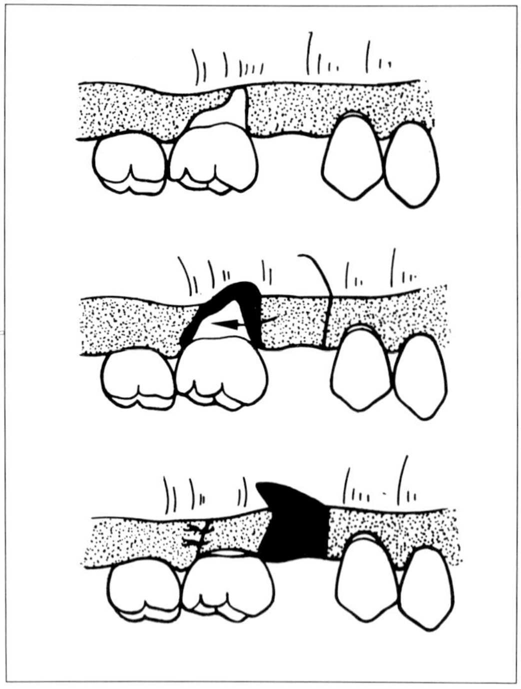

Fig. 66   The edentulous area pedicle graft utilises tissue from an adjacent saddle area, which can be apically and laterally positioned to cover an area of isolated recession.

Free gingival grafts

Free autogenous grafts have been used with great success for many years in plastic surgery. Their application in periodontal therapy is more recent and can be attributed to *King* and *Pennel* (1964) and the well-documented studies of *Sullivan* and *Atkins* (1968). The particular indications for the use of free gingival grafts are where there are inadequate bands of attached gingiva, often with high muscle attachments, in the presence of a shallow vestibule. In contrast to the flap procedures mentioned above, the free gingival graft can be effectively used to deepen the vestibule as well as increasing the zone of attached gingiva. The problems associated with muscle attachments will be eliminated when these fibres are dissected away from the area covered with mature gingival tissue. The free gingival graft is unpredictable when attempts are made to cover exposed root surfaces. The graft will usually necrose over the avascular root surface unless the defect is narrow and the periodontal membrane on each side close together to provide a good blood supply. The gingival graft should also be avoided in areas requiring osseous surgery. The danger here is that lack of adjacent periosteum may compromise the revascularisation of the graft. In these cases the establishment of a functional zone of attached gingiva is usually carried out as a two-stage procedure, the graft being carried out either before or after pocket elimination.

Fig. 67 (a)   Isolated recession on a maxillary canine caused by a partial denture. (b) The edentulous area pedicle graft is used to cover the root surface that has not been restored and a good overlap is made on the stable side. (c) The final result shows an adequate zone of attached gingiva, prior to the completion of restorative procedures.

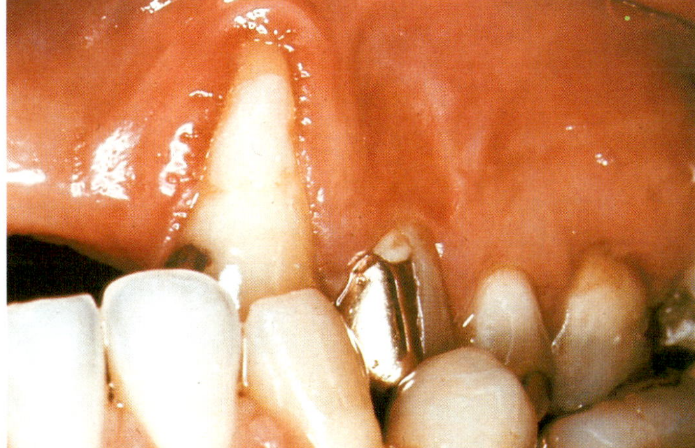

Figure 67 a

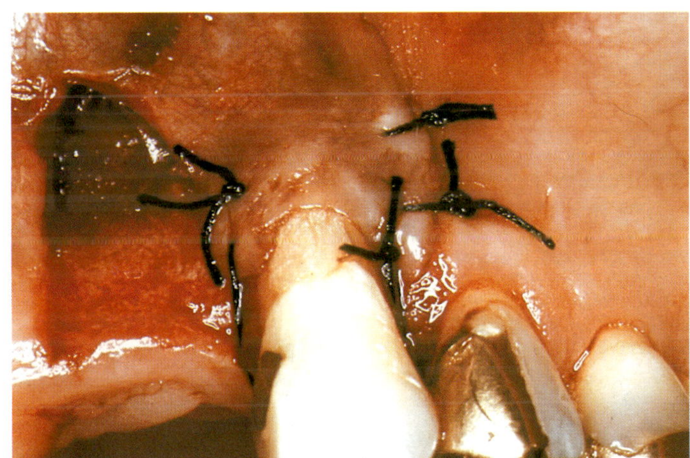

Figure 67 b

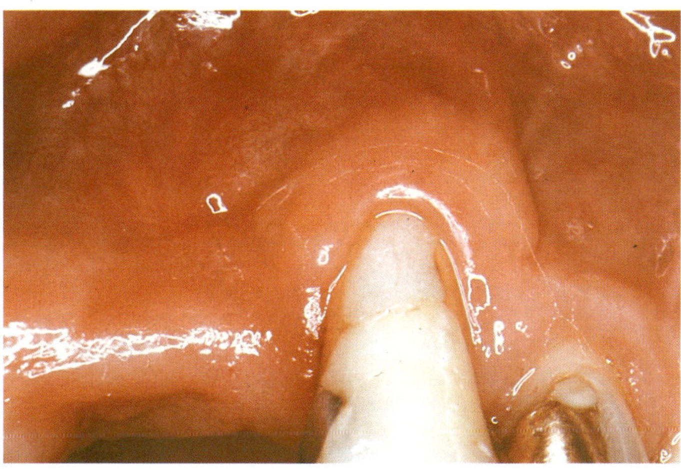

Figure 67 c

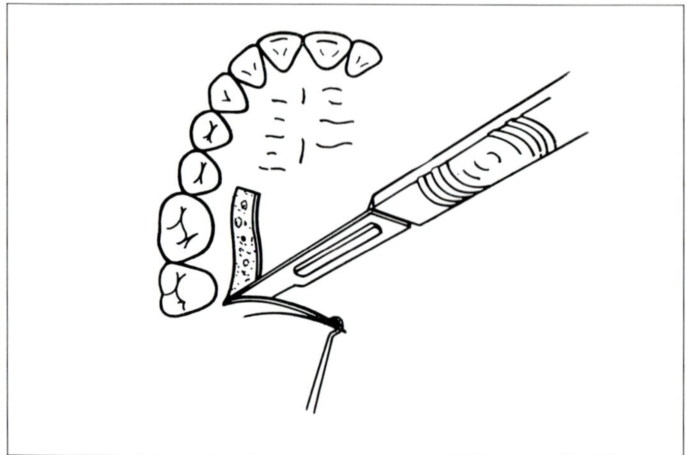

Fig. 68   A split thickness disection of graft tissue from the palate. This should be 1 to 1½ mm in thickness. The shape of the graft can be outlined with a Bard Parker No. 15 scalpel blade and either disected off using the same instrument, or a Goldman Fox No. 7 knife, which has an excellent angulation for this palatal procedure.

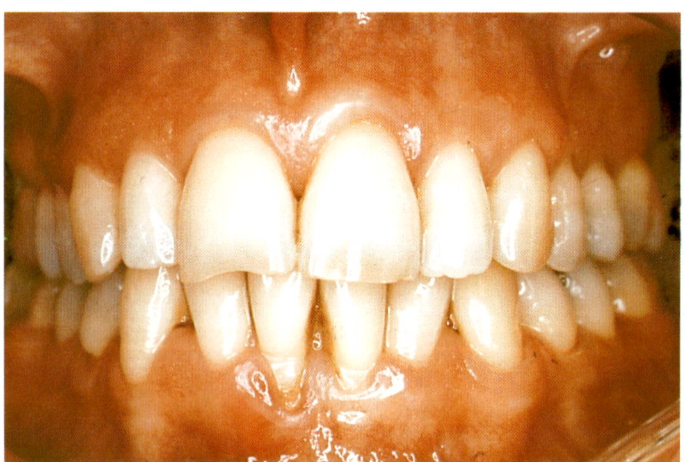

Fig. 69 (a)   Recession has occurred on the lower right mandibular incisor, leaving little or no attached gingiva. There is also a muscle pull. Some marginal tissue is still available on the lower left incisor tooth. (b) A free gingival graft has been utilised, replacing the gingival margin on the right incisor but being submarginal on the left incisor tooth.

Figure 69 a

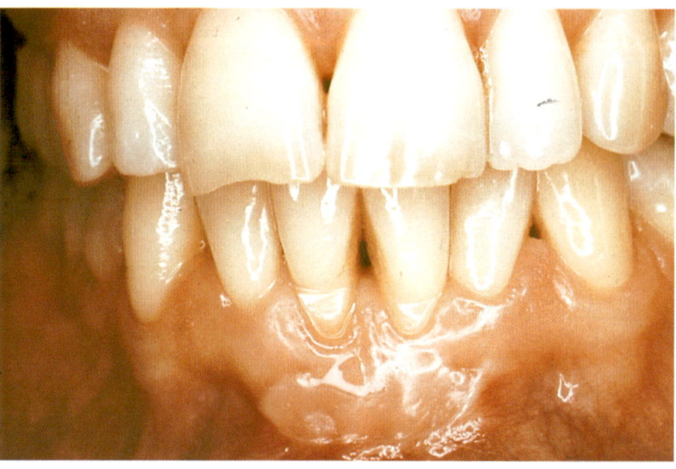

Figure 69 b

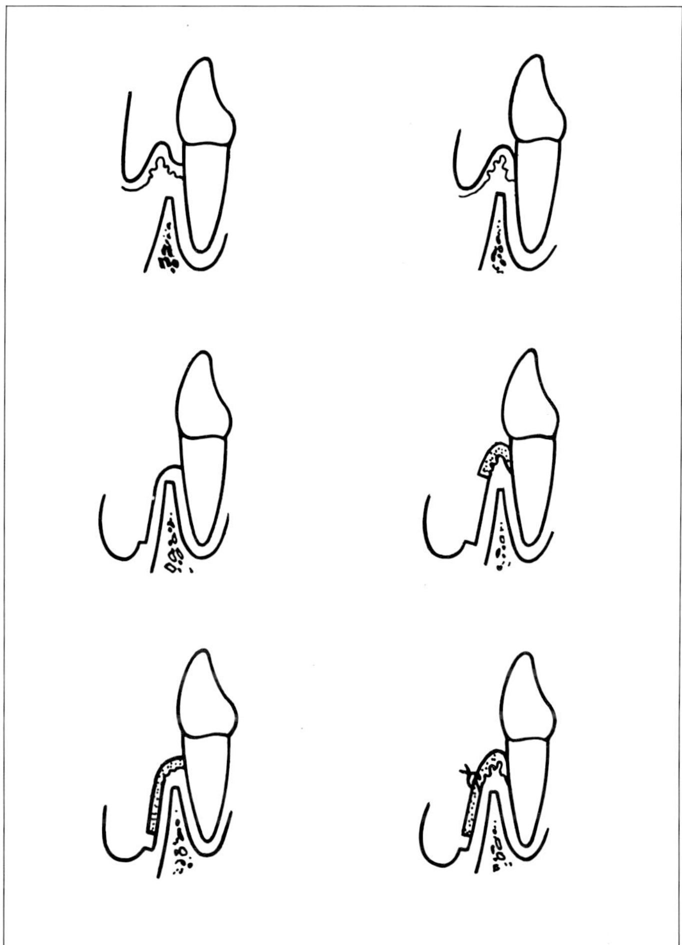

Fig. 70 Left: Where the marginal tissues are formed of mucosa, or where the gingival width is very narrow and perpetually inflamed, a marginal graft would be used to com pletely replace these tissues. Right: Where the marginal gingiva is healthy, but gingival width needs to be increased and vestibular depth is shallow, the marginal tissues can be left intact and the submarginal graft used.

Gingival grafts may be considered marginal or submarginal (Fig. 68 to 70). Where the marginal gingiva is narrow and perpetually inflamed, despite initial treatment, the graft should completely replace the marginal tissue. If, on the other hand, the gingival sulcus is clinically healthy and there is a narrow pre-existing zone of gingiva, this tissue is left *in situ,* but extended apically by means of a submarginal graft. The recipient site is prepared by means of a split thickness dissection, together with careful removal of all muscle and connective tissue down to the firm base of periosteum. The donor area for the graft is the masticatory mucosa of the hard palate and, if necessary, a foil template may be used to ensure the accurate size and shape of the graft. *Soehren et al* (1973) have suggested that the optimal thickness of gingival grafts should be 1 to 1.5 mm, based upon functional, healing, mechanical and aesthetic

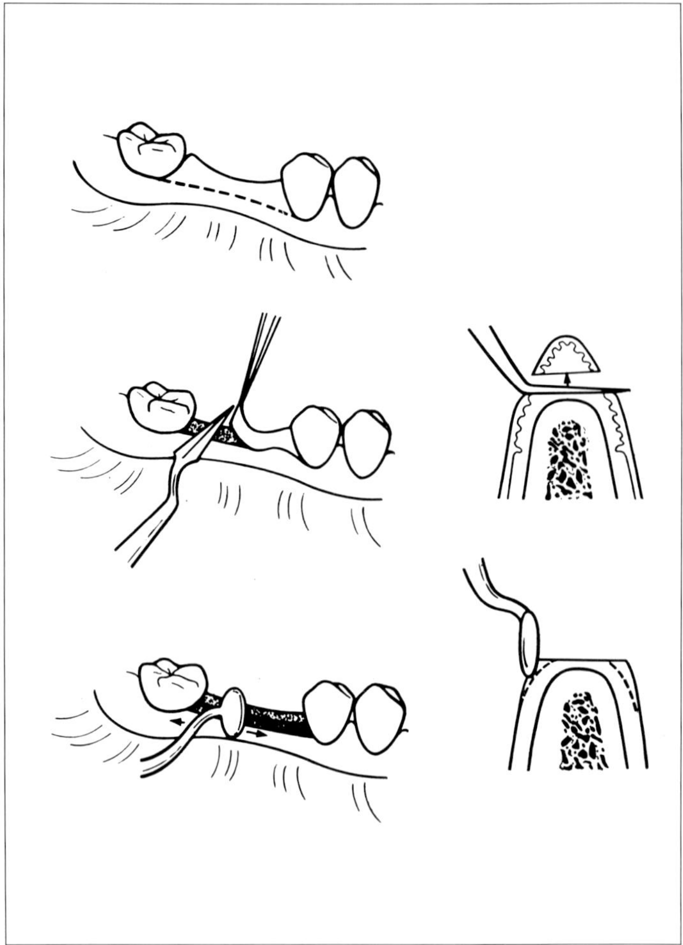

Fig. 71 A simple gingivect-omy/gingivoplasty incision can be used to correct distorted ridge areas, providing pocket depth is shallow and there is an adequate zone of attached gingiva. Either a Bard Parker No. 15 scalpel blade, or Goldman Fox No. 11 knife, can be used for the marginal resection and a Goldman Fox No. 7 knife used to scrape the tissue to provide the marginal bevelling.

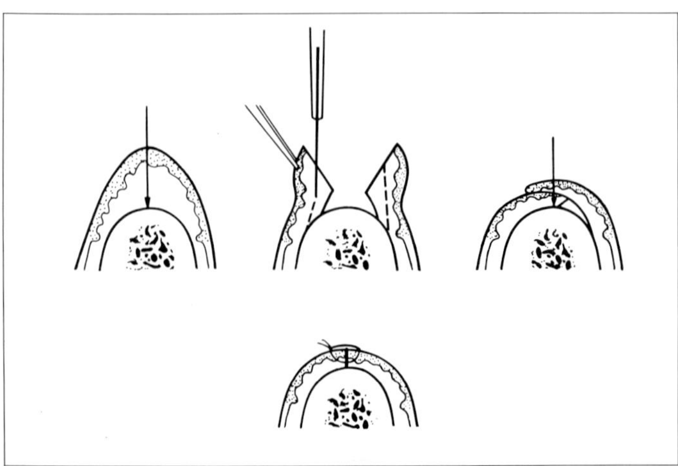

Fig. 72 If pocket depths are more severe and underlying bony deformities are present, a flap procedure should be used to eliminate pocket depths in relation to ridge areas. Where a more than adequate zone of attached gingiva is present, a linear incision is made along the crest of the ridge, the flaps partially reflected and thinned on their inner surface. The flaps are then overlapped and the excess tissue removed. The two flaps are then approximated with interrupted sutures.

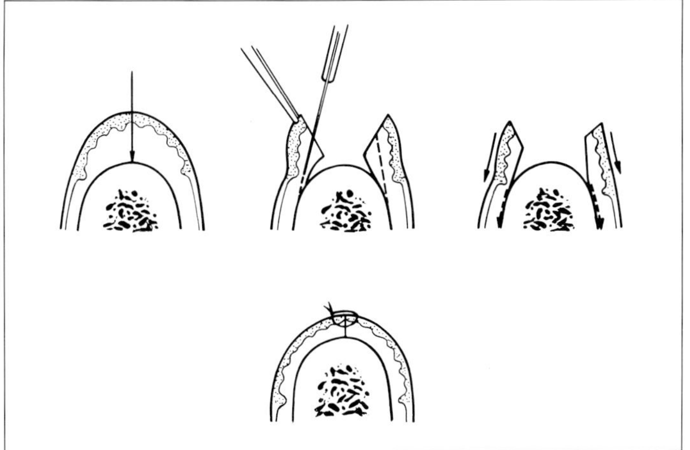

Fig. 73 Where gingival widths are barely adequate in relation to ridge areas, pocket depths should be eliminated by apically positioning the tissue, so that none of the gingival width is sacrificed. Ridgeplasty procedures should be blended in with surgery in adjacent areas.

factors. The graft should be completely immobilised during healing. Immobilisation is achieved by holding the graft under pressure for several minutes, to ensure a uniformly thin fibrin clot, then a minimal number of sutures can be inserted, or the coronal and lateral margins of the graft covered with cyanoacrylate. To reduce the area of the wound, the mucosa apical to the graft can be sutured to the underlying periosteum. On no account should it be sutured to the graft itself, because of the movement that will ensue. Both the recipient and donor sites are covered with surgical dressing.

The treatment of edentulous ridge areas

A simple gingivectomy/gingivoplasty technique can be used to correct distorted ridge areas, provided that adjacent pocket depth is shallow and there is an adequate zone of attached gingivae. The gingivectomy incision is carried right along the crest of the ridge, from one abutment tooth to the other. Following this, the ridge can be embellished by gingivoplasty either by means of scraping with the gingivectomy knife (Fig. 71) or by using a pair of surgical nippers. The removal of fibrous tissue from the crest of the ridge will produce more vertical space, so making for better and stronger pontic design.

If pocket depths are more severe and underlying bony deformities exist, a flap approach should be used. Providing there is an adequate zone of attached gingiva, two parallel and converging incisions are made along the crest of the ridge. The distance apart of these incisions will vary according to the pocket depths on the abutment teeth. The central wedge is removed and lateral wedges of tissue dissected free by undermining incisions. The flaps are then elevated as far as necessary to expose the underlying bony deformities, which can be reshaped, the flaps are then approximated and sutured (Fig. 72). Where the edentulous ridge has only a narrow zone of attached gingiva, it is wise to conserve this as far as possible. A linear

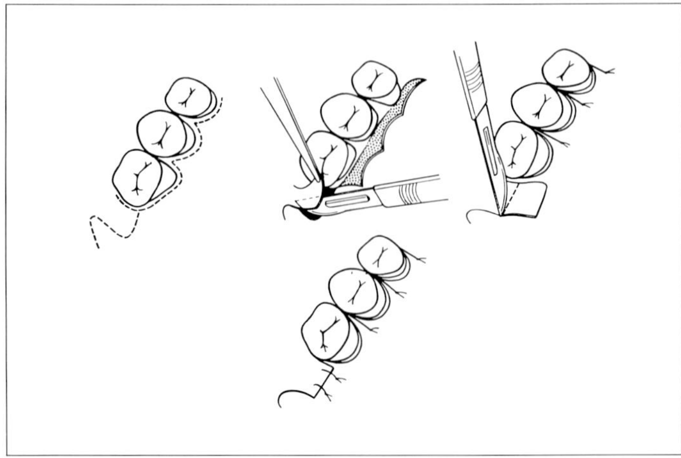

Fig. 74   A variety of incisions are available for tuberosity reduction, but one that works well is a split thickness lateral flap, reflected as part of the buccal gingival wall. The underlying area is debrided and osseous lesions treated as required and then the flap replaced over the area. The excess overlap can then be removed. Tuberosity procedures are again blended in with surgery that is being carried out around adjacent teeth.

incision is therefore made, passing along the crest of the ridge, the two flaps are elevated into a vertical plane and thinning incisions made allowing the wedges of thickened tissue to be removed. In order to facilitate the apical repositioning of the gingiva in the saddle area, the flaps are reflected beyond the mucogingival junction. Vertical relieving incisions may be necessary on the distal and mesial aspects of abutment teeth. This will depend on the periodontal procedures being carried out in adjacent areas. Following osseous surgery, the flaps are approximated and sutured. The gingival tissue in the saddle area, now occupying a more apical position, allows for an increase in clinical crown height and an optimal ridge contour for good pontic adaption (Fig. 73).

Tuberosity and retromolar areas

The presence of excessive amounts of thick fibrous tissue is common in both these areas. Pocket depths are due more to the exaggerated soft tissue morphology than to a down-growth of the epithelial attachment onto cementum. The shortened clinical crowns that result from these deformities in tuberosity and retromolar areas complicates tooth preparation, impression-taking and establishing a margin to the restoration that is supragingival. In addition, the shortened clinical crown provides inadequate retention. Surgical reduction of thickened tuberosity and retromolar areas follows the same principles as those outlined for ridge areas (Fig. 74; 75). A word of caution should be given about the excessive reduction of tuberosity tissue, because of the inherent problems that will occur if a partial denture is required at some time in the future. In these circumstances, a partial reduction of the tuberosity area may be carried out and the remaining pocket maintained by curettage. Where the first molar tooth is available, it may be more prudent to sacrifice the second molar when pocket depths related to tuberosity areas are excessively deep and involve the furcation.

Fig. 75 Pocket reduction in retromolar areas can be achieved by a split thickness flap distal to the last molar tooth. This allows the underlying connective tissue to be removed and exposure and treatment of osseous deformities. The flap is then collapsed back over the area and the excess tissue removed. This form of surgery is again blended in with surgical procedures in adjacent areas.

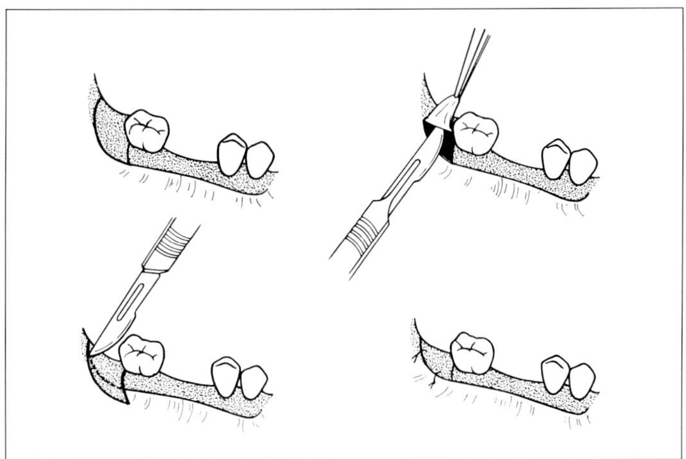

The management of periodontal abnormalities by root removal

The pattern of alveolar and supporting bone loss in periodontal disease may be unequal, even in relation to the different roots of a molar tooth. Removal of the offending root or roots will allow the tooth to be retained and, if necessary, to function as an abutment (Fig. 76 a, b). In some instances the roots of posterior teeth are in close proximity, making for difficulties in oral hygiene and treatment. This type of situation is often found where the distobuccal root of the first maxillary molar flares towards the mesiobuccal root of the second maxillary molar (Fig. 77 a, b). In addition to the problems of plaque control, no space remains for an adequate embrasure if these teeth are to be restored. The removal of one or both of these roots will allow for a manageable embrasure form. Following periodontal disease, the furcation areas of molar teeth may become exposed. Such areas are not amenable to plaque control and are often the site of

periodontal abscess formation. Such teeth are therefore not satisfactory as abutments. Removal of one root in relation to mandibular molar teeth, or one or two roots in relation to maxillary molars (Fig. 78 a, b), will allow access to these areas and carefully designed restorations will allow for adequate plaque control.

The maintenance problem

The inherent susceptibility of the periodontal tissues to recurrent disease must always be borne in mind. However, many studies have now demonstrated that it is possible, by comprehensive plaque control programmes, to prevent the progression of periodontitis (*Lovdal et al* 1961; *Lightner et al* 1971; *Lindhe* and *Nyman* 1975; *Hirschfeld* and *Wasserman* 1978; *Knowles et al* 1979).
Nyman and *Lindhe* (1979) reported on a 5 to 8 year study evaluating the potential

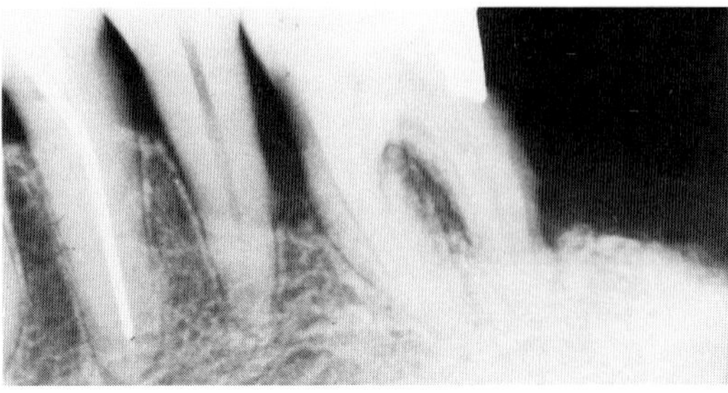

Figure 76 a

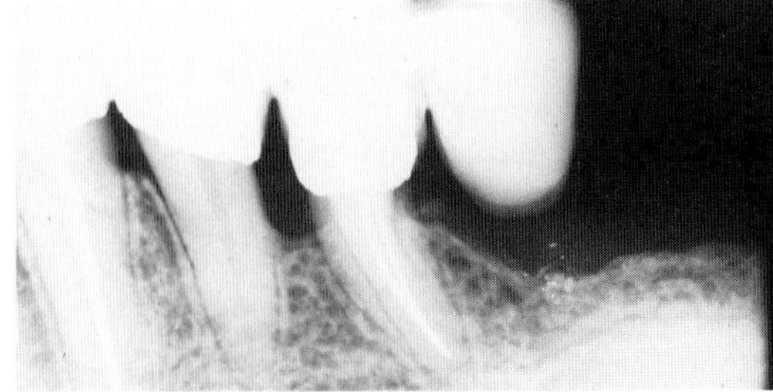

Figure 76 b

Fig. 76 (a)   A mandibular molar tooth with extensive periodontal destruction distally. The mesial root of the molar is retained and treated endodontically, the distal root removed by hemisection. (b) Following periodontal therapy, the mesial root provides excellent support for fixed bridgework.

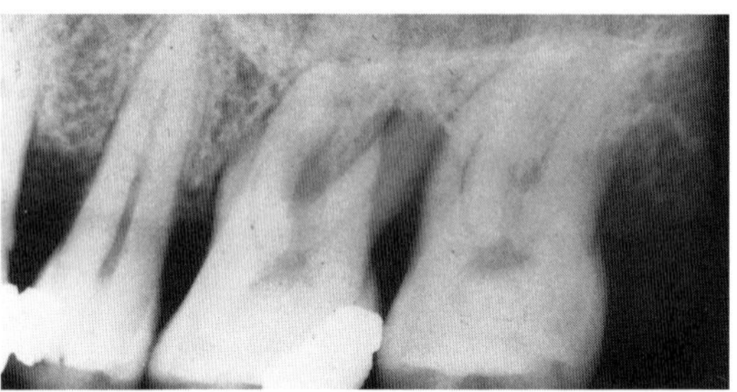

Figure 77 a

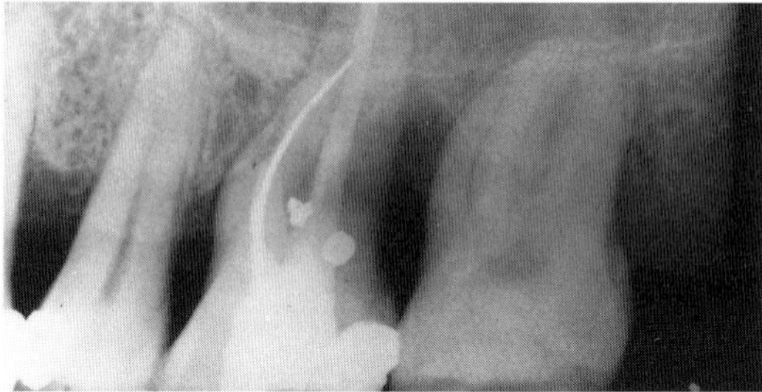

Figure 77 b

Fig. 77 (a)   Vertical alveolar bone loss is associated with the close proximity of the distobuccal root of the first molar and the mesiobuccal root of the second molar. (b) Root amputation of the distobuccal root of the first molar, together with endodontic therapy, will often allow for definitive pocket elimination. In some instances the mesiobuccal root of the second molar may also need removal.

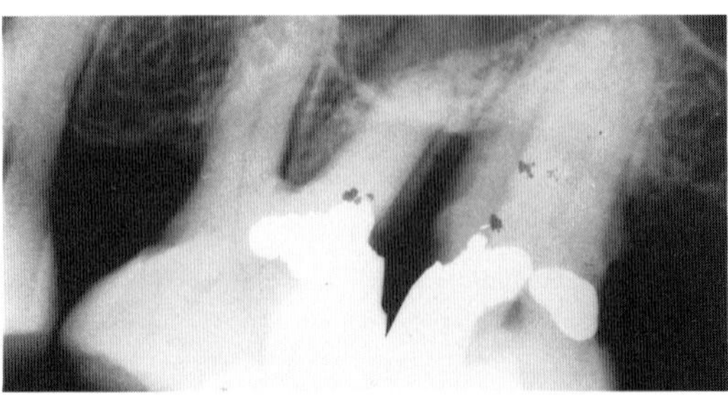

Figure 78 a

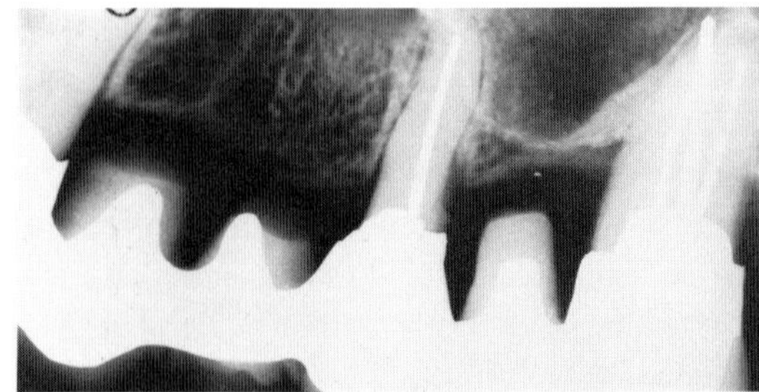

Figure 78 b

Fig. 78 (a)   Furcation involving maxillary first molar. The furcation could be probed through from buccal, mesial and distal aspects. (b) The mesiobuccal root with good bony support is retained as an abutment for a fixed bridge. The remaining two roots are sectioned and removed during periodontal surgery in this quadrant of the mouth.

72

for maintaining teeth with advanced periodontal problems in extensive prosthodontic cases. Fifty patients who were willing to accept periodontal treatment, including tooth extractions, periodontal surgery and prosthetic treatment, and who were also capable of maintaining optimal plaque control and were willing to appear every 3 to 6 months for maintenance care, were evaluated. Results showed a stable situation, using the parameters of plaque index, gingival index, pocket depth, attachment level and marginal alveolar bone height. In a classic study, *Axelsson* and *Lindhe* (1981) treated 90 patients with advanced periodontal disease. Scaling and plaque control procedures in well-motivated patients were followed by periodontal surgery to correct pocket depths. Two months after the completion of surgery the patients were divided into two groups.

Patients in the second group were maintained on a 2 to 3 month recall programme. When the results were compared over 3 and 6 years, the patients that were maintained on a carefully designed recall programme were able to maintain unaltered attachment levels. In contrast, patients who were not maintained in a supervised programme showed signs of recurrent periodontitis. A retrospective study by *Hirschfeld* and *Wasserman* (1978) assessed the results of treatment and continuous recall of patients in a private practice for periods of up to 50 years. The standard of plaque control in these patients would not be considered to be as perfect as those described in the Gothenberg studies (*Axelsson* and *Lindhe* 1981) and yet the results were excellent, despite the changing philosophies of treatment over this long span of time.

When planning partial dentures and restorations, it is essential that the design facilitates plaque control procedures. Crown margins should be kept supragingival, proximal areas should allow proper cleansing and the denture materials should be placed as far away from the marginal gingivae as possible. The problems of oral hygiene may be further compounded by restorations with precision attachments that distort the anatomy of abutment teeth. Despite the greatest care in the planning and execution of treatment, the results of periodontal therapy may result in anatomical deformities that are difficult to maintain. Available information has shown that gingivitis can be prevented buccally and lingually by the correct use of a toothbrush (*Lindhe* and *Koch* 1967), but the effect of the toothbrush alone has only a limited effect in interdental areas. A series of studies (*Gjermo* and *Flotra* 1970; *Wolffe* 1976; *Nyak* and *Wade* 1977) has shown that ancillary methods of interdental cleaning are absolutely essential if periodontal health is to be maintained. The choice of which agent to use seems to depend on the individual needs and capabilities of the subject in question. Thus, wood sticks, floss, proxa-brushes and interspace brushes were all of value, though none demonstrated a clear superiority. However, in wide open interproximal areas following periodontal destruction, the interdental brush proved to be the most efficient.

The well-worn phrase 'that familiarity breeds contempt' could not be more apt than when applied to the problems of maintenance. Dentists, by nature, are attracted to new patients with new and taxing problems and are often negligent about picking up the subtle tissue changes that may occur in patients who have been under their care over a long period. In the true sense of the word, periodontal disease is never cured but is only controlled, and there will be instances when further treatment will be required, possibly of a surgical nature. It is perhaps better to discuss these possibilities with the patient at the end of the treatment phase, rather than explain them at one of the recall appointments. The frequency of maintenance treatment should be based on tissue response. A frequent recall (every 2 to 4 months) is needed by patients whose plaque formation is heavy and where oral hygiene procedures, despite constant motivation, remain only moderate. On the other hand, patients who have excellent plaque control abd form monimal deposits on their teeth, can be seen at yearly intervals.

Periodontal probing in areas that are presenting problems should be carried out at each recall visit. A full periodontal probing should only be required every year. Particular attention should be paid to furcation involvements and areas of gingival recession should be re-assessed; tooth mobilities and occlusal relationships should also be recorded. A full mouth, long cone, radiographic survey need only be repeated once every 3 years. However, in areas of particular concern, a more frequent assessment may be required.

References

Axelsson P. and Lindhe J. (1981).
The significance of maintenance care in the treatment of periodontal disease. J. Clin. Periodont., 8: 281.

Barrington E. P. (1981)
An overview of periodontal surgical procedures. J. Periodont., 52: 518.

Bergman B., Hugoson A. and Olsson C. O. (1977)
Caries and periodontal status in patients fitted with removable partial dentures. J. Clin. Periodont., 4: 134.

Brown I. S. (1973)
The effect of orthodontic therapy on certain types of periodontal defects. I: Clinical findings. J. Periodont., 44: 727.

Carlsson S. E., Hedegard B. and Koivumaa K. K. (1965).
Studies in partial dental prosthesis. IV. Final results of a 4-year longitudinal investigation of dentogingivally supported partial dentures. Acta odont. scand., 23: 443.

Cohen B. (1959).
Morphological factors in the pathogenesis of periodontal disease Brit. Dent. J., 107: 31.

Cohen D. W. and Ross S. E. (1968).
The double papillae repositioned flap in periodontal surgery J. Periodont., 39: 65.

Corn H. (1964).
Edentulous area pedicle graft in mucogingival surgery. Periodontics, 2: 229.

Derry, A. and Bertram V. (1970).
A clinical survey of removable partial dentures, after two years usage. J. Prosth. Dent., 16: 721.

DeTrey E. and Bernimoulin J. R. (1980).
Influence of free gingival grafts on the health of the marginal gingiva. J. Clin. Periodont., 7: 381.

Eissmann H. F., Radke R. A. and Noble W. A. (1971).
Physiologic design criteria for fixed dental restorations. Dent. Clin. N. Amer., 15: 543.

Gjermo P. and Flotra L. (1970).
The effect of different methods of interdental cleaning. J. Periodont. Res., 5: 230.

Glavind L. (1977).
The effect of monthly professional mechanical tooth-cleaning on periodontal health in adults J. Clin. Periodont., 4: 100.

Grupe H. and Warren R. (1956).
Repair of gingival defects by sliding lateral flap. J. Periodont., 27: 92.

Hirschfeld L. and Wasserman B. (1978).
A long-term survey of tooth loss in 600 treated periodontal patients. J. Periodont., 49: 225.

King K. and Pennel B. (1964).
Free Autogenous Gingival Grafts. Paper presented at the Annual Meeting of the Philadelphia Society of Periodontology.

Knowles J. W., Burgett F. G., Nissle R. R. (1979).
Results of periodontal treatment related to pocket depth and attachment level. J. Periodont., 50: 225.

Koivumaa K. (1956).
Changes in periodontal tissues and supporting structures connected with partial dentures. Suom. hammaslaak. toim., 52: Suppl.l.

Koivumaa K., Hedegard B. and Carlsson G. (1960).
Studies in partial denture prosthesis. I. An investigation of dentogingivally supported partial dentures. Suom. hammaslaak. toim., 56: 248.

Lang N. P., Cumming B. R. and Löe H. (1973).
Tooth brushing frequency as it relates to plaque development and gingival health. J. Periodont., 44: 396.

Lang N. P. and Löe H. (1972).
The relationship between the width of keratinized gingiva and gingival health. J. Periodont., 43: 623.

Leon A. (1975).
A Clinical Study of the Effect of Cl. II. Amalgam Fillings on the Periodontium. M.D.S. Thesis, University of London.

Lightner L. M., O'Leary T. J., Drake B. D., Cramp P. P. and Allen M. F. (1971).
Preventive periodontic procedures: results over 46 months. J. Periodont., 42: 555.

Lindhe K. and Koch G. (1967).
The effect of supervised oral hygiene on the gingivae of children: Lack of prolonged effect of supervision. J. Periodont. Res., 2: 215.

Lindhe J. and Nyman S. (1975).
The effect of plaque control and surgical pocket elimination on the establishment and maintenance of periodontal health. A longitudinal study of periodontal therapy in cases of advanced disease. J. Clin. Periodont., 2: 67.

Löe H., Theilade E. and Jensen S. B. (1965).
Experimental gingivitis in man. J. Periodont., 36: 177.

Lovdal A., Arno A., Schei O. and Waerhaug J. (1961).
Combined effect of supragingival scaling and controlled oral hygiene on the incidence of gingivitis. Acta odontol. scand., 19: 537.

Magnusson I., Runstad L., Nyman S. and Lindhe J. (1983).
A long junctional epithelium, a locus minoris resistentiae in plaque infection. J. Clin. Periodont., 10: 333.

Marcum J. S. (1967).
The effect of crown marginal depth upon gingival tissues. J. Prosth. Dent., 17: 479.

Miyasato M., Crigger M. and Egelberg J. (1977).
Gingival condition in areas of minimal and appreciable width of keratinized gingiva. J. Clin. Periodont., 4: 200.

Newcomb J. M. (1974).
The relationship between the location of subgingival crown margins and gingival inflammation. J. Periodont., 45: 151.

Nyak R. P. and Wade A. B. (1977).
The relative effectiveness of plaque removal by the Proxa brush and rubber cone stimulator. J. Clin. Periodont., 4: 128.

Nyman S. Rosling B. and Lindhe J. (1975).
The effect of professional tooth cleaning on healing after periodontal surgery. J. Clin. Periodont., 2: 80.

Nyman S. and Lindhe J. (1979).
A longitudinal study of combined periodontal and prosthetic treatment of patients with advanced periodontal disease. J. Periodont., 50: 163.

Parkinson C. D. (1976).
Excessive crown contours facilitate endemic plaque niches. J. Prosth. Dent., 35: 424.

Ramfjord S. P. (1959).
Indices for prevalence and incidence of periodontal disease. J. Prosth. Dent., 35: 424.

Ramfjord S. P., Knowles J. W., Nissle R. R., Schick R. A. and Burgitt F. G. (1973).
A longitudinal study of periodontal therapy. J. Periodont., 44: 66.

Ramfjord S. P. and Nissle R. R. (1974).
The modified Widman flap. J. Periodont., 45: 601.

Rosling B., Nyman S., Lindhe J. and Jern B. (1976).
The healing potential of the periodontal tissues following different techniques of periodontal surgery in plaque free dentitions. A two year clinical study. J. Clin. Periodont., 3: 233.

Silness, J. (1970).
The periodontal condition in patients treated with dental bridges. III. The relationship between the location of crown margins and periodontal conditions. J. Periodont. Res., 5: 225.

Sockransky S. S. (1970).
The relationship of bacteria to the etiology of periodontal disease. J. Dent. Res., Supplement No. 2.

Soehren S. E., Allen A. L., Cutright D. E. and Seibert J. S. (1973).
Clinical and histologic studies of donor tissues utilized for free grafts of masticatory mucosa. J. Periodont., 44: 727.

Sullivan H. and Atkins J. (1968).
Free autogenous gingival grafts. II. Principles of successful grafting. Periodontics, 6: 121.

Suomi J. D., Greene J. C., Vermillion J. R., Doyle J., Chang J. J. and Leatherwood E. C. (1971).
The effect of controlled oral hygiene procedures on the progression of periodontal diseases in adults. Results after the third and final year. J. Periodont., 42: 152.

Tomlin H. R. and Osborne J. (1961).
Cobalt chromium partial dentures. A clinical survey. Brit. Dent. J., 110: 307.

Valderhaug J. (1972).
Prepaver ingsgrensens beliggenhet krone/bro synspunkter. Norske Tandlaegeforen. Tidende, 82: 386.

Wennstrom, J. and Lindhe, J. (1983).
Plaque induced gingival inflammation in the absence of attached gingiva in dogs. J. Clin. Periodont., 10: 266.

Wheeler R. C. (1962).
Complete crown form and the periodontium. J. Prosth. Dent., 11: 722.

Widman L. (1920).
The operative treatment of pyorrhea alveolaris, a new surgical method. Stockholm 1918. Reviewed in the Brit. Dent. J., SI: 293.

Wolffe G. N. (1976).
An evaluation of proximal surface cleansing agents. J. Clin. Periodont., 3: 148.

Yuodelis R. A., Weaver J. D. and Saphos G. (1973).
Facial and lingual contours of artificial complete crown restorations and their effect on the periodontium. J. Prosth. Dent., 29: 61.

Chapter 3

The Occlusal Surfaces

The occlusal surfaces influence jaw movements, effect jaw postures and determine masticatory movements. The forces of mastication and occlusion are transmitted through these areas. The occlusal surfaces of a restoration are its working surfaces and need to be planned with care and constructed with accuracy.

Dentures are normally constructed to place artificial teeth in the mouth. It is surprising, therefore, that in practice one so often finds these artificial teeth added apparently as an afterthought. Components of partial dentures may interfere with the articulation of the opposing teeth. By their irregularities these opposing teeth may play havoc with the denture when eccentric jaw movements are attempted. Had these problems been diagnosed, correction at an early stage of treatment would have been relatively straightforward. Instead, we all too frequently see desperate and mutilating 'corrections' in which an attempt is made to adapt a prosthesis to a hopeless situation. At best, the prognosis, function and appearance of the restoration is jeopardised. Bearing in mind the time, care and cost involved in extensive restorations, a cavalier attitude to the occlusal surfaces is hard to justify.

Important as it may be, careful analysis of individual diagnostic casts alone is inadequate. These casts must be correctly related to one another, requiring an intermaxillary record. Since the intermaxillary record may involve a change in vertical dimension, a facebow should be employed. Even if centric relation were recorded at the vertical relation of occlusion, the facebow would still be necessary as an aid in the assessment of lateral jaw movements. Furthermore, the infra-orbital marker will relate the occlusal plane to the Frankfort plane, a factor that may help in planning the appearance of the restoration. Precise hinge axis location is not always necessary so that relatively simple facebows like the Dentatus, Hanau, or Whipmix will suffice. *Matsumoto* (1976) has classified deficient occlusions into three groups.

Group 1: The vertical dimension of occlusion is determined by occlusal stops.

Group 2: No occlusal stops, but teeth present in both jaws.

Group 3: Teeth present in one jaw only.

Depending on the patient's dentition, the vertical dimension of occlusion may be assessed by:

1. Direct measurement
2. Indirect measurement.

The vertical relation of occlusion

If this essential relationship is determined by the natural teeth, a major difficulty is overcome. One can proceed as follows:

1. Direct apposition of casts

This simple and accurate method may be employed where there are adequate teeth remaining in contact to make the existing jaw relationship obvious. One proviso is essential: a previous occlusal analysis in centric relation and the correction of any interferences.

2. Overlay occlusal rims

This procedure may be used where there are widely spaced occlusal stops, but insufficient teeth present to allow direct cast apposition. The Dawson-type occlusal rim is constructed on the upper cast covering the premolar and molar teeth. It should not touch the areas representing the mucosa. This wax is chilled and cut away from the buccal cusps so that the seating of the cast in the record is easily checked.

3. Mucosal-borne occlusal rims

Unfortunately the remaining occlusal stops are often closely spaced, particularly where distal extension spaces are present. In these circumstances the occlusal rim will need to be mucosal-supported and closely adapted to the edentulous area. Hard wax bases will suffice, if handled with care. A soft recording index, such as fast-setting stone or zinc-oxide, is desirable. Record bases supported by mucosa are particularly prone to distortion and errors in jaw relation recording owing to the forces that may be exerted by the opposing natural teeth. A shortage of vertical space in the edentulous area may well become apparent at this stage so that a little extra time spent planning early on will be well rewarded later. Far better to spend a few extra moments early in the therapy, than to be faced with hours of frustration later on.

Unlike a complete denture, in which the condylar pathway is virtually the only factor outside the operator's control, the partial denture will have to conform to an established occlusal plane. Careful jaw relation recordings will show the modifications necessary to the opposing teeth.

Without occlusal stops the problem is more complex. Efforts at measuring the vertical relation of occlusion by maximum biting force, or other means, have not yet proved reliable in clinical practice. It is therefore necessary to make indirect assessments by first measuring the vertical relation of rest.

The vertical relation of rest

The original *Brodie* and *Thompson* concept (1942, 1946) of a stable vertical dimension of rest throughout life was convenient for prosthodontics as removal of the teeth was not considered to affect the rest position of the mandible. Unfortunately, the theory has not stood the test of time. *Nairn* (1976) has pointed out that removal of teeth or occlusal stops is often followed by the adoption of a new rest position, usually with the jaws closer together. *Tallgren*

(1967) showed that dentures can be constructed to a variety of occlusal vertical dimensions all demonstrating an inter-occlusal (freeway) space. Demonstrations of inter-occlusal space were not by themselves reliable guides to the occlusal vertical dimension of the dentures.

Factors influencing the vertical dimension of rest may include higher centres, mechanoreceptor activity in the periodontal ligament, oral mucosa and temporomandibular joint, together with possible monosynaptic stretch reflexes. *Möller* (1976) has put forward evidence suggesting that the rest position is subject to a servo-control mechanism. *Yemm* (1976), however, postulated that the position is determined by the tendency of structures to come to physical rest because of their visco-elastic properties.

Whatever the outcome of these controversies the best the clinician can achieve is to seat his patient comfortably and upright. An assessment should be made with the minimum of fuss and with no more than one occlusal rim in the mouth. The occlusal rims are mucosal-borne and usually constructed of extra-hard base wax.

With the vertical dimension of rest established, an inter-occlusal space needs to be provided. As a general rule, this space will measure about 4 mm in the first premolar region—slightly larger for patients with Angles Class II, Division II malocclusions and slightly smaller for those with Class III malocclusions. Swallowing and phonetic guides are often useful.

Patients who have only roots present in one jaw are treated as edentulous. The occlusal rims cover the roots.

Where teeth are present, jaw relation problems may be considered in two situations:

1. Teeth present in both jaws
2. Teeth present in one jaw alone.

In both situations, overerupted or tilted teeth may complicate the determination of the occlusal plane. To overcome these problems, steps will need to be cut in the opposing occlusal rim but not through the entire width. In this way a recess for the tooth can be provided while the occlusal plane level is maintained (Fig. 79). The manner in which the anterior section of the rim is cut will help decide both labial support and appearance (Fig. 80). It will clearly show irregularities of the occlusal plane requiring correction.

Far from being of assistance, non-occluding teeth present in both jaws complicate jaw relation recordings. First of all there may well be glancing contacts in terminal hinge closure, resulting in a forward thrust. Unusual wear facets are a valuable clue in this respect. Diagnosing these small glancing contacts can be more difficult than it sounds. Apart from the problems of guiding the mandible into centric relation, marking the initial contact is complicated by the fact that neither ribbon nor articulating paper is particularly effective in marking highly polished surfaces. In order to obtain accurate results the surfaces must be dry and the marking paper held in a suitable holder (Fig. 81), otherwise there is the danger of it wrinkling and giving false marks. If this problem is not readily eliminated, the centric relation record must be made at a deliberately increased vertical dimension. The second complication arises from the possible irregularities of both upper and lower arcades of teeth. Extra time and care will be required in the trimming of the rims.

Overdentures require particularly careful

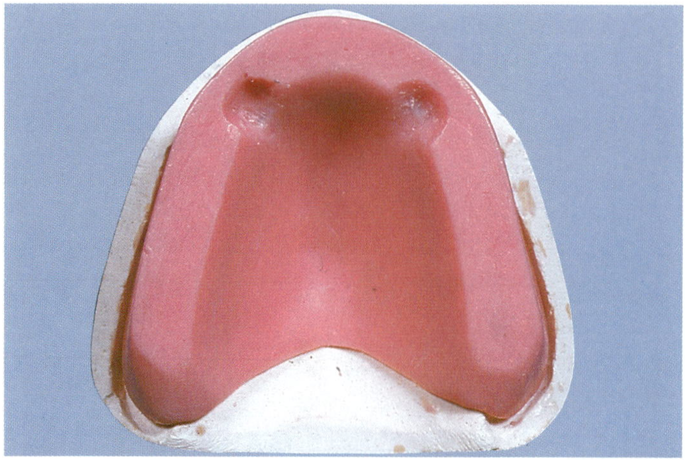

Fig. 79 Recesses for the opposing teeth allow the occlusal plane to be determined at the vertical relation of occlusion.

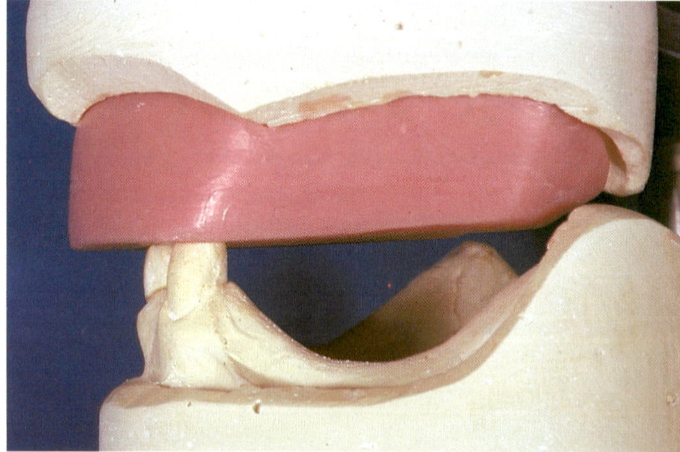

Fig. 80 The upper rim should be adapted to determine labial support.

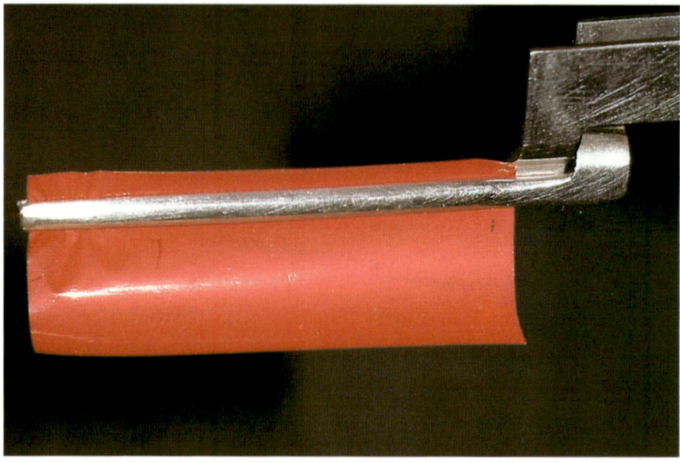

Fig. 81 A holder for ribbon or articulating paper is essential for accuracy. Without it, wrinkling of the marker is likely to give false contacts.

assessment of vertical space. There must be sufficient room for roots, copings and, possibly, attachments, together with an adequate thickness of denture base material and artificial teeth; all this without jeopardising the strength of the denture.

When discussing antero-posterior relations, two important terms require definition: 'centric relation' and 'centric occlusion'. *Nairn* (1974) has pointed out the difficulties in terminology that stem from a reluctance to use words in the sense of their meaning only. Terms are only names for things, each can only be a name for one thing.

Centric relation is the most posterior relation of the mandible to the maxilla that can be recorded by the operator at the chosen vertical dimension. To use this term does not mean that you wish to build a dentition to this jaw relationship. This is simply a relationship of one jaw to another and can be taken as a reference point. Centric relation is usually recorded at the vertical relation of occlusion. There are, however, many circumstances where a deflective (interceptive) occlusal contact may guide the mandible forwards. *Kass* and *Knap* (1974) have explained that vertical deflective contacts close to the arc of closure make a disproportionate deflection; nevertheless, once identified, minimal adjustments are required. In these and other similar circumstances, it will be necessary to record centric relation at an increased vertical relation and to assume a hinge closure from this point.

On the other hand, centric occlusion is a tooth-to-tooth relationship defined as 'the relationship between opposing occlusal surfaces that results in maximum intercuspation and/or planned contact'. Once

this important difference is understood, various conflicting opinions that have existed in the past may be expressed as follows:

1. Centric occlusion (of the teeth) should coincide with centric (jaw) relation.
2. The cusp/fossa relationship of the opposing teeth should allow a small area of freedom forward and lateral to centric relation.
3. Centric occlusion should coincide with a mandibular position 2 mm anterior to centric relation.

The relations of the opposing cusps are three-dimensional and it is an oversimplification to think in simple two-dimensional terms. Furthermore, there is a limit to the accuracy that even the most exacting clinical techniques can achieve in the mouth and this must be remembered when evaluating optimistic claims—particularly when these claims are unsubstantiated.

Studies with cineradiographs, cinefilms and magnetic sensors confirm that the masticatory cycle is based on centric occlusion. The chewing cycle commences with an opening phase, an almost ballistic movement, followed by closure in a lateral occlusion. The teeth then slide over one another, or may be slightly separated by food, as they travel back to centric occlusion.

Ahlgren (1976) divided the masticatory cycle into three components: opening phase, closing phase and intercuspal phase. The opening movement rarely goes straight down but deviates to one side, usually the working side. He found that each individual had a characteristic pattern of mandibular movements in chewing, but there was variation between consecutive chewing cycles. Those with normal occlusions showed simple and well coordinated masticatory movements, whereas those with malocclusions had an irregular and complicated pattern of movements.

Extreme vertical overlap produced an almost vertical chewing stroke. The effect of tough food was to widen the chewing cycle, so that the occurrence of tooth contact glide during the closing phase depended on the type of food and occlusion. Tooth contacts in centric occlusion were to be found in most chewing cycles, and it was at this point that maximum force was exerted for about 100 msec.

The findings are corroborated if one examines masticatory function with a device like the Kinesiograph*. The anatomy of the contacting cusp sections in chewing can be mirrored in the chewing cycle. Furthermore, it is interesting to note variations in the mandibular speeds reached. Using similar foods, subjects with stable occlusions appear to reach far higher speeds than those with obvious irregularities. Maximum speed is normally reached midway through the opening and closing phases and can exceed 200 mm/sec. *Matsumoto* (1976) made clasp-retained and attachment-retained dentures for the same subjects. He found higher chewing speeds for attachment-retained dentures. He felt that this higher chewing speed was a result of the better retention of attachment-retained dentures.

Recent findings have, therefore, substantiated earlier work by Boos (1959) who felt that powerful biting was more comfortable close to centric occlusion, and Trapozzano

* Myotronics Research Inc., Seattle, Washington, USA.

(1960) and Woelfel et al (1962) who described the influence of occlusal surfaces on the masticatory cycle.

Neill and Howell (1983) have further demonstrated the influence of the occlusal surfaces upon the masticatory cycle. Poorly defined cuspal anatomy can lead to wide, irregular and inefficient chewing movements. The dwell time at, or close to, centric occlusion is affected by the stickiness of the food. Voluntary swallowing contacts are also based on centric occlusion; but what of involuntary swallows?

Brewer (1963) has shown that complete denture-wearers may make between 180 and 1300 nonmasticatory occlusal contacts per hour. Although these contacts are transient, there is direct tooth-to-tooth contact with no intervening 'shock-absorbing' bolus. Therefore, it is important that the teeth meet evenly when these small, subconscious, nonmasticatory movements are made.

Graf and *Zander* (1963) used minute radio transmitters built into bridge pontics to show that contacts are made only in centric relation while swallowing food or preparing to do so, but not while actually chewing. Contacts in centric occlusion occurred mainly during chewing, although some nonmasticatory contacts took place as well. They suggested that some of these latter contacts were the result of an initial contact in centric relation, followed by a slide forward.

Involuntary swallowing movements and other nonmasticatory contacts appear to occur in centric relation, although this was not borne out by *Glickman* and co-writers (1969). These investigators pointed out that tooth contacts in swallowing were of longer duration than those in chewing, and work by *Schärer et al* (1967) suggests similar conclusions.

Butler and *Zander* (1968) reported tooth contacts in centric relation during both chewing and swallowing, following occlusal adjustment.

The centric occlusion of many young adult patients does not coincide with centric relation (*Posselt* 1952), and it is possible that involuntary movements may result in an initial contact followed by a forward mandibular slide. Unlike artificial teeth, however, natural teeth are supported by a periodontal ligament that incorporates extremely sensitive mechanoreceptors.

Hodge and *Mahan* (1967), while agreeing that occlusal slides occur, point out that most occlusal research has been carried out on dental students who tend to have a greater number of restorations than an equivalent group of patients. These authors suggest a potential iatrogenic cause for the occlusal slide. *McCollum* and *Stuart* (1955) stated that people with well-formed dental arches and well-aligned and well-shaped teeth do not have a forward occlusal slide. However, the number of patients falling into this category must be comparatively small.

Care should be taken when diagnosing a discrepancy between centric occlusion and centric relation because, when the subject slowly opens his mouth, what appears to be a distinct posterior movement may be due to the fact that the teeth are moving on the arc of a circle. This movement may result in sliding contact of the inclined planes of the teeth, giving rise to a subjective feeling of posterior movement (*Zola* and *Rothschild* 1961). *Aarstad* (1954) described the wear facets on cusp inclines resisting retrusive forces and found that many of these facets were tangential to the posterior hinge arc of closure.

Some types of apparent forward slides result from interferences to the most posterior hinge path of closure, but do not affect the final mandibular position when the teeth meet (*Zola* and *Rothschild* 1961; *Hodge* and *Mahan* 1967). In these cases, elimination of the interferences will not alter the horizontal overlap (overjet) of the incisors. Other types of interference do, in fact, guide the mandible to a more protruded position, often with a lateral component.

In order to examine the occlusion, a reliable method of establishing centric relation has to be found. There are, of course, many methods available. *Dawson's* method (1974) has been found to give consistent results:

The patient is inclined and the neck extended. The operator, seated behind the patient, stabilises the patient's head between his forearm and ribcage. The four fingers of each hand are placed either side on the lower border of the mandible. The thumbs are placed in light contact with one another over the symphysis. With a gentle touch, the jaw is moved through small arcs and manipulated into centric relation. The fingers exert upward pressure and the thumbs downwards and backwards. If there has been any tenderness in the temporo-mandibular joint regions the resistance to closure will become progressively greater as the teeth come towards each other. Slowly, the closing arc allows the teeth to approximate until the initial contact is made. With the mandible held in this manner, the movement is repeated. The patient is then asked to keep the jaw in that position for a second and then squeeze the teeth together. The direction in which the mandible moves is noted. The initial contact can be marked by drying the teeth and placing ribbon between them. The ribbon should be held in a special holder to minimise the hazards of false marks.

When making the interocclusal centric relation record, the wax record is placed over the occlusal surfaces of the upper teeth and the mandible manipulated by the method described above. The lower teeth occlude with the wax record and are not permitted to touch their antagonists.

Mounted diagnostic casts are essential when prosthodontic therapy is contemplated. It is, however, difficult to give hard and fast rules for the correction of forward slides as their effects will vary. Abnormal wear facets, particularly on anterior teeth, are often found. Difficulty with chewing, or temporo-mandibular pain dysfunction syndrome, together with a deviation in opening and positive pterygoid signs, are other possible occurrences. In many instances the cause is easily found and eliminated. However, there can be little excuse for interfering with the occlusion of the natural teeth without good reason.

Schuyler (1935) and *Ramfjord* and *Ash* (1983) suggested that a degree of freedom should be allowed in the cusp/fossae relationships of the natural teeth. At one time it was felt that movements of 1–2 mm should be allowed forward and lateral from a position corresponding with centric relation before the cusp reached an inclined plane. Problems of terminology, and those of representing a three-dimensional object in two have possibly contributed to the controversy these ideas still arouse. In expert hands the degree of freedom allowed

seems to average 0.2 mm. Bearing in mind that this figure is approaching the accuracy that can be achieved with cemented castings, a great deal of earlier argument appears to have been quite unnecessary.

In those patients whose centric occlusion coincides with centric relation, no problem is presented. The following paragraphs are devoted to those patients who can retrude their mandibles behind the position corresponding with centric occlusion.

The small-span Tooth-Supported Prosthesis

Anyone who has seen the havoc wrought by well-intentioned but unskilled 'prophylactic' adjustments would think twice about recommending such a procedure. However, it would be unfair to blame failings of the execution upon the technique. Suffice to say, one should be aware of the hazards. Nevertheless, there can be little excuse for interfering with a natural dentition without due cause.

A short slide involving multiple even contacts seldom produces problems, while the elimination of such a slide is difficult and requires postgraduate training. Problems that do arise are often caused by single or small number of contacts. Ironically, these are usually the easiest to locate and eliminate. Common culprits are restorations, a third molar and a slightly rotated upper first molar, or the mesial surface of the palatal cusp of the upper first premolar.

Many small restorations can therefore be made in centric occlusion, but diagnostic casts mounted in centric relation are a valuable aid a decision-making. Where occlusal corrections are required, these must be completed before tooth preparation is begun.

Complete dentures, distal extension dentures, and large-span fixed prostheses

The occlusion of any of these restorations is best made to coincide with centric relation. In an unequivocal fashion, *Nairn* (1974) has summarised the arguments as follows: 'It is difficult to find convincing evidence for any of the views that are held, but the matter can be largely resolved on the grounds of practicability'. He goes on to point out that if you have to rebuild the occlusion, there is no practical alternative to building an even occlusion of maximum intercuspation with the mandible in its most retruded position. This is the only position which the dentist can find and repeat, and this is a practical necessity. There may be a better place for the mandible in each case, but at present there is no way of finding it.

One or two of these points may be challenged today, but the basis of the statement holds good.

Recording centric relation can be difficult in those patients in whom loss of posterior occlusal support has resulted in a forward mandibular posture. The apparent forward thrust of the mandible may be accentuated by a decreased vertical relation of occlusion. Nevertheless, if one fails to record centric relation, there is a danger that the patient may assume a more retruded posture after the restoration has been completed. Where a fixed prosthesis is con-

cerned, this would involve remaking the entire restoration. Transitional restorations are particularly useful in situations like these. No matter how carefully jaw relations are made, an additional step is required for partial dentures when an altered cast technique has been employed. This usually applies to distal extension bases. Before the trial insertion of the artificial teeth, the cast of the corrected base should be related to the opposing dentition. This particular jaw relation cannot normally be made until the framework has been cast and the secondary impression made.

Lateral and protrusive contacts

An adjustable articulator will be required to establish the shape of the artificial occlusal surfaces. The articulator should ensure that correct separation of the teeth occurs, when necessary, and that desired contacts can be obtained.

Adjustable articulators are often misused when attempting to copy jaw movements. Sliding the teeth sideways or forwards from centric occlusion is useful in establishing pathways of contact and the way in which the teeth disclude. However, it can hardly be termed 'normal physiological movement'. During mastication the teeth are separated when eccentric movements are made, so that the timing of components of lateral movement is insignificant. The eccentric movement will have been completed before the teeth contact. Attempting to mimic masticatory movements in the reverse sense can give a misleading impression of the vectors of forces applied (*Nairn* 1974).

DePietro (1977) has suggested that the Frankfort mandibular plane angle might be a useful guide in assessing the type of disclusion required in a subject's dentition. In his study, 112 subjects with anterior guided disclusion had an FMA of 24°, or less, while those with group function had FMAs of 24°–40°. He has also put forward the idea that a low FMA angle and, therefore, natural disclusion is associated with higher biting forces than those with higher FMA angles and group function.

The actual requirements of lateral contacts will vary, but can be divided into fixed prostheses, distal extension dentures and complete dentures.

Fixed prostheses

During protrusive movements, anterior guidance should separate the remaining teeth, while throughout lateral movements the teeth on the nonworking side should part. On these aspects, at least, there seems little disagreement.

Opinion varies as to whether there should be even sliding contact between all the cusps on the working side, or whether the canines should lift the working side cusps out of occlusion. The idea of the 'cuspid-protected occlusion' is based on the concept that the shape and size of the canine is particularly well adapted to resist lateral loads. It should, therefore, lift the other working side cusps out of occlusion as the jaw is moved to one side, thereby protecting these cusps and preventing contacts on the side as well.

However, the canines could only protect the occlusion by cuspal guidance, and if this continually occurred a high rate of wear could be expected. Many patients seem to adapt to canine rise by assuming a more vertical chewing cycle, and it is in this indirect manner that the occlusion is protected. Among the applications of this type of occlusion are the situations in which porcelain covers part of the occlusal surfaces.

In several respects the anthropological and functional aspects of canine protection might be questioned. Indeed, it might be argued that this concept is merely a rationalisation of a clinical procedure based on necessity (*Nairn* 1974). It certainly is a convenient arrangement of artificial occlusal surfaces and simplifies the elimination of nonworking contacts with little evidence to show that it does any harm. On the contrary, the bulk of clinical evidence points the other way and one can look for reassurance to the fact that many natural dentitions appear to have this type of articulation. The majority of fixed prostheses appear constructed in this manner and give satisfactory service. On the other hand, it would not be possible to provide this canine protection where these teeth are weak, missing, or where there was a Class III malocclusion present.

Distal extension dentures

Here a compromise must be reached between the functions the appliance can serve and the necessity to reduce to a minimum rotational loads applied to the denture base. While a narrow artificial occlusal table should limit the leverage of loads applied, it is wise to allow only 1.5 – 2.00 mm of working side contact of the artificial teeth, after which the guidances of the natural teeth should be allowed to take over. Where anterior natural teeth remain, the canine teeth should normally lift the artificial teeth out of contact as soon as lateral movement is begun. No contacts of natural or artificial teeth should take place on the nonworking side. Protrusive contacts will normally be made on the anterior teeth.

A functional path recording is favoured by some operators when a distal extension denture occludes against natural teeth. The wax record on the denture base is carved by opposing cusps and a template then cast corresponding with the paths travelled by these cusps. By adjusting the denture teeth to occlude with the template, the cuspal relationships in centric relation and eccentric relations are determined. The template needs to be handled with care and made of the hardest artificial stone or it will be easily worn, or damaged, and the result unsatisfactory.

Complete dentures

The presence of a complete denture alters the situation because of the need to make it as stable as possible. There may be a complete upper and lower denture, a complete upper denture opposed to a natural dentition, or a complete upper denture opposed to a natural dentition and a partial lower denture. The requirements are similar; only the method of achieving the goal varies.

Even contact is required at centric occlusion, which in these cases must always coincide with centric relation. Lateral movements should produce even contact on the working side and simultaneous contacts on the nonworking side. These nonworking side contacts are required for stability of the complete denture. For a similar reason, anterior contact should be accompanied as far as possible by posterior contacts when the mandible is protruded.

These requirements can be met quite simply with complete upper and lower dentures, for the positioning and alignment of the posterior teeth is in the hands of the operator. Where natural teeth are present it becomes more difficult to incorporate them within this occlusal pattern, yet it is particularly important that it be achieved owing to the powerful displacing forces that can be exerted. For this reason, diagnostic casts should always be made, in order to assess the amount of natural tooth substance to be removed. Narrowing of the natural occlusal surfaces should accompany this grinding. The occlusal reshaping may have to be carried out in two stages, for it is difficult to determine the precise contours required until all the artificial teeth have been set up. The main occlusal reshaping should be planned on the diagnostic cast and be carried out before denture construction is begun. Further occlusal corrections may be required if it proves impossible to accommodate the natural teeth within the final occlusal pattern, in which case a new impression and jaw relation record will be subsequently required. Methods of recording jaw relationships vary; the essential factors are that the centric relation record be correct and that lateral and protrusive movements produce even contacts. To achieve this, it is imperative that occlusal corrections to the natural teeth be completed before the final jaw relation records are made and that the occlusal rims be constructed on the master cast and be stable in the mouth.

For the purpose of this discussion, movements of the mandible have been described as moving laterally or forwards with the teeth in contact. Again it must be pointed out that these types of movement are not physiological and should rarely take place. Normal movements are, in the reverse sense, those with a separation of the teeth preceding any lateral or forward movement.

Materials for artificial teeth

Where dentures are to be constructed, thought should be given to the material of which the occlusal surfaces are to be made.

For many brought up with vacuum-fired porcelain teeth, there is seldom an acceptable substitute. Porcelain teeth have an unrivalled appearance, are straightforward to arrange, and have a negligible rate of wear. Unfortunately they are prone to damage, but the greatest restriction is limitation of vertical space. Owing to the need for retaining pins, or the diatoric design, there is a limit to the adjustment possible. This severely limits their applications to partial dentures, overdentures and complete dentures with space restrictions.

Considerable improvements have now been made to cross-linked acrylic resin teeth. Both from the point of appearance and wear resistance, recent products have shown amazing improvements. Most partial dentures, particularly those with attach-ments, will require acrylic resin teeth. For similar reasons, acrylic resin teeth are indicated for most overdentures. They are also convenient to employ for many complete dentures. If after several years the teeth need to be replaced, this can hardly be described as catastrophic. Inserting silver alloy restorations in the occlusal surfaces of acrylic resin artificial teeth appears to reduce the rate of wear and provides good clinical results.

Acrylic resin teeth may be opposed to porcelain, provided the glaze of the porcelain teeth is not disturbed. The coefficient of friction between this combination is less than that of opposed acrylic resin surfaces, so that the rate of wear should be correspondingly reduced. Since adjustments can be made to only one of the occluding surfaces, this arrangement can be difficult to use in practice.

Improved masticatory efficiency has always been claimed for specialised metal inserts in artificial teeth. Now that the problems of appearance, balancing the articulation and preventing accidental tongue biting seem to have been overcome (*Levin* 1977), this type of metal insert is likely to prove popular.

Where natural and artificial teeth oppose each other, gold is the material of choice for the artificial occlusal surface. Acrylic resin teeth are reduced in height to allow a gold occlusal surface to be waxed-upon them. The wax is then removed, invested, cast and subsequently joined to the resin teeth to form the occlusal surface. The gold occlusal surface can be contoured to fine limits to provide a stable occlusion. It is appearance that limits its usefulness, although cost, weight and space must be considered as well.

Occlusal surfaces of crowns

The merits of gold surfaces for denture teeth apply equally well to crowns, with considerable additional advantages. The delicate details possible with gold allow the development of an articulation that is both functional and stable. Gold produces few problems when opposed to natural teeth and is usually the material of choice. It also requires less vertical space than any technique that requires a second material to be introduced on the occlusal surface.

Once again, it is appearance rather than other factors that may limit the usefulness of gold. Porcelain occlusal surfaces are difficult to construct with accuracy. Adequate vertical space must be provided for the material and sufficient space allowed for it to be carried onto the lingual surface of the tooth. Best results are achieved when significant anterior guidance can be provided. It had been felt that the hardness of porcelain might damage opposing natural teeth, and there is evidence of a degree of wear taking place. Monasky (1971) showed the rate of wear to be virtually self-limiting. The explanation rests with the production of an improved glaze on the porcelain surface and a corresponding reduction in the coefficient of friction between the two surfaces. Gold, however, had no such effect on the porcelain. Opposing gold surfaces may, therefore, be quite severely damaged in time by porcelain.

Careful treatment planning should include the occlusal surfaces of the restoration. The amount of space available, the opposing surfaces, and the loads that may be applied are all factors that need to be taken into account. A little care at an early stage makes the construction of a restoration simpler, for the amount of space available for gold, attachments, artificial teeth and facings can be clearly seen and difficulties anticipated. Furthermore, the completed restoration will work better, require minimal adjustments and provide the patient with the service he deserves.

References

Aarstad T. (1954).
The Capsular Ligaments of the Temporomandibular Joint and Retrusion Facets of the Dentition in Relationship to Mandibular Movements. Akademisk Forlag, Oslo.

Adams S. H. and Zander H. A. (1964).
Functional tooth contacts in lateral and in centric occlusion. J. Amer. Dent. Assoc., 69: 465.

Ahlgren J. (1976).
Masticatory movements in man. In Mastication. (Anderson D. J. and Matthews B. eds.) John Wright, Bristol.

Alexander P. C. (1963).
Analysis of cuspid protective occlusion. J. Prosthet. Dent., 13: 2, 309.

Applegate O. C. (1965).
Essentials of Removable Partial Denture Prosthesis. 3rd Edn., pp 299–314, Saunders, Philadelphia and London.

Bergman B. and Ericson S. (1973).
The effect of increasing the morphologic face height in full denture restorations on the width of the intra-articular space in the temporomandibular joint. Acta Odontol. Scand., 31:75–88.

Beyron H. L. (1954).
Characteristics of functionally optimal occlusion and principles of occlusal rehabilitation. J. Amer. Dent. Ass., 48: 648.

Boos R. H. (1959).
Vertical centric and functional dimensions recorded by gnathodynamics. J. Amer. Dent. Ass., 59: 682.

Brewer, A. A. (1963).
Prosthodontic research and progress at the School of Aerospace Medicine. Prosthet. Dent., 13: 1: 49.

Brill N., Schubeler S. and Tryde G. (1962).
Influences of occlusal patterns on movements of the mandible. J. Prosthet. Dent., 12: 2, 255.

Butler J. H. and Zander H. A. (1968).
Evaluation of two occlusal concepts. Parodont. Acad. Rev., 2: 5.

Clayton J. A., Kotowitz W. E. and Zahler J. M. (1971).
Pantographic tracings of mandibular movements and occlusion. J. Prosthet. Dent., 25: 4, 389.

Colman A. J. (1967).
Occlusal requirements for removable partial dentures. J. Prosthet. Dent., 17: 2, 155.

D'Amico A. (1958).
Canine teeth: normal functional relation of the natural teeth of man. J. S. Calif. Dent. Ass., 26, 6, 49, 127, 175, 194, 299.

Dawson P. E. (1973).
Temporomandibular joint pain-dysfunction problems can be solved. J. Prosthet. Dent., 29: 1, 100.

Dawson P. E. (1974).
Evaluation, Diagnosis and Treatment of Occlusal Problems. C. V. Mosby Co., St. Louis, Mo.

DePietro G. J. (1977).
A study of occlusion as related to the Frankfort-mandibular plane angle. J. Prosthet. Dent. 38: 4, 452.

Dyer E. G. (1973).
Importance of a stable maxillomandibular relation. J. Prosthet. Dent., 30: 3: 241.

Emslie R. D. (1954).
Malocclusion and periodontal health. A periodontist's viewpoint. Euro. Orthodont. Soc. Trans., 254.

Funakoshi M., Fujita N. and Takehana S. (1976).
Relations between occlusal interference and jaw muscle activities in response to changes in head position. J. Dent. Res., 55: 4, 684.

Gazit E. and Lieberman M. A. (1973).
The intercuspal surface contact area registration: an additional tool for evaluation of normal occlusion. Angle Orthod., 43: 96.

Gibb C. H., Suit S. R. and Benz S. T. (1973).
Masticatory movements of the jaw measured at angles of approach to the occlusal plane. J. Prosthet. Dent., 30: 3, 283.

Gillings B. R. D., Graham C. G. and Duckmanton N. A. (1973).
Jaw movements in young adult men while chewing. J. Prosthet. Dent., 29: 6: 616.

Gillings B. R. D., Kohl J. T. and Zander H. A. (1963).
Contact patterns using miniature radio transmitters. J. Dent. Res., 42: 177.

Glickman I., Pameijer J. H. N. and Roeber F. (1968).
Intraoral occlusal telemetry: a multifrequency transmitter for registering tooth contacts in occlusion. J. Prosthet. Dent., 19: 1, 60.

Glickman I., Pameijer J. H. N., Roeber F. and Brion M. A. M. (1969).
Functional occlusion as revealed by miniaturised radio transmitters. Dent. Clin. N. Amer., 13: 667.

Graf H. and Zander H. A. (1963).
Tooth contact patterns in mastication. J. Prosthet. Dent., 13: 6, 1055.

Hildebrand G. Y. (1931).
Studies in the masticatory movements of the human lower jaw. Skand. Arch. Physiol., 61: 190.

Hobo S., Shillingburg H. T. and Whitsett L. D. (1976).
Articulator selection for restorative dentistry. J. Prosthet. Dent., 36: 7, 35.

Hodge L. C. and Mahan P. E. (1967).
A study of mandibular movement from centric occlusion to maximum intercuspation. J. Prosthet. Dent., 18: 1, 19.

Hoffman P. G., Silverman S. and Garfinkel L. (1973).
Comparison of condylar position in centric relation and in centric occlusion in dentulous subjects. J. Prosthet. Dent., 30: 4, 582.

Kass C. A. and Knap F. J. (1974).
Analysis of occlusion before and after occlusal adjustment. J. Prosthet. Dent., 32: 2, 163.

Kurth L. E. (1942).
Mandibular movements in mastication. J. Amer. Dent. Ass., 29: 1769.

Lauritzen A. G. (1951).
Function, prime object of restorative dentistry: a definitive procedure to obtain it. J. Amer. Dent. Ass., 42: 523.

Levin B. (1977).
A review of artificial posterior tooth forms including a preliminary report on a new posterior tooth. J. Prosthet. Dent., 38: 1, 3.

Long J. H. (1973).
Locating centric relation with a leaf gauge. J. Prosthet. Dent., 29: 6, 608.

Lucia V. A. (1961).
Modern Gnathological Concepts, pp. 293–294. C. V. Mosby, St. Louis. Mo.

Mann A. W. and Pankey L. D. (1960).
Oral Rehabilitation: I. The use of the P. M. instrument in treatment planning and in restoring the lower posterior teeth. J. Prosthet. Dent., 10: 1, 135.

Mann A. W. and Pankey L. D. (1960).
Oral rehabilitation: II. Reconstructions of the upper teeth using a functionally generated path technique. J. Prosthet. Dent., 10: 1, 151.

Markovic M. A. and Rosenberg H. M. (1973).
Corrected laminagraphic evaluation of the TMJ in 100 MPD patients. Int. Assoc. Dent. Res., Abst. No. 70.

Matsumoto J. M. (1976).
Personal communication.

McCollum B. B. (1958).
Consideration of the mouth as a functioning unit as the basis of dental diagnosis. J. S. Calif. Dent. Ass., 5: 268.

McCollum B. B. and Stuart C. E. (1955).
A Research Report: Basic Course for the Postgraduate Course in Gnathology, pp. 91–95. Scientific Press, South Pasadena.

Mehringer E. J. (1973).
Function of steep cusps in mastication with complete dentures. J. Prosthet. Dent., 30: 1, 367.

Millstein P. L., Clark R. E. and Kronman J. H. (1973).
Determination of the accuracy of wax interocclusal registrations. Part II. J. Prosthet. Dent., 29: 1, 40.

Möller E. (1976).
Evidence that the rest position is subject to servo control. In Mastication. (Anderson D. J. and Matthews B. eds.) John Wright, Bristol.

Monasky G. E. (1971).
Studies on the wear of porcelain, enamel and gold. J. Prosthet. Dent., 25: 3, 299.

Nagasawa T. and Tsuru H. (1973).
A comparative evaluation of masticatory efficiency of fixed and removable restorations replacing mandibular first molars. J. Prosthet. Dent., 30: 3, 263.

Nairn R. I. (1974).
Maxillomandibular relations and aspects of occlusion. J. Prosthet. Dent., 31: 4, 361.

Nairn R. I. (1976).
The concept of occlusal vertical dimension and its importance in clinical practice. In Mastication. (Anderson D. J. and Matthews B. eds.) John Wright, Bristol.

Neill D. J. and Howell P. G. T. (1983).
Kinesiograph studies of jaw movement using the Commodore Pet microcomputer for data storage

and analysis. Proc. Brit. Soc. for the Study of Prosthet. Dent.

Paffenbarger G. C., Sweeney W. T. and Bowen R. L. (1967).
Bonding porcelain teeth to acrylic resin denture bases. J. Amer. Dent. Ass., 74: 1018.

Pameijer J. H. N., Glickman I. and Roeber F. E. (1968).
Intraoral occlusal telemetry: II. Registration of tooth contacts in chewing and swallowing by intraoral electric telemetry. J. Prosthet. Dent., 19: 1, 151.

Pankey L. D., Mann A. W. and Schuyler C. H. (1964).
The teaching manual for the P-M-S philosophy of occlusal rehabilitation. The Occlusal Rehabilitation Seminar.

Posselt U. (1952).
Studies in the mobility of the human mandible. Acta Odont. Scand. Supp., 10: 10, 19.

Powell R. N. (1963).
Tooth contact during sleep. Thesis. University of Rochester.

Preiskel H. W. (1967).
Considerations of the check record in complete denture construction. J. Prosthet. Dent., 18: 2, 98.

Preiskel H. W. (1970).
Bennett's movement. A study of human lateral mandibular movement. Brit. Dent. J., 129: 372.

Preiskel H. W. (1971).
The canine teeth related to Bennett's movement. Brit. Dent. J., 131: 312.

Ramfjord S. P. (1961).
Bruxism, a clinical and electromygraphic study. J. Amer. Dent Ass., 62: 21.

Ramfjord S. p. and Ash M. M. (1983).
Occlusion. 3rd Edn. W. B. Saunders Co. Philadelphia, USA.

Ramfjord S. P., Berry H. M., Charbeneau G. T., Lee R. E., Pavone B. W. and Phillips R. W. (1974).
Report of the committee on scientific investigation of the American Academy of Restorative Dentistry. J. Prosthet. Dent., 32: 2, 198.

Roth R. H. (1973).
Temporomandibular pain-dysfunction and occlusal relationships. Angle Orthod., 43: 136.

Schärer P., Stallard R. E. and Zander H. A. (1967).
Occlusal interferences and mastication: An electromyographic study. J. Amer. Dent. Ass., 62: 21.

Schuyler C. H. (1935).
Fundamental principles in the correction of occlusal disharmony, natural and artificial. J. Amer. Dent. Ass., 22: 1193.

Schuyler C. H. (1961).
Factors contributing to traumatic occlusion. J. Prosthet. Dent., 11: 4: 708.

Schweitzer J. M. (1962).
Masticatory function in man. J. Prosthet. Dent., 12: 2, 262.

Schweitzer J. M. (1963).
Concepts of occlusion: A discussion. Dent. Clin. N. Amer., 649.

Shore, N. A. (1959).
Occlusal Equilibration and Temporomandibular Joint Dysfunction, pp 143–145. Lippincott, Philadelphia.

Sicher H. (1949).
Oral Anatomy, p. 171. C. V. Mosby, St. Louis, Mo.

Sicher H. (1951).
Functional anatomy of the temporomandibular joint. In The Temporomandibular Joint. (Sarnat B. ed.) C. C. Thomas, Springfield, Illinois.

Stallard H. and Stuart C. E. (1961).
Elementary tooth guidance in natural dentition. J. Prosthet. Dent., 11: 3, 474.

Tallgren A. (1967).
The effect of denture wearing or facial morphology: a 7-year longitudinal study. Acta Odont. Scand., 25: 563.

Trapozzano V. R. (1960).
Test of balanced and nonbalanced occlusions. J. Prosthet. Dent., 10: 3, 476.

Weinberg L. A. (1973).
Temporomandibular joint function and its effect on centric relation. J. Prosthet. Dent., 30: 2, 176.

Wilkie N. D., Hurst T. L. and Mitchell D. L. (1974).
Radiographic comparisions of condyle-fossa relationships during maxillomandibular registrations made by different methods. J. Prosthet. Dent., 32: 5, 599.

Woelfel J. D., Hickey J. C. and Allison M. C. (1962).
Effects of posterior tooth form on jaw and denture movement. J. Prosthet. Dent., 12: 5, 922.

Yemm R. (1976).
The role of tissue elasticity in the control of mandibular resting posture. In Mastication. (Anderson D. J. and Matthews B. eds.) John Wright, Bristol.

Zander H. A. and Hurzeler B. (1958).
Diagnosis of occlusal disharmonies. J. S. Calif. Dent. Ass., 26: 382.

Ziebert G. J. and Knap F. J. (1973).
Effect of jaw guidance on retruded stroke as recorded in the sagittal plane. J. Prosthet. Dent., 29: 3, 262.

Zarb G. A., Bergman B., Clayton J. A. and Mackay H. F. (1978).
Prosthodontic Treatment for Partially Edentulous Patients. C. V. Mosby Company, St. Louis, Mo.

Zola A. and Rothschild E. A. (1961).
Condyle positions in unimpeded jaw movements. J. Prosthet. Dent., 11: 5, 873.

Chapter 4

Distal Extension Prostheses

Thanks to modern endodontics and periodontics, many distal abutments can be saved where, years ago, an extraction would have been necessary. Hemisected molar abutments can prove particularly useful. Even when an abutment has been lost, a small space does not automatically dictate the construction of a prosthesis.

In planning a distal extension prosthesis, support and retention are among the greatest problems to be overcome. However, the criteria of success include careful patient selection, evaluation and education, together with a highly trained operator supported by suitable technical resources. Compare this with the haphazard prescription and careless construction often found and it is small wonder at the disappointing results of the longterm surveys carried out over the last decade or so (*Carlsson et al* 1961, 1962; *Rantanen et al* 1972). The conclusions of these surveys indicate that far from *DeVan's* maxim of 'preserving what remains', the majority of removable prostheses actively contribute to the demise of their supporting structures. Considering the problems and cost of denture construction, this is an undertaking requiring planning with discretion and completion with care.

However, more optimistic results have been reported by *Derry* and *Bertram* (1970) and, more recently, by *Schwalm, Smith* and *Erickson* (1977). Well-made dentures provided for properly motivated and instructed patients showed remarkably good results at follow-up examination.

The reasons for making a restoration may vary from appearance to the prevention of abnormal jaw postures, but a surprising feature of denture construction is that the artificial teeth are all too often added as an afterthought once the framework has been found to fit. The entire restoration has only been made to carry these artificial teeth into the mouth. If these factors were considered at the outset one would not see, so frequently, evidence of last minute gross occlusal corrections where frantic efforts had been made to accommodate artificial teeth where inadequate space exists.

Loss of posterior occlusion may lead to a forward thrust of the mandible, giving the patient a prognathic look. This apparent forward thrust may arise in two ways:

1. Decreasing the vertical relation of occlusion results in the mandible rotating upwards and forwards. Efforts at correcting this malocclusion by increasing the vertical relation of occlusion alone are not always successful. They may result in the problems of limited interocclusal space that used to be associa-

ted with the immediate post-Costen era.

2. The prognathic appearance results from an anterior translation of the mandible, and a forward posture is assumed by the patient in an effort to provide some occluding surfaces and possibly to improve appearance as well. A prosthesis made to this prognathic posture, and restoring the occlusion to this jaw relationship, will cause problems when the patient, now with posterior occlusion restored, assumes centric relation. Since the condyle translates posteriorly and upwards, this results in a premature posterior occlusal contact.

Opposing natural teeth

The new prosthesis may occlude with natural teeth, artificial teeth, or both. As a result of tooth loss, opposing natural teeth may overerupt and, in extreme cases, there may be little or no room between them and the edentulous ridge. *McArthur* and *Turvey* (1979) have described a maxillary segmental osteotomy for extremely difficult problems in this respect. Using their technique the entire maxillary posterior segment is repositioned.

More conservative measures are normally indicated and work well, provided they are planned beforehand. Mounted diagnostic casts are invaluable. Overeruption is usually accompanied by tilting so that one or two of the cusps become unduly prominent. For example, overerupted upper molars appear to tilt buccally so that the mesiopalatal cusps become prominent. Even if it were possible to find room for a denture, such a cusp would play havoc

with it when the mandible was moved from side-to-side. It is necessary to assess the opposing dentition and decide whether or not some reshaping of the natural teeth is warranted. Occlusal reshaping may involve just reshaping a cusp; on the other hand, it may require isolated extractions, the provision of crowns, or the construction of a prosthesis. Planning the occlusal surfaces is important and cannot be carried out by guesswork.

Opposing dentures

An opposing complete denture will place comparatively little load on the denture base. It is assumed that a lower distal extension prosthesis is planned to oppose an upper complete denture since few lower dentures will survive opposed to natural upper teeth. However, there are other problems to be considered. The upper complete denture defines the occlusal plane, and this may not be satisfactory for the new lower prosthesis. Furthermore, the new lower restoration will alter the shape of the lower occlusal surface; it hardly gives the patient good service to provide him with a complex lower prosthesis that makes his existing upper denture completely unstable. It is generally wiser to remake the opposing denture. The extra time required is not great, but it simplifies the treatment and gives a far better result. The same may hold true for an opposing partial denture, since it defines the posterior section of the occlusal plane. In most situations, it is quicker and better to remake an opposing denture, rather than attempt to accommodate the artificial and natural teeth of the new restoration to a prosthesis probably made by someone else under entirely different oral conditions.

The occlusal load applied to the denture base will be influenced by the shape and size of the artificial teeth on the denture base, the opposing dentition, and by the patient himself. It is difficult to make a quantitative assessment of this load, but it is apparent that a strong muscular man will probably apply more force to his teeth than a frail elderly woman.

Opposing natural teeth might also be expected to exert greater forces than opposing artificial teeth. By keeping the artificial occlusal table as small as possible, the bolus penetration forces necessary for mastication will be reduced. Furthermore, if the occlusal table is kept narrow and short, the leverage effects of those forces will be reduced as well (Figs. 82, 83).

There is another point to be considered when removable and fixed prosthesis are present in the same arch and possibly with natural teeth as well. It is quite possible to produce nonworking interferences, by subtracting guidance from one side as well as overbuilding or overcontouring the other. For example, automatically using zero cusp teeth on every denture could result in contralateral nonworking interferences if the anterior guidance were restricted. It is therefore important to relate the arrangement of artificial teeth and their cusp angles to the remaining dentition.

Support

Cantilevered extensions

Support to resist occlusal forces may be obtained entirely from the abutment teeth. *Nyman* and *Lindhe* (1976, 1979) have been remarkably successful in constructing distal extension cantilevers on fixed prostheses. The patients were carefully selected, placed on a rigorous plaque control programme, and the prosthodontic work carried out to a high standard. While these experts were able to demonstrate excellent results, not all operators have been so fortunate and the general principles should be further considered. The cantilevered extension from a fixed prosthesis is neat, and particularly useful where an opposing complete denture is concerned. When natural teeth are in opposition, the loads applied can be considerable. In these circumstances, even a short cantilevered extension may have a limited prognosis. Lower restorations are particularly prone to dislodgement due to the lingual inclination of the displacing forces (*Schweitzer et al* 1968; *Henderson et al* 1970). Nevertheless, there are still many situations in which a short cantilevered extension is all that is required. *Izikowitz* (1966, 1971) and *Hildebrand* (1968) have described fixed prostheses for which additional support was obtained from the mucosa, but this is a method that has failed to gain wide acceptance.

Implants

Until recently there was little evidence to suggest that intraosseous or subperiosteal implants were surrounded by any-

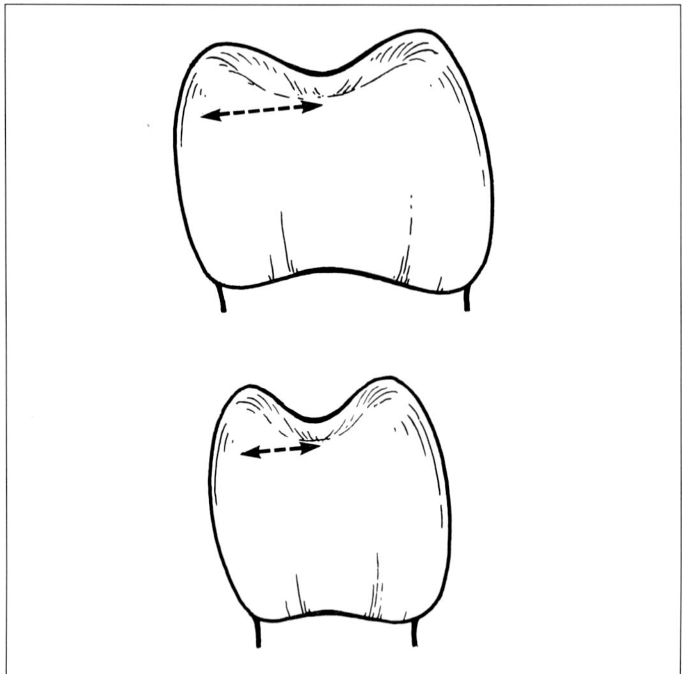

Fig. 82 The force required to penetrate a bolus of food is reduced if the occlusal table is kept narrow. The torques resulting from masticatory and non-masticatory contacts are also lessened.

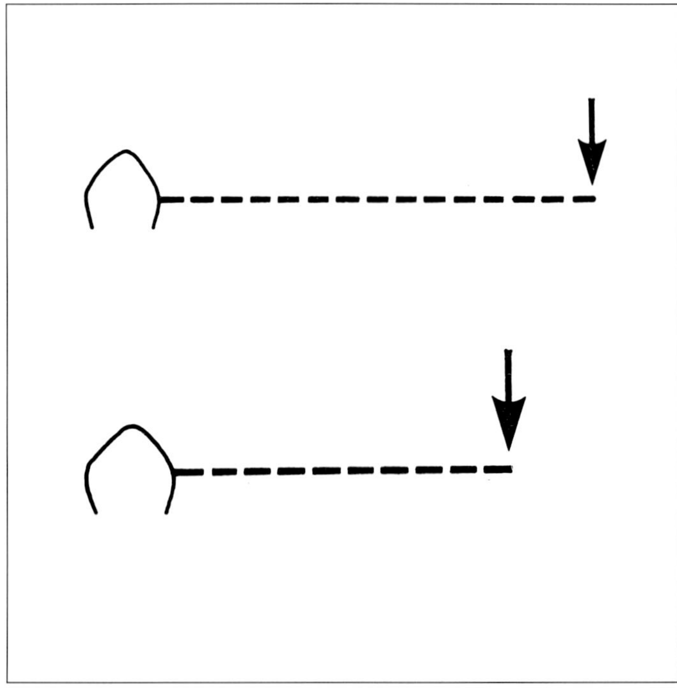

Fig. 83 A short artificial table reduces the occlusal leverages exerted by vertical and horizontal loads.

thing other than fibrous tissue. The major problem rested naturally, as it still does, with the transition from the internal to the external environment (*Johns* 1976). It seemed only a matter of time before the downgrowth of epithelium succeeded in exteriorising the implant. This was disappointing in view of the obvious value of an artificial distal abutment.

Work in 1983 by *Hansson et al, Bergman, Lekholm* and *Branemark* has shown exciting possibilities using pure titanium implants. The implants were left unloaded and buried for a period exceeding 3 months before being uncovered and connected to fixed prostheses. The system, known as the osseointegration method, involves very careful insertion of the implant with a specialised technique. Investigations up to 7 years later have lead to the conclusion that implants of pure titanium are integrated into both human and animal tissue. When the implants were cut out, a strong bond was noticed between the bone and the metal surface of the implant; possibly due to the deposition of a very fine oxide layer on the titanium itself.

While the aesthetic results, the plaque control facility and the prosthodontic techniques leave considerable room for improvement the potential is enormous and we look forward to the day when many of the problems of the distal extension space may be virtually eliminated.

Tooth and mucosal support

The majority of distal extension prostheses require support from the teeth and from the mucosa. The ideal abutment might consist of all the natural teeth splinted together, but effective support from the mucosa can be obtained only by covering the largest possible area.

Compared with the natural teeth, the mucosa of the denture-bearing area is relatively displaceable. *Steiger* (1959) suggested that, under load, the mucosa may be displaced by an amount four to twenty times greater than a healthy natural tooth. Fortunately, these are matters that can be measured. No matter how wide the mucosal coverage of the denture, on theoretical considerations it will have a tendency to rock under occlusal load. This tendency to rock is more noticeable in lower dentures due to the limited amount of mucosal coverage that is possible. The denture base tends to sink under load until the forces resisting this movement are equal to the displacing forces. It would seem likely that mucosal resistance would become more effective and require less movement of the denture base if its impression surface were made to correspond with the shape of the mucosa when subjected to slight displacing loads. However, mere suggestion of such a thought would, in the past, have divided clinicians into those who believed in the sanctity of the load-free shape of the mucosa and those who believed in deliberately applying some load. Somewhat puzzling was the undeniable fact that experienced and competent clinicians from either camp could produce excellent results, sometimes indistinguishable from one another. Only a close look at modern research will show that these clinicians were probably achieving similar results with their differing techniques, despite their avowed diverging aims.

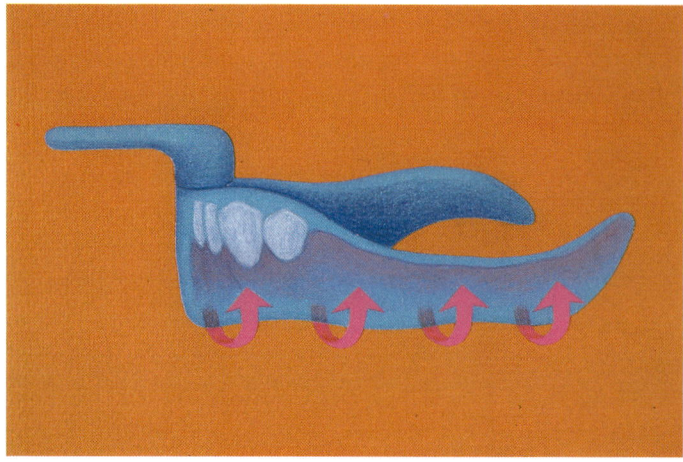

Fig. 84 Frequently overlooked is the rate at which impression material escapes around the border of the tray. A correctly adapted and extended tray is essential.

Matsumoto (1970), following on the work of *Rehm* (1962), demonstrated the loads required to cause slight mucosal displacement during impression procedures. Provided the border seal is adequate, the adaptation of the tray to the mucosa is an important factor in the result. If two flat plates are brought together with a viscous material between them, the rate of flow of the material varies as the 5th power of the distance between the plates. Halve the distance between the plates and 32 times the load is required to produce the same rate of flow. To simplify the issue, imagine that a close-fitting tray is made without any space between the tray and the mucosa. If the tray is then seated in the mouth and there is subsequently impression material left in it, some displacement of the mucosa must have occurred.

A failing of some previous research has been the lack of a time-base when measuring mucosal displacement. The influence of the impression material on the mucosa depends not only on its viscosity, but at the rate at which it escapes around the border of the tray (Fig. 84). Border moulding of the tray is therefore important. Apart from the viscosity of the impression material, other factors involved are the rate of force application and the physical properties of the mucosa.

Recent work has clarified understanding of the mucosa's physical properties. The mucosa itself appears to behave as a visco-elastic material (*Picton* and *Wills* 1978). If a load is applied for a short time the mucosa will deform elastically; if the load is sustained the mucosa will flow up to a point (Figs. 85 and 86). *Picton* and *Wills* also demonstrated that the underlying bone behaved as an elastic material.

Water's 1975) theoretical analysis also lends weight to arguments favouring secondary impression techniques, or those with a closely adapted tray. He points out that under normal circumstances the tray will not be inserted parallel to the mucosa, nor will the impression material be adapted to the shape of the mucosa. Flow of the

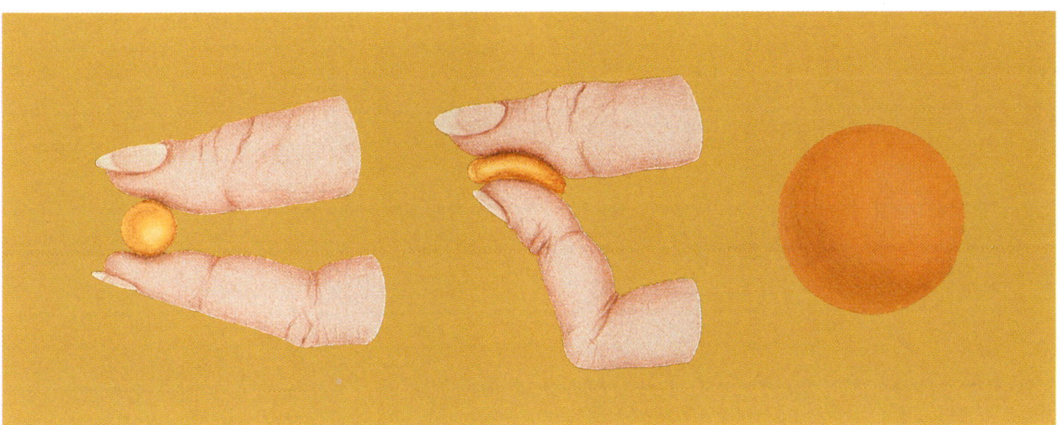

Fig. 85   Load applied for a short period allows elastic recoil.

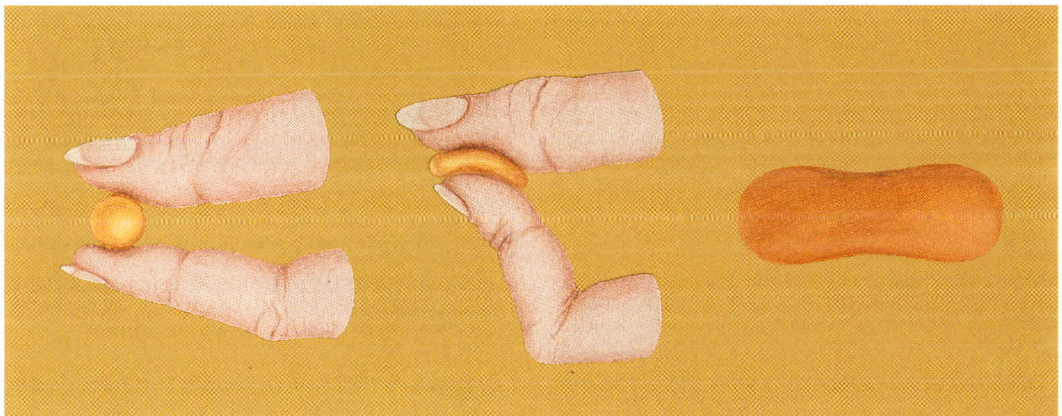

Fig. 86   Loads applied for a longer period result in plastic deformation.

impression material will occur first at any contact areas, and away from those areas where pressure is highest. Only when the impression material is in contact over the whole area with mucosa, and the latter is parallel to the tray, will the flow be radial from the centre of the tray. *Sieweke et al* (1977) have shown that custom-made trays should be spaced by approximately 2 mm around the abutment teeth to give the most accurate results. *Craig* and *Farah* (1978) feel that the most important factor in distributing stresses correctly to the mandible is a healthy, firm and uniform mucosa with a removable partial denture base well adapted to it. They point out that the abutment tooth, together with its periodontal ligament, helps in converting the compressive force on a tooth into a tensile force in bone. *Maxfield* and others (1979) have

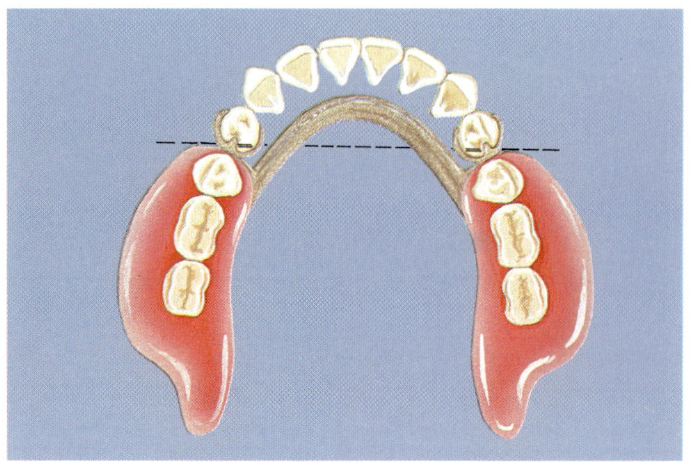

Fig. 87 Clasp-retained distal extension dentures tend to rotate around the distal occlusal rest under occlusal load.

shown that dentures processed onto an altered cast produced the least applied force on the abutments during mastication.

Trays spaced by more than 4 mm may produce completely different results, particularly when reversible hydrocolloid or alginates are used. For example, *Holmes* (1965) found that denture base movement ranged from 0.11 mm, using a functional wax impression, to 0.9 mm when an alginate impression had been employed.

One argument levelled against fluid wax is that cooling the impression from mouth temperature to room temperature might introduce significant dimensional changes. An assessment of the coefficient of expansion of Korecta Wax No. 4* yielded a figure of approximately $1.93 \times 10^{-3}/°C$. These figures were obtained in the Department of Prosthetic Dentistry, Guy's Hospital, and checked through the range 21 °C–

37 °C. It seems unlikely, therefore, that this factor would produce clinically significant changes in the impression. Nevertheless, the material appears to be falling from favour among operators who substitute a zinc-oxide based material.

The removable prosthesis gains support from some form of occlusal rest or attachment. The design of these structures influences the forces to which the abutment teeth will be subjected, and affects the manner in which the base may tend to move when under load.

A clasp-retained distal extension partial denture tends to rotate around its distal occlusal rests when subjected to load. Figure 87 shows a common design of this type of prosthesis. Since the vertical components of the occlusal loads are applied distal to the long axes of the teeth, there will be a marked tendency for the teeth to be tilted backwards.

The tilting effect of the distally placed loads would be accentuated with the clasp de-

* Korecta Wax, D & R Miner Dental, 14 Lavina Court, Orinda, USA.

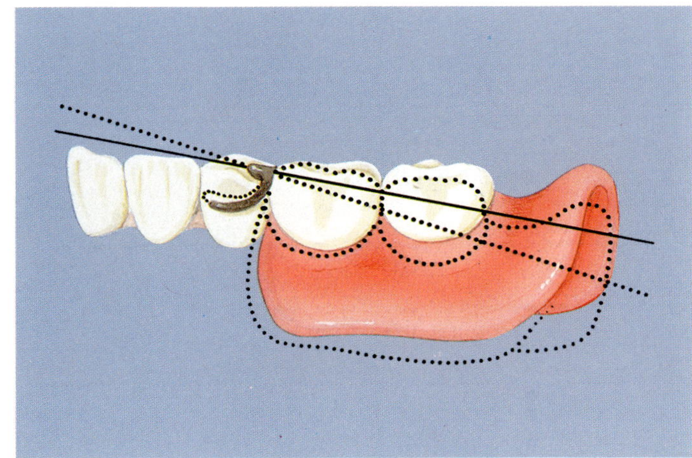

Fig. 88 Tilting effects on the abutment teeth are increased if rigid clasp arms are employed.

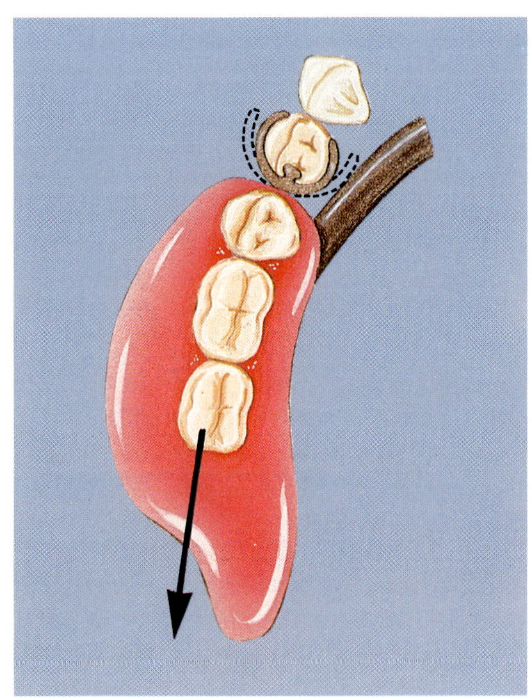

Fig. 89 Where possible, posterior displacing forces should be resisted by a rigid component of the denture framework. In this instance, there will be a tendency for the clasp arms to open when distally inclined forces are applied.

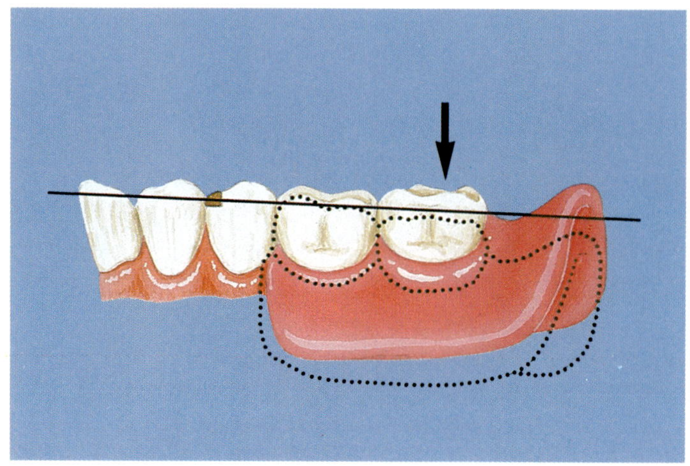

Fig. 90   A mesially placed occlusal rest showing favourable load distribution.

sign illustrated (Fig. 87). By engaging the mesial undercut, the clasp acts on the 'bottle-opener' principle (Fig. 88).

Model experiments confirm the drawbacks associated with a distal occlusal rest. The proximity of the rest to the denture base results in the base rotating around a small radius when it is displaced towards the mucosa. *Kratochvil* (1963) has found a tendency for the base to move forward under load. However, the distal section of the base will tend to sink more than the mesial section and cause uneven load distribution to the mucosa. The tilting potential upon the distal abutment will be accentuated by a poorly designed clasp (Fig. 88). Another drawback is that the entire clasp unit is poorly adapted to resist posterior displacing forces (Fig. 89). When sticky foods are chewed, the posterior section of the denture base has a tendency to rotate around the free end of the clasp, unless an effective indirect retainer is incorporated.

Placing an occlusal rest on a canine is particularly difficult due to the shape of the palatal surfaces of these teeth. *Wong* and others (1982) have described an interesting prefabricated rest seat that can be bonded directly to the tooth substance, thereby simplifying the design and construction of the prosthesis. At the time of writing, only model experiments have been carried out.

The mesial occlusal rest has several worthwhile advantages (Fig. 90). Work by *Nally* (1963), *Thompson, Kratochvil* and *Caputo* (1977), together with other model experiments, confirm that the mesially positioned rest results in a more apical resolution of forces applied vertically to the artificial teeth. Not only is the direction of the force more favourable, but the available bone support is generally better mesially. Furthermore, the increased radius of rotation provides a more equitable load distribution. Buttressing by the anterior teeth should prevent any tendency to tilt the abutment mesially, while distal displacement of the denture is counteracted by a rigid component of the partial denture framework. The chances of tipping the abutment distally are reduced still further as the retainer will have a tendency to disengage under load.

The mesial rest, guide plane, I-bar clasp

The mesial rest, guide plane, I-bar clasp design is a particularly interesting development of the gingivally approaching clasp. *Kratochvil* (1963) developed the early clasp assembly, while *Krol* (1973) modified the design and named it the RPI bar clasp. When used for distal extension prostheses, the assembly has the following features:

1. Occlusal rest placed mesially on the most distal abutment.
2. I-shaped bar clasp engaging the mid-buccal aspect of the abutment tooth.
3. Guide planes, distal and distolingual, with abutment tooth and adjacent mucosal contact provided by the vertical plate (and its extension) on the denture.

This comparatively simple system has obvious merit and should be considered where circumstances permit. *Demer* (1976) has described minor differences of design. All three clinicians place importance on potential movement of the denture base. *Kratochvil* constructs a full length guide plane (Fig. 91) that is subsequently relieved in the mouth to prevent torque or binding. Disclosing paste is used for this purpose. *Krol* (Fig. 92) has 2–3 mm of contact with the guide plane, the section below this point being relieved. The con-

tact point is made good with the artificial tooth of the denture, but a small V-shaped space is left underneath (Fig. 93). The *Demer* modification moves the guide plane mesiolingually so that the proximal plate contacts at the survey line only.

This ingenious and effective system requires an adequate zone of attached gingivae to be covered by the gingivally approaching retainer and a sulcus depth of about 5 mm. Individual retainers need to be identified as being in tooth-supported or extension situations. Provided the jaw relations and base extension are correct, engagement of distal undercuts appear to produce no undue problems, despite the warnings of the original designs. Inlays or crowns may be used with contours designed to provide the rest seats, guide planes and undercuts that are necessary.

So far, the position of the rest has been discussed; equally important is the depth of the rest seat. *Cecconi* (1974) analysed loads applied to a laboratory model through intracoronal precision attachments and deep (semi-precision) rests. He pointed out that many unsubstantiated claims are made for precision attachments including:

1. Occlusal forces directed parallel to the long axes of abutment teeth.
2. Even distribution of lateral stresses.
3. Prevention of movement or tipping of the abutment teeth.

Cecconi found that the depth of the rest seat was the all important factor in prevention of abutment mobility, when distal extension situations were considered. The deeper rests significantly reduced tilting movements, precision units acting in a sim-

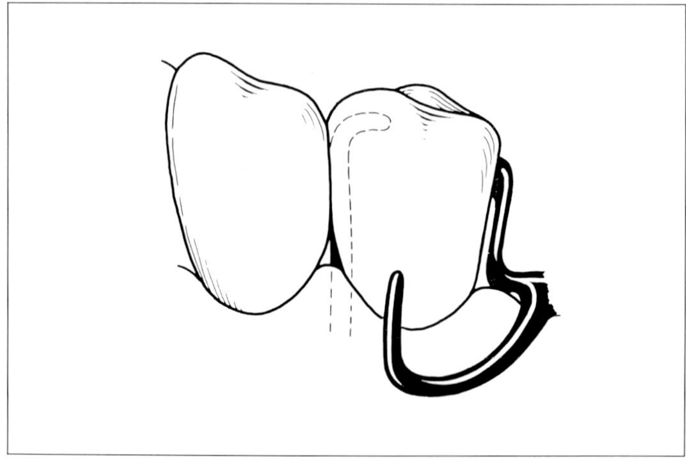

Fig. 91 The Kratochvil designed retainer with maximum contact between denture base and distal guide plane. Subsequent relief is provided at the lower extremity.

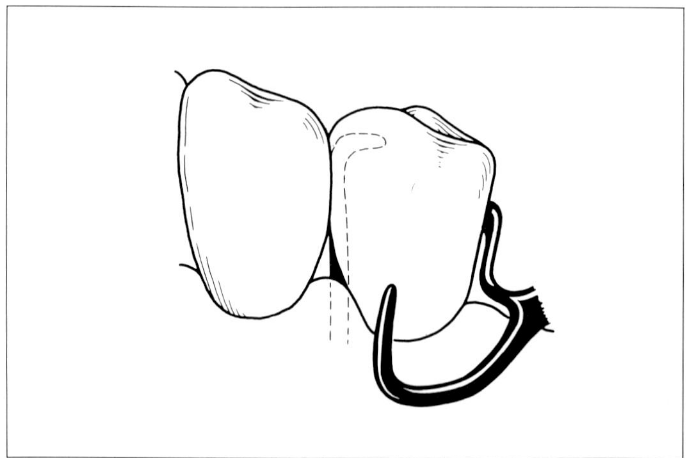

Fig. 92 The Krol modification. The occlusogingival contact between denture base and guide plane is restricted to about 3 mm.

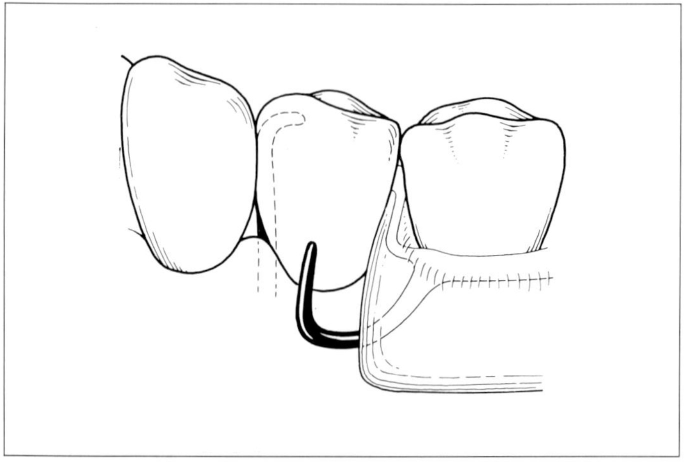

Fig. 93 The artificial denture tooth determines the contact area.

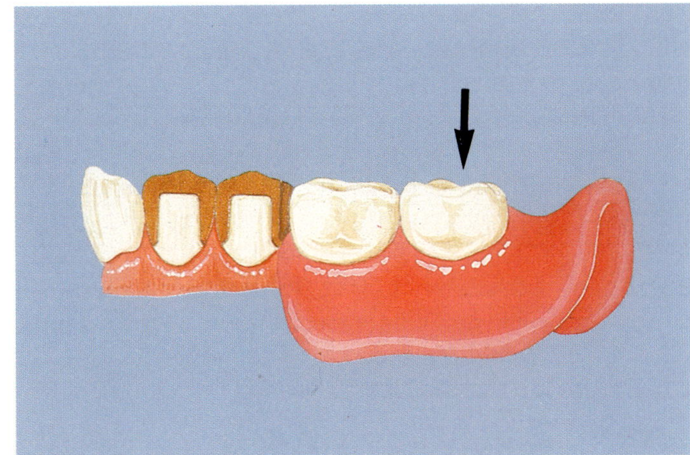

Fig. 94 Intracoronal attachments may apply loads closer to the long axes of the abutments.

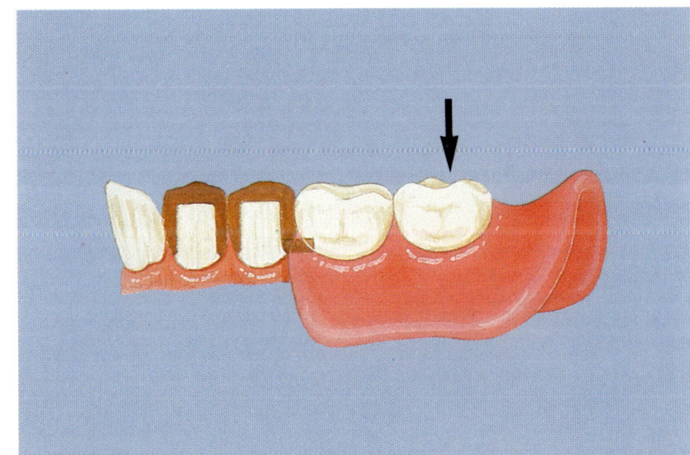

Fig. 95 Vertical loads applied through extracoronal attachments will be distal to the long axes of the abutment teeth.

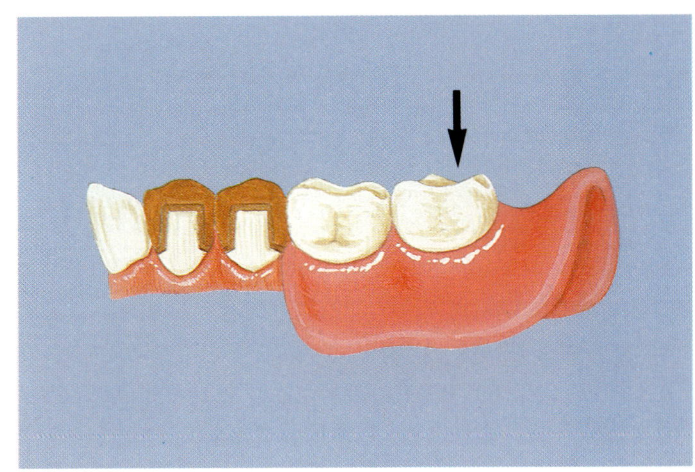

Fig. 96 Telescopic crowns appear to offer considerable advantages in vertical load distribution. In practice, these advantages may not be so clear-cut.

ilar manner. Where they must differ is in the mechanism and effectiveness of retention. Intracoronal attachments are usually placed distally on the abutment adjacent to the space (Fig. 94). Despite the advantage confirmed by their depth, vertical load distribution is still distal to the long axes of the teeth. This problem is accentuated with extracoronal attachments (Fig. 95). Telescopic crowns might appear to offer some advantages in this respect, but these are often theoretical rather than real (Fig. 96). If the connection between fixed and removable sections of the prosthesis were absolutely rigid, the positioning of the joint would not affect load distribution. However, not even the removable prosthesis itself can be considered absolutely rigid for clinical purposes, let alone the comparatively small junction between the two components.

The problems of off-centre vertical loads become more acute when attachments are cantilevered behind the distal abutment. Intracoronal attachments may be employed in this manner. Extracoronal attachments are notorious in this respect and for this reason should not be placed distal to a cantilevered pontic.

In view of the loads that might be applied, it is wise practice to employ splinted abutments of at least two connected teeth.

Stress-breaking

So far the discussion has involved load distribution to the mucosa and to the teeth. Many attachments allow a certain degree of movement between the components: for this reason they are known as 'stress-breakers'. This is a misleading term for, at best, all these devices can do is to transfer load from one structure to another. 'Load distributor' is probably more descriptive, and 'stress director' would be an alternative term (*Mensor* 1972). If the total load is too great, no amount of 'stress-breaking' is going to help.

Another point should be considered. These devices transfer load from the teeth to the edentulous ridge. Up to a point, the periodontal ligament is better able to resist these loads than the edentulous ridge.

A host of ingenious devices have been designed to allow movement between the denture base and the natural teeth. Analysis of the action of these devices is difficult, and one frequently suspects they do not achieve the results intended by their inventors—particularly after a certain amount of wear has occurred. Hinges, for example, might allow pure hinge movement while new, but are prone to wear after use in the mouth and allow lateral movement. Lateral or rotational play within an attachment may severely reduce the cross-arch support provided by the major connector.

It might be argued that, on theoretical considerations, some slight movement of the denture base must occur under load and that the tendency for the base to rotate could be eliminated by allowing movement in a vertical direction. A hypothetical attachment, allowing movement in this direction alone, is illustrated (Fig. 97). However, it can be seen that simple vertical movement would apply even loading only in situations where the entire mucosa were of even displaceability and, presumably,

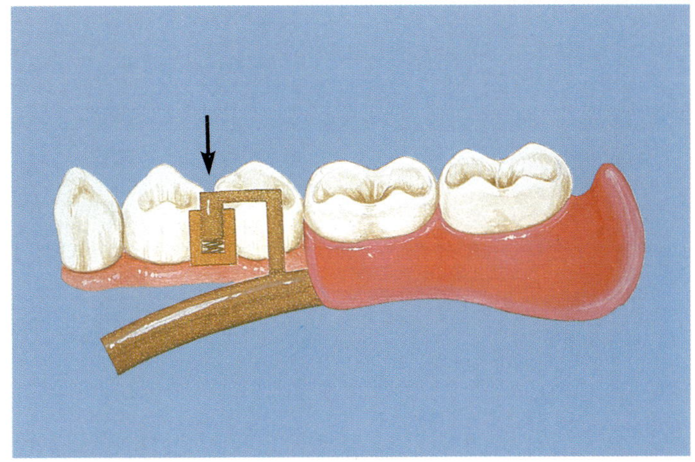

Fig. 97 A hypothetical attachment allowing movement simply in a vertical direction. Even load distribution to the mucosa occurs only when the entire mucosa is of even displaceability, while denture base movement relative to the papilla behind the distal abutment tooth may cause damage.

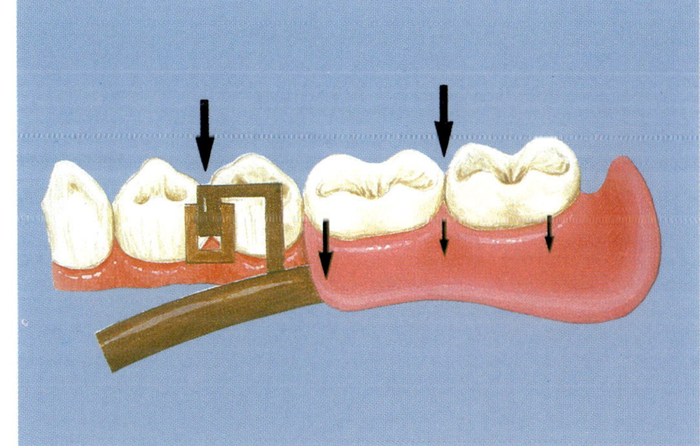

Fig. 98 Loss of the spring, or lack of resilience, can remove tooth support for the denture base. Unless springs are regularly checked, damage to the gingivae and edentulous ridges may ensue.

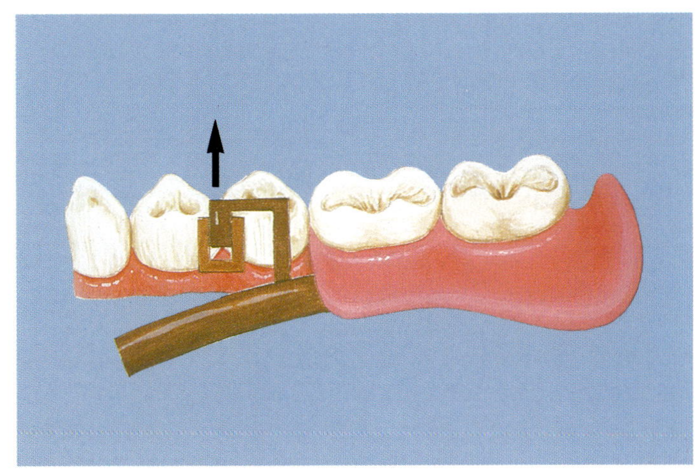

Fig. 99 An incorrect replacement spring may not permit the attachment to engage and will lift the denture base out of contact with the mucosa.

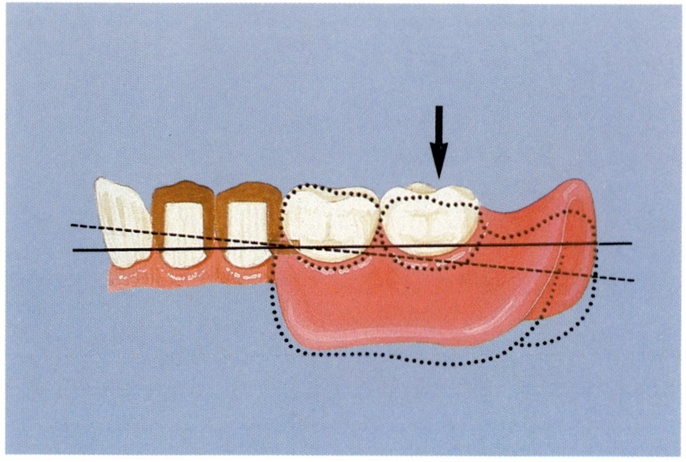

Fig. 100 A hinge may limit denture base movement adjacent to the abutments, but load distribution may be uneven.

thickness; furthermore, a food bolus contacting an off-centre section of the base might jam the attachment. The spring-loaded device immediately reduces the effective support from the abutment teeth, and denture base movement relative to the papilla behind the distal abutment tooth is likely to be increased. Damage to this papilla is a common finding among patients treated with an attachment of this type that has not been maintained regularly. Failure to change the spring regularly will result in permanent deformation of the spring that, in turn, leads to the denture becoming entirely mucosal-borne (Fig. 98). On the other hand, if the spring is incorrectly seated, the attachment may not engage and the denture base will be lifted out of contact with the mucosa (Fig. 99).

Although a hinge in the position illustrated in Figure 100 would not permit significant movement of the denture base adjacent to the abutment teeth, load distribution would be uneven. Some attachments allow both vertical and hinge movements, thereby combining the advantages and drawbacks that have been discussed. The alignment of hinges is discussed in Chapter 7. The distal projection, however, is likely to complicate plaque control problems. Furthermore, a hinge out of alignment with the edentulous ridge is likely to require considerable buccolingual space (Fig. 101).

It would be too dogmatic, however, to insist that the connection between denture and abutment teeth should be rigid for every prosthesis that is made. There are situations where the number, distribution and condition of the remaining teeth cannot form a sufficiently strong abutment to withstand exceptional loads that might be applied to them by an attached distal extension prosthesis. It is here that a very slight degree of freedom of movement may be allowed between denture base and abutment teeth. This slight, potential movement should be considered as a safety valve and it must be stressed that a correctly de-

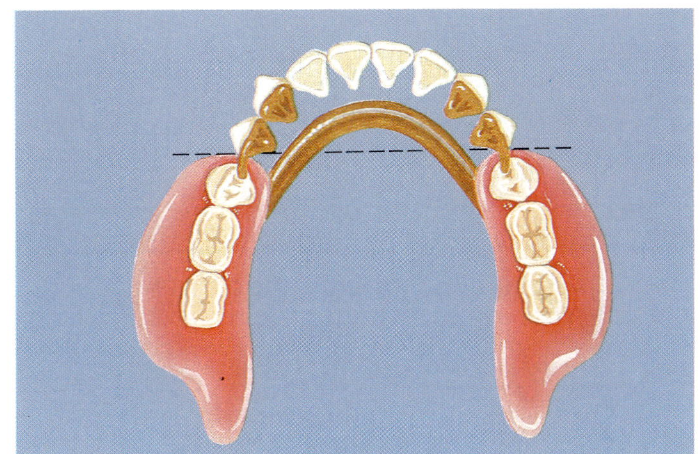

Fig. 101 The distal projection of an extracoronal attachment will complicate plaque control. When twisted out of alignment with the edentulous ridge, buccolingual space requirements are increased.

signed and constructed denture has only the minimal tendency to move. A prosthesis that constantly moves serves little purpose apart from causing damage to the abutment teeth, their supporting structures and possibly hastening bone resorption of the edentulous areas. Boitel*, for example, found that vertical movements of the denture base of about 0.4 mm produced significant damage to the distal gingival papillae of the abutment teeth. It is, therefore, unnecessary to introduce mechanical complexities in order to allow the denture base a large range of undesirable and potentially damaging movements.

For the majority of restorations, a comparatively straightforward and rigid connection can be used, provided the denture is stable.

There is, of course, no such thing as a rigid denture. All materials possess some inherent flexibility. Apart from major connectors, *Heckneby* (1969) has pointed out that the levels of transverse and sagittal flexibility of acrylic resin denture bases may well reach clinical significance.

Path of insertion

When a partial denture is in position, it may be withdrawn along its path of insertion, or it may be rocked and rotated out of place. Proximal tooth surfaces bearing a parallel relationship to one another guide the denture while it is being inserted or removed. A correctly designed clasp-retained partial denture restoring a bounded space should incorporate effective guiding planes from the abutments. If precise frictional contacts between denture base and abutment teeth are obtained, there will

* Personal communication.

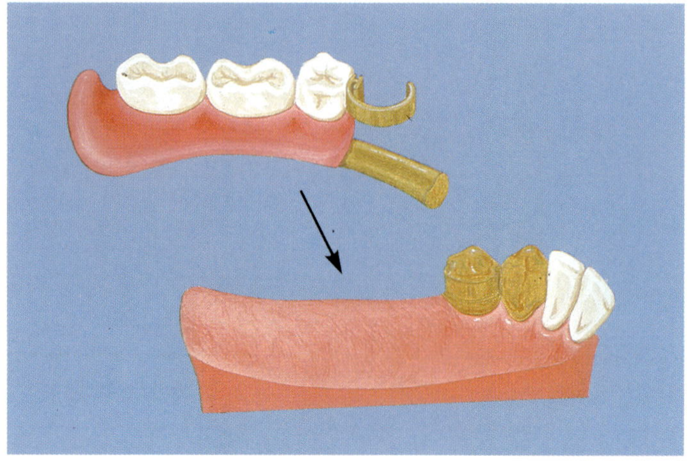

Fig. 102   The distal extension prosthesis usually requires a path of insertion approaching the distal aspects of the abutments.

be no spaces into which the gingivae can proliferate or food stagnate. The guiding planes prevent the denture being rocked or rotated out of place, for it can only move along its path of insertion. Since the tips of the retaining clasps are placed in undercuts relative to this path, removal of the denture can be achieved only by deformation of the clasp arms. The longer the guide plane, the more effective it will be. Where distal extension dentures are concerned, *Kratochvil* (1963) and *Krol* (1973) have suggested that proximal guide planes be limited to about 2 mm. Where clasp retention is considered, there is some advantage in the lingual surfaces of abutment teeth having surfaces parallel to the proximal guide planes. Apart from increasing the surface area of contact, it may also help overcome a theoretical hazard of clasp design—unopposed lateral force application when the denture is inserted. *Stern* (1975) has pointed ed out that as the denture is inserted, the retention arm contacts the surface above until it is completely seated, when it becomes passive. If the bracing arm contacts the tooth all the time the clasp is exerting a load, no lateral components will be exerted on the abutment teeth.

Mucosal contours, as well as those of the teeth, need to be considered, particularly when attachments are to be employed. Few attachments allow the partial denture to be rocked and rotated into position. A distal extension prosthesis usually requires a path of insertion approaching from the distal aspect of the abutments (Fig. 102). This path allows maximum contact between the denture base and the distal abutment, while also permitting the base to enter the retromylohyoid fossae—areas frequently undercut to an approach path at right-angles to the occlusal plane. Anterior removable prostheses often require a path of insertion with an approach from the labial aspect.

Retention

The retention of a denture depends on its ability to resist displacement away from its supporting structures. In this discussion, retention is the degree of resistance of the prosthesis to removal in a direction opposite to that of its insertion. Retention can be provided by both clasps and attachments, but the mechanism by which they act is different.

The clasp achieves retention by means of its flexible tip placed in an undercut. This clasp tip should be passive when the prosthesis is in position, although this ideal state may not always occur in practice. Nevertheless, an unseating force is required to cause deformation of the clasp before the denture can be removed, and this force is a measure of the retention provided by the clasp.

This state of affairs exists where the path of withdrawal is determined precisely.

Apart from the presence of adequate guide planes, the clasp can be effective only where a suitable undercut relative to this path can be engaged. Not only the undercut depth, but its location is important. *Avant* (1971) has pointed out that both the undercut depth and its distance below the survey line exert important influences on retention.

Take two undercuts of the same size, one placed near the survey line, the other close to the gingivae. The work required to remove the dentures constructed would be the same. But work is the product of the force and the distance through which it acts. The clasp near the survey line does not need to travel very far, but the force required for its movement is considerable. Retention is a measure of force, not work, and so the clasp near the survey line will provide greater retention than its counterpart closer to the gingivae (Fig. 103). The clasp near the survey line may have a bracing arm nearer the occlusal surface than the clasp close to the gingival margin.

In the majority of situations, the clasp will be the retainer of choice. Recent developments with the bar (gingivally approaching) retainer makes possible a neat and effective unit. An adequate guide plane, undercut and sulcus depth is required. Whether or not the guide plane should reach the gingival margin is a point at issue. However, as a matter of principle, the less effective the guide plane the more cumbersome the retaining arm must be. Occlusally approaching clasp arms are more rigid, simpler to make, but may interfere with appearance. For a detailed examination of clasp retainers, the reader is referred to *McCraken's Removable Partial Prosthodontics (Henderson* and *Steffel* 1981) or *Neill* and *Walter* (1983).

Unlike clasps, attachments provide their retention by frictional contacts or by mechanical locks. Some units employ both. The retention provided is usually extremely effective and achieved irrespective of the contours of the natural teeth.

Indirect retention

Movement of a distal extension base away from its supporting tissues may occur as a rotation about an axis, or as a displacement of the entire denture along its path of insertion. Movement along the path of insertion should be prevented by the direct retainers, but rotational movements present a problem.

When the denture base is tilted away from the mucosa, the denture tends to rotate around the direct retainers (Fig. 104). It tends to rotate, in fact, about an axis passing through the tips of the distal retaining clasps which are, therefore, virtually powerless to prevent this movement. However this rotational movement can be prevented by rigid components of the denture base placed anterior to the axis of rotation, on the principle of the Class 2 lever. The indirect retainer replaces the clasp tip as the centre of rotation and the clasp tip is thereby placed in an undercut relative to this movement, which it can then prevent (Fig. 105). *Nairn* (1966) felt that clasps placed in distal undercuts of abutment teeth might be ineffective when used in conjunction with indirect retainers, as they might not be in undercuts relative to rotational movements around the indirect retainer (Fig. 106). However, if the cast was surveyed with a nose-down tilt, as should normally be the case for distal extension prostheses, the clasp should well be able to resist this movement.

An indirect retainer can be effective only if it is placed some considerable distance anterior to the direct retainers. When only anterior teeth remain, the distance between direct and indirect retainers must be small and thus there is little to prevent the denture base separating from the mucosa. A clasp-retained denture in the situation illustrated (Fig. 107) would have a tendency to drop away from the mucosa posteriorly. For this reason many prosthodontists, in the past, preferred to construct complete immediate replacement dentures for similar situations.

Berg and *Caputo* (1978) examined the differing anterior rests available with distal extension prosthesis. Horizontal force components, particularly those that were

Fig. 104 Unless an effective indirect retainer is incorporated, there is little to prevent the posterior sections of the denture bases rotating around the free ends of the clasps.

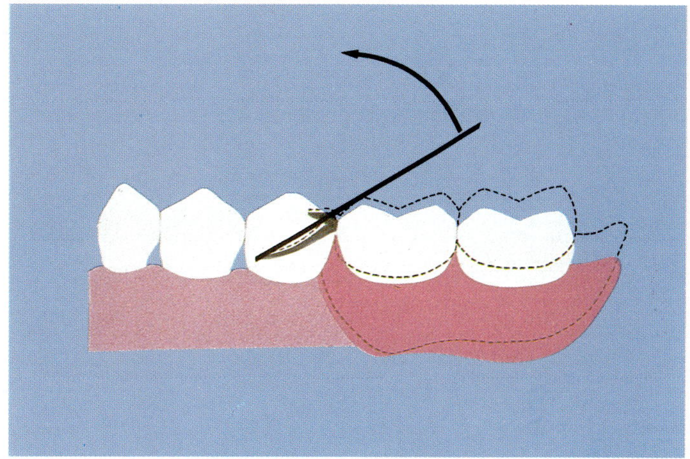

Fig. 105 The indirect retainer replaces the clasp tip as the centre of rotational movement of the saddle away from the mucosa. The clasp tip is thereby placed in an undercut relative to the movement which it can then prevent.

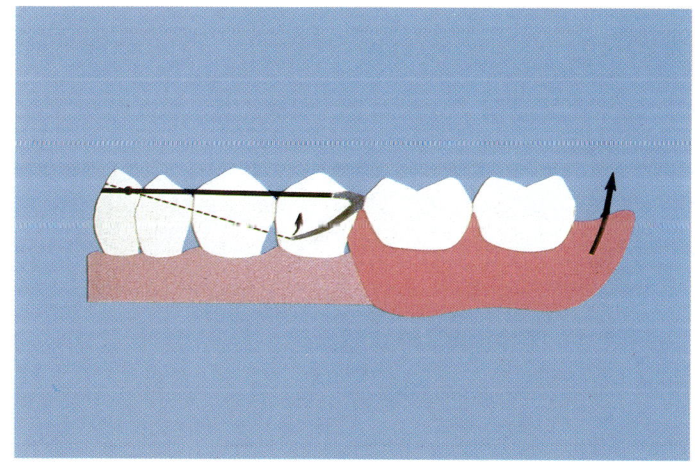

Fig. 106 Clasps placed in some distal undercuts might be ineffective when used in conjunction with indirect retainers as they may not be in undercuts relative to rotational movements around the indirect retainer. This problem should not arise if the cast is surveyed with a 'nose-down' tilt.

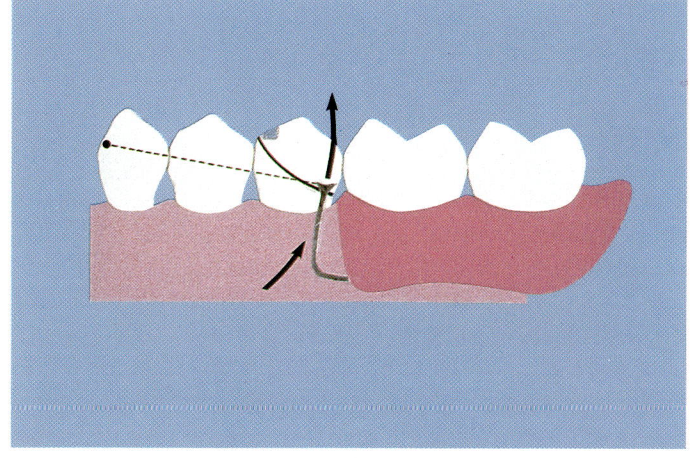

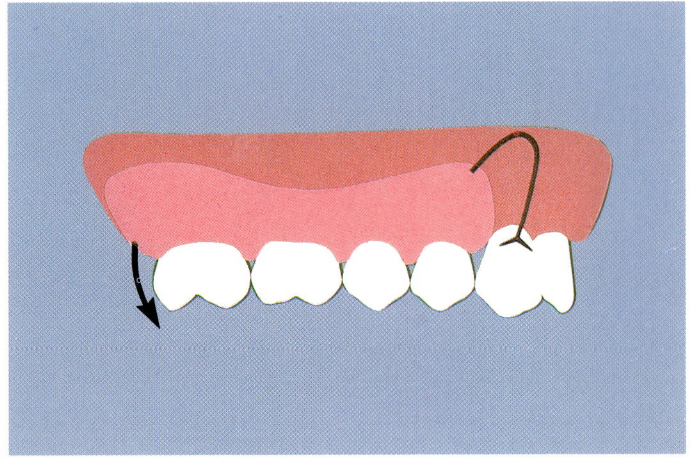

Fig. 107   As a result of lack of indirect retention, a clasp-retained denture has a tendency to drop away from the mucosa posteriorly.

antero-posteriorly inclined, produced the most widely dispersed and intense stress patterns. Loads to the anterior base and the central incisors produced the greatest transmission of stress to other components in the arch. Distobuccally directed loads on the extension base affected the immediate canine abutments. Proximal plates gave gross stability to the removable prosthesis, thereby lessening stress in any one region. This was particularly true for isolated canine abutments when affected by loadings on the distal-extension base.

Positive anterior rests function as direct transmitters of force to the lingual inclines of the anterior teeth and to anterior tooth-borne bases, so that positive rests throughout the arch are significant in restraining the anterior teeth. The central incisors benefit somewhat more than the canine.

Positive anterior rests were shown to be an essential element of design when considering stress distribution with a removable partial denture involving anterior teeth.

Attachments have great advantages with respect to indirect retention. Intracoronal units possess such a precise path of insertion that there is little opportunity for the denture base to rotate. Some extracoronal attachments incorporate effective tilt-stopping devices, but with others additional components need to be added to the denture framework.

Attachments normally require splinted abutments and involve additional complications, compared with clasps. Nevertheless, their invisible and most effective retention together with their ability to resist tilting and other displacing forces make attachments useful where the clasp might be ugly and inoperative.

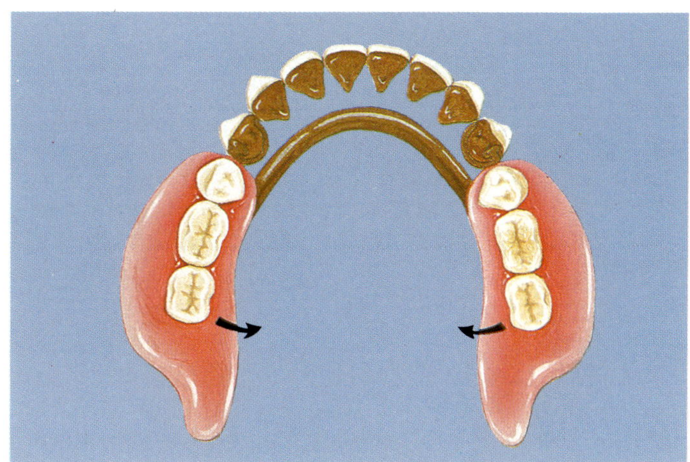

Fig. 108   The major connector should prevent any tendency for the denture bases to whip.

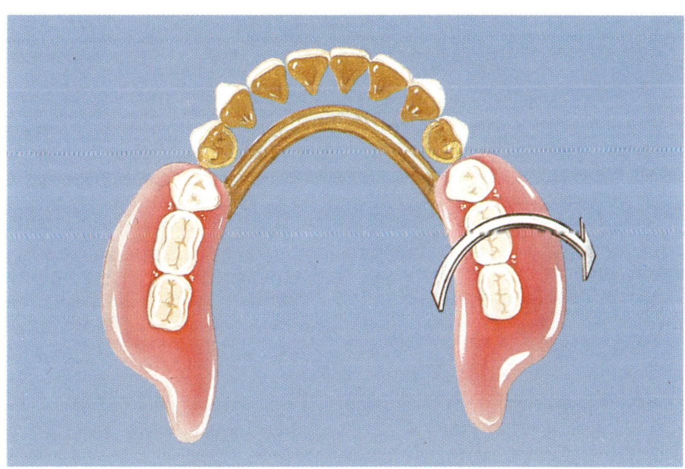

Fig. 109   A bilateral prosthesis is able to resist horizontal loads with the teeth and mucosa of both sides of the jaw. Rotational loads applied to one side are resisted by the retainers of the opposite side acting with a considerable mechanical advantage.

Connectors

If the distal extension base is to resist forces applied in all directions, as indeed it must, additional support from other quadrants of the mouth is nearly always necessary. By distributing lateral loads, the major connector prevents any tendency for the denture base to whip (Fig. 108). Another example of how the major connector functions concerns forces applied through the buccal cusps of the artificial teeth. These forces may cause the entire prosthesis to rotate (Fig. 109). Attachments or clasps on the side of the applied force resist with a poor mechanical advantage. Direct retainers on the opposite side of the arch can resist these forces with an appreciable mechanical advantage.

The major connector can only serve these functions if it is comparatively rigid. Space limitations of the mouth and the restricted

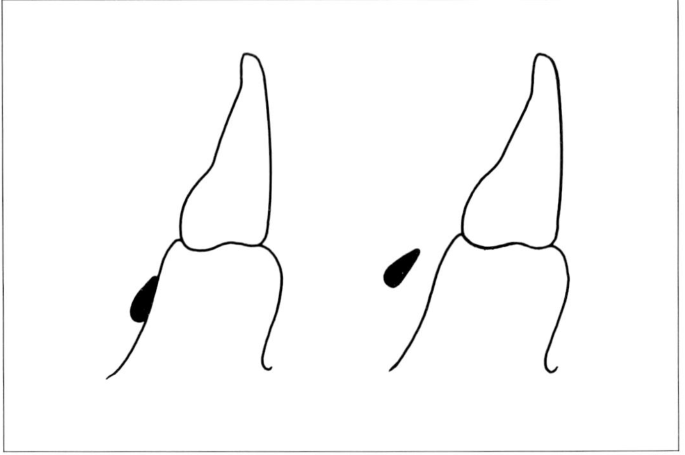

Fig. 110   Where vertical space restrictions are present, it may be possible to space the lingual bar from the mucosa.

stiffness of the materials available today make it virtually impossible to construct the major connector of a lower distal extension prosthesis that will not flex by at least 0.3 mm when subjected to loads of 10 kg. For example, *Bates* (1966) reported base deflections of 0.65 mm when subjected to 1.2 kg. In practice, it is extremely difficult to evaluate the stiffness or load/deflection characteristics of a cast lingual bar, with an irregular and variable cross-section and whose geometrical shape is determined by the characteristics of the patient's jaw. Since any significant flexing of the connector will degrade the benefit of cross-arch support, the major effort should be directed at producing a connector of adequate stiffness, not the reverse.

Lingual bars are popular lower connectors when attachments are employed as there is seldom need for additional indirect retainers. Unfortunately, the space available for the bar is often limited. Short lingual sulcus depth can be overcome by spacing the bar lingually from the mucosa (Fig. 110). Within the limitations of patient tolerance, this has the additional advantage of reducing the length of the major connector and decreasing the radius of curvature, factors that contribute to its tortional rigidity. Where space restrictions apply, the higher modulus of elasticity (stiffness) of chrome compared with gold has obvious advantage.

The designs of upper major connectors generally pose less of a problem. Where support is required, the plate is the obvious choice otherwise the strength inherent in a ring-type connector is to be preferred (Fig. 111). Where patient tolerance dictates a posterior palatal strap, the design is weakened (Fig. 112). Choice of materials and the cross-section of components becomes critical in this situation. The anterior palatal bar, or horseshoe, manages to combine most of the drawbacks of the

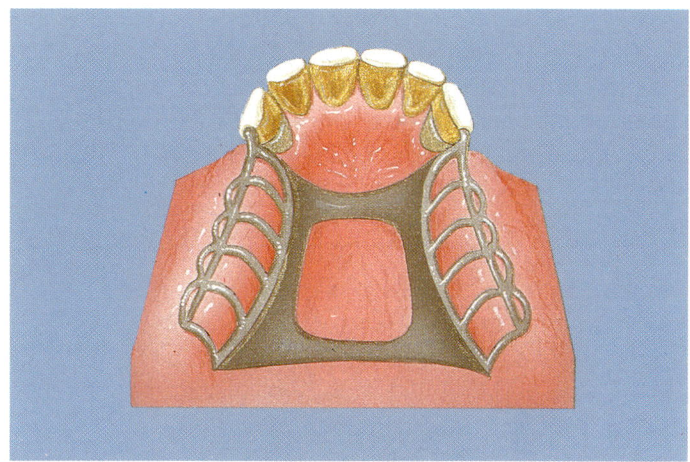

Fig. 111 The strength inherent in a ring-type design is to be preferred.

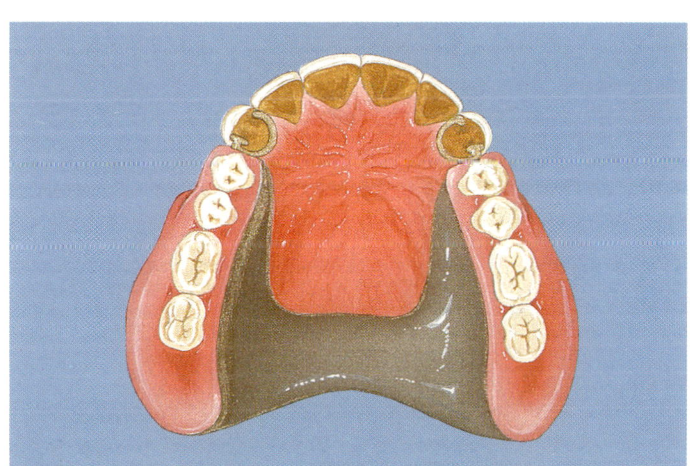

Fig. 112 Where patient tolerance dictates a palatal strap, the design is weakened.

rings and bars with few advantages, save where an inoperable torus exists.

Any design that involves coverage of gingival margins will place the gingivae at risk. *Hobkirk* and *Strahan* (1979) have reinforced the well-established prosthodontic maxim of ensuring minimal coverage of the gingival areas by the prosthesis. Their conclusions were that where such coverage is unavoidable, the prosthesis should be well-fitting and cross the gingival at right angles, if possible.

Chrome cobalt alloys have obvious advantages where spans are long and space is restricted. There are, however, drawbacks some of which are peculiar to attachment-retained restorations.

Whereas a good connector can be cast in any laboratory capable of constructing the abutment crowns, chrome cobalt alloys require special facilities. It is also extremely difficult to produce a chrome casting that will fit the intricacies of milled bracing arms or other prepared components. Problems arising from differential hardness of gold and chrome cobalt are frequently over-rated; it is the adaptation that is so hard to produce. Soldering chrome cobalt alloys to precious metal components requires skill as the attachments are easily damaged in the process. On the other hand, certain extracoronal attachments, like the Dalbo, can be buried in the denture base acrylic resin and require no bracing arm. Chrome cobalt alloys produce no problems with these types of unit. The lower stiffness of a hard yellow gold alloy requires the cross-section of the connector to be about 25% thicker than one made in chrome cobalt. There is one final point. In considering technical problems it is all too easy to forget the patient. There are still many patients who, despite the extra bulk required, prefer gold.

Even supposing that a rigid major connector could be constructed, heat-cured acrylic resin has only about one-seventieth the stiffness of chrome cobalt. *Heckneby* (1969) has shown that the denture base itself is quite capable of flexing by 0.3 mm under occlusal load.

For practical purposes, it is therefore almost impossible to produce a denture that will resist occlusal and masticatory forces without these slight movements and that should be all that is required––under normal circumstances at least. There seems little point in weakening the structure to allow a range of uncontrolled, unnecessary and potentially damaging movements that complicate construction and maintenance of the restoration.

The unilateral distal space

A removable prosthesis restoring such a space normally requires support from the teeth on both sides of the arch. Without this support, the denture and its abutments stand little chance of resisting forces causing the base to whip (Fig. 113), or those tending to rotate it around a sagittal axis (Fig. 114). Support from the other side of the arch makes the base stable, and damaging torques on the abutments will be eliminated.

Joining the two sides of the arch make it tooth-supported on one side and tooth and mucosal-supported on the other. It used to be argued that under occlusal load the tooth and mucosal-supported part of the prosthesis might be displaced more than the tooth-supported section, thereby introducing unfavourable forces on the abutments. Ingenious attachments were, in fact, developed that allowed different movements on the two sides of the prosthesis. Many dentures are still made in this way. However, one must not forget that movement occurring between the denture base and the major connector, or between the abutment crowns and bases, reduce support from the teeth and the effectiveness of cross-arch bracing. Impression techniques, jaw relations and maintenance therapy are more difficult when a movement potential exists. For these reasons, prostheses restoring unilateral spaces are usually best made with comparatively rigid attachments, if indeed attachments are indicated.

The clasp-retained prosthesis is usually to be recommended where there is no missing tooth on the opposite side of the arch to the distal space. Adequate guiding

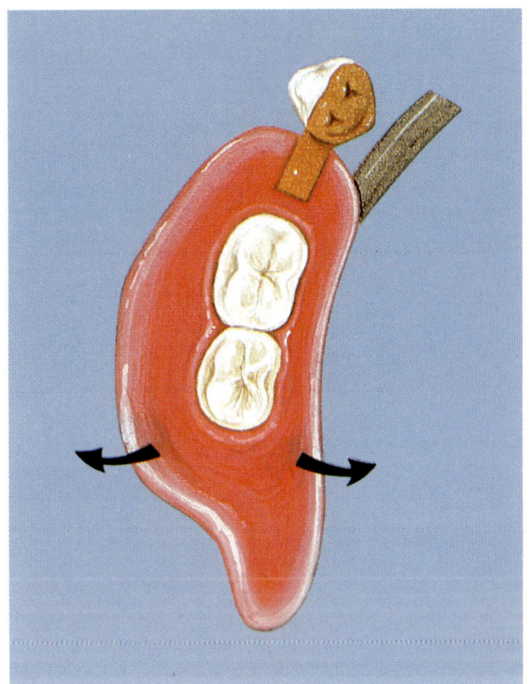

Fig. 113 Without cross-arch support the prosthesis stands little chance of resisting the forces causing the base to whip.

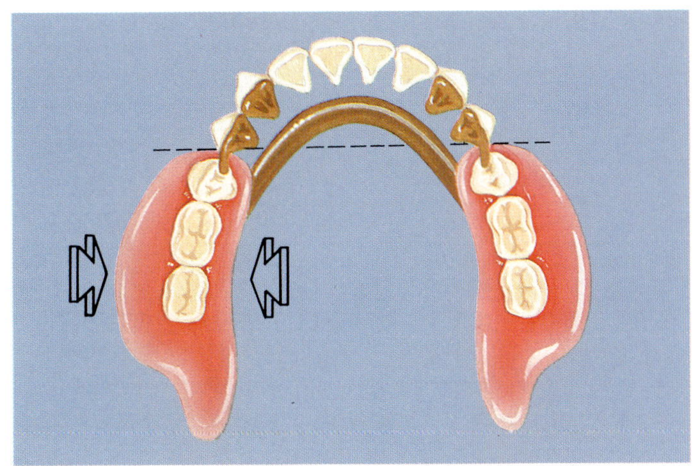

Fig. 114 The major connector will prevent the base rotating around a sagittal axis.

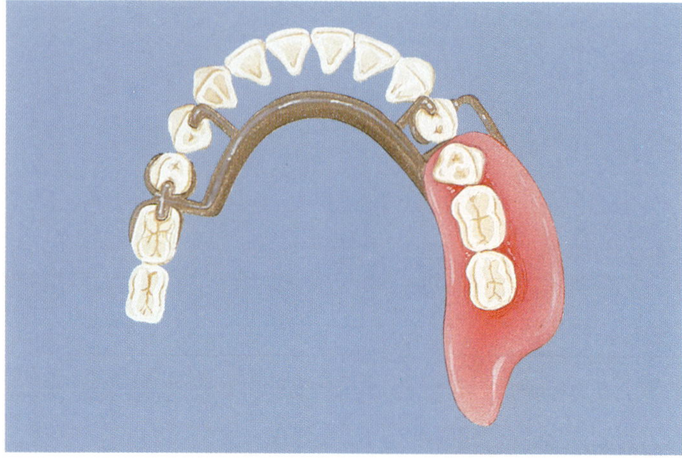

Fig. 115   A clasp-retained denture may be preferable for some unilateral spaces. The extensive tooth preparation required for an attachment-retained prosthesis may not be offset by its marginal advantages in retention and stability.

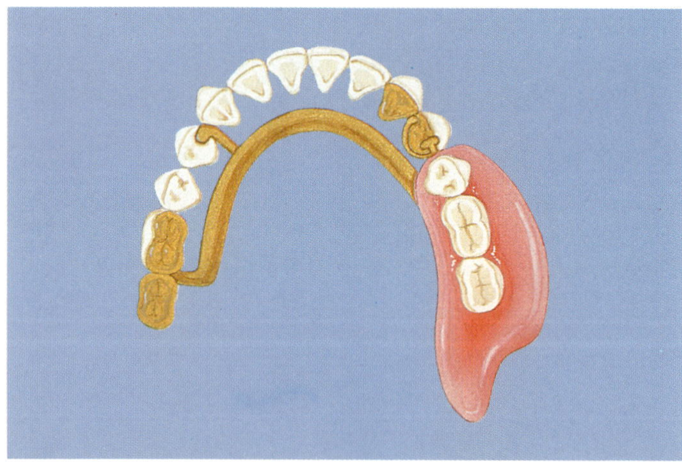

Fig. 116   Joined telescopic crowns may be employed where no space exists on one side of the arch.

planes can be provided, usually producing effective clasp retainers that are economical, neat and require little or no preparation of the abutments (Fig. 115).

Where the abutment teeth in any case require large restorations, attachments have much to offer. If no space is present on one side of the arch, it might be tempting to place an attachment between two adjacent splinted crowns, but this is not rec-ommended as it almost invariably necessitates an encroachment on the proximal space. Joined telescopic crowns are usually recommended in these situations (Figs. 116 to 118). A minimum of two splinted crowns is normally required on this side of the mouth and these may need to be devitalised if lingually inclined. The walls of the inner copings must be aligned with attachments on the side of the arch.

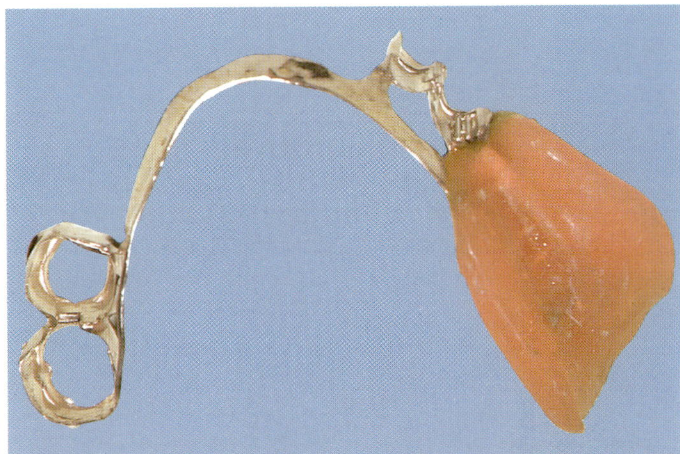

Fig. 117   Impression surface of denture showing telescopic crowns.

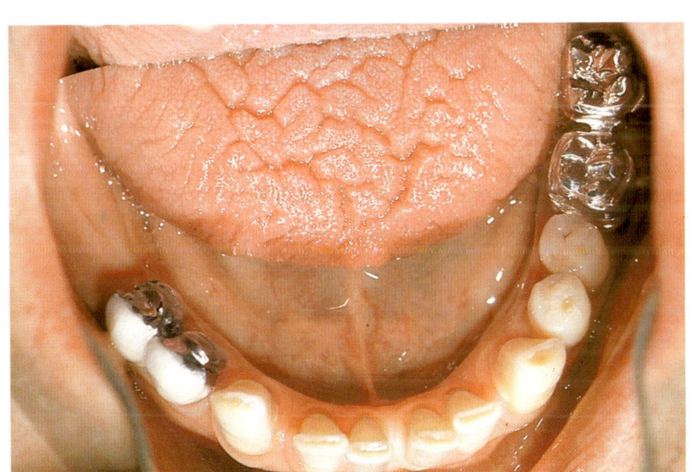

Fig. 118   Inner sections of the crowns in the mouth. (Viewed through a mirror.)

Intracoronal attachments can be employed when teeth are missing on both sides of the arch. It might then be tempting to design a prosthesis with attachments in the teeth adjacent to the spaces. However, intracoronal attachments require box preparations in the abutments. Since the intracoronal units need to be aligned with one another, a path of insertion virtually at right angles to the occlusal plane may need to be selected. This path of insertion may prevent the extension of the denture base to gain the mucosal support it needs (Fig. 119).

A modification of this technique, and one to be preferred, is to construct a fixed prosthesis across the bounded space (Figs. 120 and 121). An intracoronal unit can then be placed buccolingually within this prosthesis. Neither the size nor the alignment of

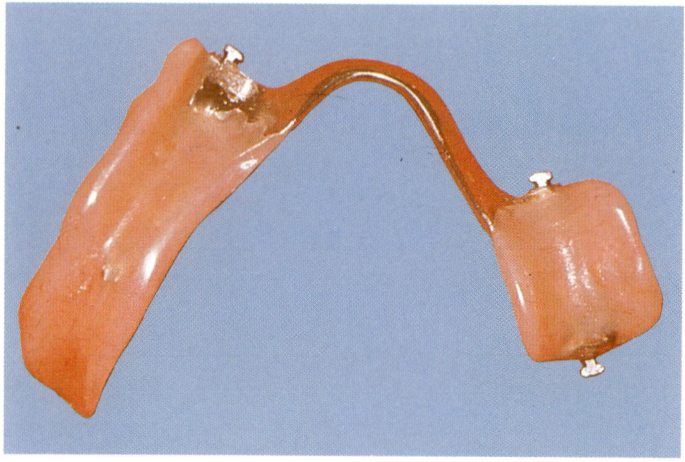

Fig. 119 Inadequate extension of the denture base resulting from a path of insertion at right-angles to the occlusal plane.

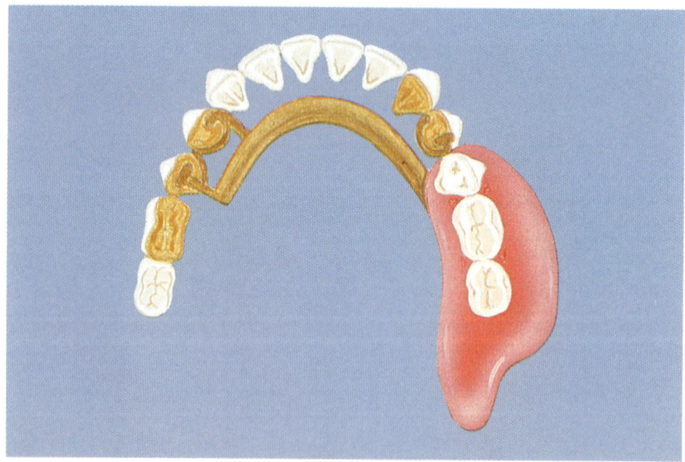

Fig. 120 Where there is a space on the opposite side to the distal extension, the denture can gain support from an attachment placed buccolingually in a bridge restoring the gap.

the attachment is limited by pulpal considerations, and the distal abutment is permanently splinted.

An intracoronal retainer within a pontic can be difficult for the patient to remove. An additional handling point should be combined with an indirect retainer. The indirect retainer is necessary to reduce loads falling on the lateral surface of the attachment, and to contribute to the stability of the denture.

A neat and simple indirect retainer would take the form of an occlusal rest attached to a minor connector and recessed within the contour of one of the mesial abutment crowns. Lingual bracing arms can be milled and modified to carry out similar roles.

The fixed prosthesis restoring the bounded space may take the form of a bar unit. The bar unit becomes more valuable when the bounded space is long, for some mucosal support can be gained for the prosthesis (Fig. 122).

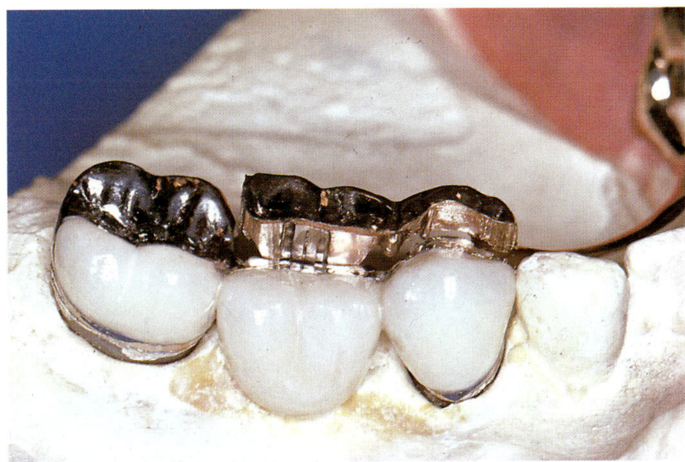

Fig. 121 Attachment placed buccolingually in pontic. Note the indirect retainer that also acts as an additional handling point.

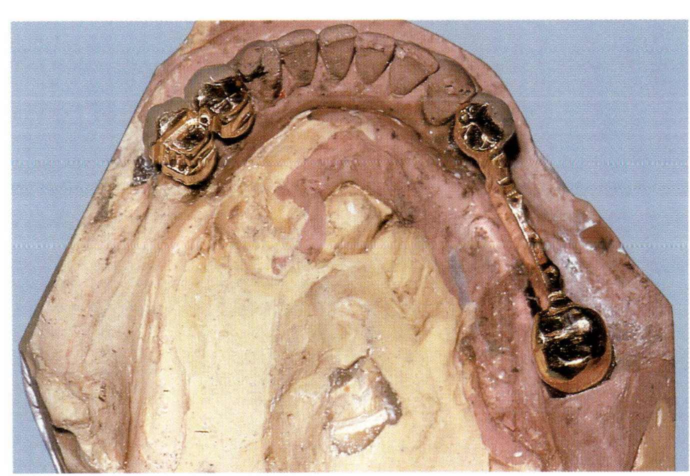

Fig. 122 The fixed prosthesis may take the form of a bar unit.

Missing anterior teeth

As a general rule, anterior teeth should not be added to bilateral distal extension dentures. No matter how well the prosthesis is made there is always a tendency for it to rotate around the abutments (Fig. 123). Where possible, the anterior space should be restored by a fixed prosthesis. Alternatively, a bar can be used to span the anterior edentulous gap, thereby splinting the abutments either side.

The check record

The importance of accurate jaw relations has been stressed throughout the text. When a distal extension denture opposes a complete denture there are apparent practical difficulties in making a check record, yet it is particularly important that this be carried out.

A remount cast is made for the upper denture and a new facebow record taken. The upper denture and its remount cast can

125

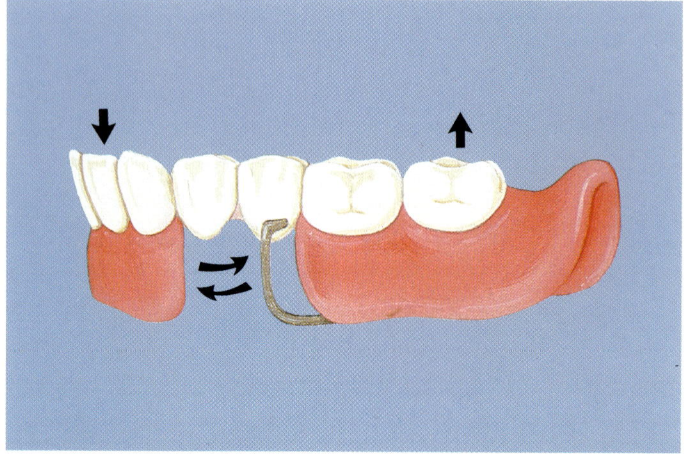

Fig. 123 An anterior base results in a tendency for the prosthesis to rotate around its abutments. Where possible an anterior fixed prosthesis should be constructed, or the abutments connected by a bar.

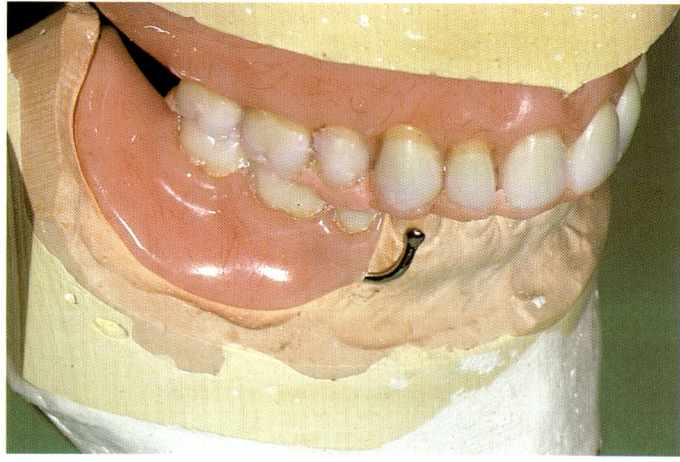

Fig. 124 Lower partial denture remounted on an articulator by means of a check record.

now be mounted on the articulator. A record rim of extra hard wax is then applied to the upper denture and, after suitable warming, the centric relation record made, with the teeth just failing to contact. By dampening the lower natural and artificial teeth, one can ensure that the rim stays adhered to the upper denture.

If the lower master cast has been destroyed, an impression of the entire lower dentition is made removing the denture in the impression. The cast of this impression is subsequently mounted on the articulator using the centric relation record (Fig. 124). It is then possible to perfect the occlusion and articulation without the possible complication of denture base movement.

To summarise, the clasp retainer is still the retainer of choice for the majority of removable prostheses, being comparatively cheap, effective, straightforward to use, and requiring the minimum of preparation of the abutment teeth. However, the shape, number, or distribution of the natural teeth does not always allow the effective use of clasps, and it is here that attachments are particularly valuable. For the intermediate situations, the practitioner must weigh carefully the mechanical advantages of attachments and the better appearance against the tooth preparation required and the extra cost involved. The need to provide better distal extension prostheses has been recognised, and attachments have much to contribute to this end.

References

Applegate O. C. (1955).
The partial denture base. J. Prosthet. Dent., 5, 5: 636.

Applegate O. C. (1959).
Essentials of Removable Partial Denture Prosthesis. 2nd Edn. Saunders, Philadelphia.

Atwood D. A. (1962).
Some clinical factors related to rate of resorption of risidual ridge. J. Prosthet. Dent., 12, 3: 411.

Avant W. E. (1971).
Factors that influence retention of removable partial dentures. J. Prosthet. Dent., 25, 3: 265.

Bates J. F. (1963).
Retention of cobalt-chromium partial dentures. Dent. Pract., 14: 168.

Bates J. F. (1966).
Studies related to the function of partial dentures. The functional strain in cobalt-chromium dentures: a preliminary report. Brit. Dent. J., 5: 79.

Bates J. F. (1970).
Partial Denture Construction: A Laboratory Manual. John Wright, Bristol.

Berg T. and Caputo A. A. (1978).
Anterior rests for maxillary removable partial dentures. J. Prosthet. Dent., 39, 2: 139.

Bergman B. (1983).
Evaluation of the results of treatment with osseo-integrated implants by the Swedish National Board of Health and Welfare. J. Prosthet. Dent., 50: 1, 114.

Braden M. (1976).
Personal Communication.

Branemark P. I. (1983).
Osseointegration and its experimental background. J. Prosthet. Dent., 50: 3, 399.

Brodie A. G. and Thompson J. R. (1942).
Factors in the position of the mandible J. A. D. A., 29: 925-941.

Carlsson G. E., Hedegard B. and Koivumaa K. K. (1961).
Studies in partial dental prosthesis. II: An investigation of mandibular partial dentures with double extension saddles. Acta Odont. Scand., 19: 215.

Carlsson G. E., Hedegard B. and Koivumaa K. K. (1962).
Studies in partial dental prosthesis. III: A longitudinal study of mandibular partial dentures with double extension saddles. Acta Odont. Scand., 20: 95.

Carlsson G. E., Hedegard B. and Koivumaa K. K. (1965).
Studies in partial dental prosthesis. IV: Final results of a 4-year longitudinal investigation of dentogingivally supported partial dentures. Acta Odont. Scand., 23: 443.

Carlsson G. E. and Person G. (1967).
Morphologic changes of the mandible after extraction and wearing dentures. Odontologisk Revy, 18: 27.

Cecconi B. T. (1974).
Effect of rest design on transmission of forces to abutment teeth. J. Prosthet. Dent., 32, 2: 141.

Cecconi B. T., Asgar K. and Dortz E. (1971).
The effect of partial denture clasp design on abutment tooth movement. J. Prosthet. Dent., 25, 1: 44.

Cecconi B. T., Asgar K. and Dortz E. (1972).
Cusp assembly modifications and their effect on abutment tooth movement. J. Prosthet. Dent., 27, 2: 160.

Christensen F. T. (1962).
Mandibular free-end denture. J. Prosthet. Dent., 12, 1: 111.

Clayton J. A. and Jaslos C. (1971).
A measurement of clasps forces on teeth. J. Prosthet. Dent., 25, 1: 21.

Cooper H. (1967).
Precision attachment bridgework. Postgrad. Course, Univ. Michigan.

Craig R. G. and Farah J. W. (1978).
Stresses from loading distal extension removable partial dentures. J. Prosthet. Dent., 39, 3: 274.

Dahl, G. (1963).
Mechanical principles of superplants. Acta Odont. Scand., 21: 515.

Demer W. J. (1976).
An analysis of mesial rest-1-bar clasp designs. J. Prosthet. Dent., 36, 3: 243.

Derry A. and Bertram U. (1970).
Clinical survey of removable partial dentures after 2 years usage. Acta Odont. Scand., 28: 581.

Eames W. B., Sieweke J. C., Wallace S. W. and Rogers L. B. (1979).
Elastomeric impression materials: effect of bulk on accuracy J. Prosthet. Dent., 41, 3: 304.

Ellinger C. W., Rayson J. H. and Henderson D. (1971).
Single complete dentures opposed to natural teeth. J. Prosthet. Dent., 26, 1: 4.

Faust H. E. (1967).
Precision attachment bridgework. Postgrad. Course, Univ. Michigan.

Frank R. P. and Nicholls J. I. (1977).
An investigation of the effectiveness of indirect retainers. J. Prosthet. Dent., 38, 5: 494.

Frechette A. R. (1956).
The influence of partial denture design on the distribution of force to abutment teeth. J. Prosthet. Dent., 6, 2: 195.

Hansson H. A., Albrektsson T. and Branemark P. I. (1983).
Structural aspects of the interface between tissue and titanium implants. J. Prosthet. Dent., 50: 1, 108.

Heckneby M. (1969).
Distribution of load with the lower free-end partial denture. Acta Odont. Scand., 27: (Supp. 52), 140.

Henderson D. and Seward T. E. (1967).
Design and force distribution with removable partial dentures: a progress report. J. Prosthet. Dent., 17, 4: 350.

Henderson D. and Steffel V. L. (1981).
McCracken's Removable Partial Prosthodontics. 6th Edn. C. V. Mosby, St. Louis, Mo.

Henderson D., Blevins W. R., Wesley R. C. and Seward T. (1970).
The cantilever type of posterior fixed partial dentures: a laboratory study. J. Prosthet. Dent., 24, 1: 47.

Hildebrand G. Y. (1968).
Fixed saddle bridges. Acta Odont. Scand., 26, 4: 435.

Holmes J. B. (1965).
Influence of impression procedures and occlusal loading on partial denture movement. J. Prosthet. Dent., 15, 3: 474.

Hobkirk J. A. and Strahan J. D. (1979).
The influence on the gingival tissues of prostheses incorporating gingival relief areas. J. Dent., 7, 1: 15.

Izikowitz L. (1966).
The superplant. Acta Odont. Scand. 24: (Supp. 47).

Izikowitz L., Molin C. and Sundberg C. (1971).
The fixed saddle-bridge—the superplant. Svensk. Tandlak. T., 64: 719.

Johns R. B. (1976).
Implants as Abutments: Proceedings of the British Society for Restorative Dentistry. J. Wright, Bristol.

Kaires A. K. (1958).
A study of partial denture design and masticatory pressures in a mandibular bilateral distal extension case. J. Prosthet. Dent., 8, 2: 340.

Kass C. A. and Knap F. J. (1974).
Analysis of occlusion before and after occlusal adjustment. J. Prosthet. Dent., 32, 2: 163.

Kratochvil F. J. (1963).
Influence of occlusal rest position and clasp design on movement of abutment teeth. J. Prosthet. Dent., 13, 1: 114.

Kratochvil F. J. and Caputo A. A. (1974).
Photo-elastic analysis of pressure on teeth and bone supporting removable partial dentures. J. Prosthet. Dent., 32, 1: 52.

Krol A. J. (1973).
Clasp design for extension-base removable partial dentures. J. Prosthet. Dent., 29, 4: 408.

Lammie G. A. and Osborne J. (1964).
The bilateral free-end saddle lower denture. J. Prosthet. Dent., 4, 5: 640.

Lee J. B. (1955).
The advantages of an oblique path of insertion in tissue-borne nonmetallic partial dentures. Brit. Dent. J., 99: 191.

Lekholm U. (1983).
Clinical procedures for treatment with osseointegrated dental implants. J. Prosthet. Dent., 50: 1, 116.

Lubespere A. and Rotenberg A. (1976).
Attachments et Prothese Combinees Ed. Julien Prelat., Paris.

Matsumoto M. (1963).
Morphological changes in the human mandible following the loss of molars and premolars. IV. (In Japanese) JJPS.,7: 183.

Matsumoto M. (1970).
An experimental investigation of analysing the influence of impression procedures in clinical techniques Bull. Tokyo Med. Dent. Univ., 17: 4.

Maxfield J. B., Nicholls J. I. and Smith D. E. (1979).
The measurement of forces transmitted to abutment teeth of removable partial dentures. J. Prosthet. Dent., 41, 2: 134.

McArthur D. R. and Turvey T. A. (1979).
Maxillary segmental osteotomies for mandibular removable partial denture patients. J. Prosthet. Dent., 42, 4: 381.

Mensor M. C. (1972).
Personal communication.

Muhlemann H. R. (1960).
Ten years of tooth mobility measurement. J. Periodont., 31: 110.

Nairn R. I. (1966).
The problem of free-end denture bases. J. Prosthet. Dent., 16, 3: 522.

Nally N. N. (1963).
Methods of handling abutment teeth in Class I partial dentures. J. Prosthet. Dent., 30, 4: 561.

Neill D. J. (1958).
The problem of the lower free-end removable partial denture. J. Prosthet. Dent., 8, 4: 623.

Neill D. J. and Walter J. D. (1983).
Partial Denture Prosthetics. 2nd Edn. Blackwell Scientific, London.

Neufeld J. O. (1958).
Changes in the trabecular pattern of mandible following the loss of teeth. J. Prosthet. Dent., 8, 4: 685.

Nyman S. and Lindhe J. (1976).
Case Report. Prosthetic rehabilitation of patients with advanced periodontal disease. J. Clin. Periodont., 3, 81: 135.

Nyman S. and Lindhe J. (1976).
Case Report. Prosthetic rehabilitation of patients with advanced periodontal disease. J. Clin. Periodont., 3, 81: 135.

Nyman S. and Lindhe J. (1979).
A longitudinal study of combined periodontal and prosthetic treatment of patients with advanced periodontal disease. J. Periodontol., 50, 4: 163.

Picton D. C. A. and Wills J. (1978).
Visco-elastic properties of the periodontal ligament and mucous membrane. J. Prosthet. Dent., 40, 3: 263.

Preiskel H. W. (1971).
Impression techniques for attachment-retained distal extension removable partial dentures. J. Prosthet. Dent., 25, 6: 620.

Rantanen T., Makila E. and Yhi-Urpo A. (1972).
Investigations of the therapeutic success with dentures retained by precision attachments. II: Partial Dentures. Suom. hammaslaak. toim., 68: 73.

Rehm H., Korber E. and Korber K. H. (1962).
Biophysikalischer Beitrag zur Problematik starr abgestutzte Freiendprothesen. Dtsch. Zahnarztl., 17: 963.

Schuyler C. H. (1953).
An analysis of the use and relative value of precision attachment and the clasp in partial denture planning. J. Proothet. Dent., 3, 5: 711.

Schwalm C. A., Smith D. E. and Erickson J. D. (1977).
A clinical study of patients 1 to 2 years after placement of removable partial dentures. J. Prosthet. Dent., 38, 4: 380.

Schweitzer J. M., Schweitzer R. D. and Schweitzer J. (1968).
Free-end pontics used on fixed partial dentures. J. Prosthet. Dent., 20, 2: 120.

Sieweke J. C., Eames W. B. and Wallace F. W. (1977).
Elastomeric impression materials: effects of bulk of accuracy J. Dent. Res., 56: (Special Issue B), 147.

Steffel V. L. (1963).
Clasp partial dentures. J. Amer. Dent. Ass., 66: 803.

Steiger A. and Boitel R. (1959).
Precision Work for Partial Dentures. Stebo, Zurich.

Stern W. J. (1975).
Guiding planes in clasp reciprocation and retention. J. Prosthet. Dent., 34, 4: 408.

Thompson J. R. (1946).
The rest position of the mandible and its significance to dental science. J. A. D. A., 33: 3, 151-180.

Thompson W. D., Kratochvil F. S. and Caputo A. A. (1977).
Evaluation of photo-elastic stress patterns produced by bilateral distal-extension removable partial dentures. J. Prosthet. Dent., 38, 3: 261.

Warren A. B. and Caputo A. A. (1975).
Load transfer to alveolar bone as influenced by abutment designs for tooth supported dentures. J. Prosthet. Dent., 33, 2: 137.

Waters N. E. (1975).
Aspects of dental biomechanics. In Scientific Aspect of Dental Materials (Von Fraunhauf J. A. ed.) Butterworths, London.

Waters N. E. (1975).
Denture foundation. A consideration of certain aspects of the displacement of, and the pressure distribution within, the mucoperiosteum J. Dent., 3, 2: 83.

Weaver S. M. (1938).
Precision attachments and their advantages in respect to underlying tissues. J. Amer. Dent. Soc., 25: 1250.

Wills D. J. and Manderson R. D. (1977).
Biomechanical aspects of the support of partial dentures J. Dent., 5, 4: 310.

Wong R., Nicholls J. I. and Smith D. E. (1982).
Evaluation of prefabricated lingual rest seats for removable partial dentures. J. Prosthet. Dent., 48, 5: 521.

Zach G. A. (1975).
Advantages of mesial rests for removable partial dentures. J. Prosthet. Dent., 33, 1: 32.

Zarb G. A., Bergman B., Clayton J. A. and Mackay H. F. (1978).
Prosthodontic treatment for partially edentulous patients. C. V. Mosby Co., St. Louis, Mo.

Zoeller G. N. and Kelly W. J. (1971).
Block form stability in removable partial prosthodontics. J. Prosthet. Dent., 26, 2: 141.

Prefabricated Attachments

Prefabricated attachments usually consist of two matched precious metal components. Since the functions served by an attachment vary with the manner in which it is used, the classification employed in this book is based upon attachment shape. The purposes for which attachments can be used are discussed in Chapters 6 and 7.

Intracoronal attachments

The two parts of an intracoronal attachment consist of a flange and a slot. The flange is joined to one section of the prosthesis and the slot unit embedded in a restoration forming part of another section of the prosthesis. These attachments usually

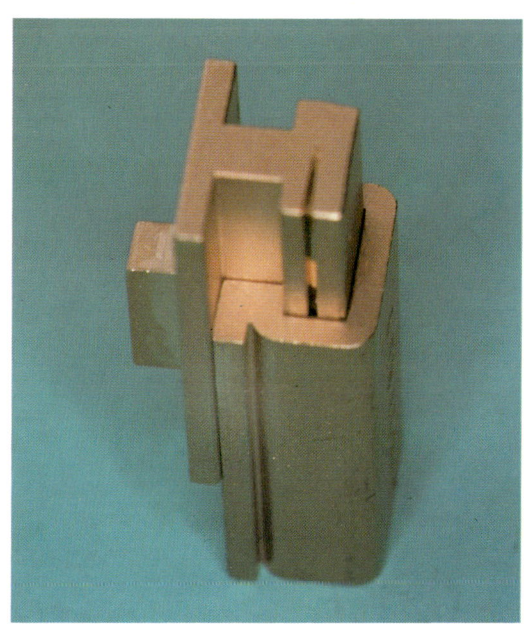

Fig. 125 The McCollum intracoronal unit. A well-tried example of a unit with entirely frictional retention.

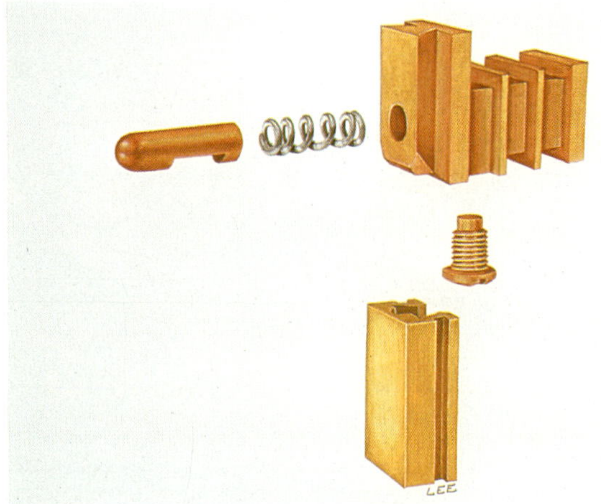

Fig. 126   The Schatzmann unit. Additional retention is provid-ed by a spring-loaded plunger.

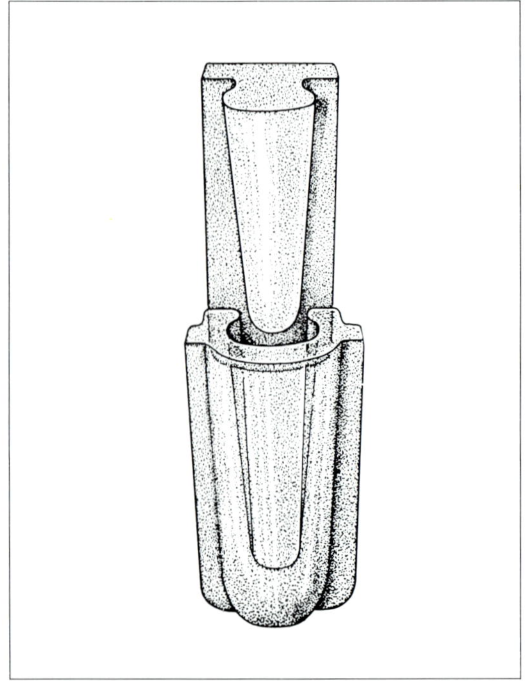

Fig. 127   Pattern for a semi-precision (tapered) intracoro-nal attachment.

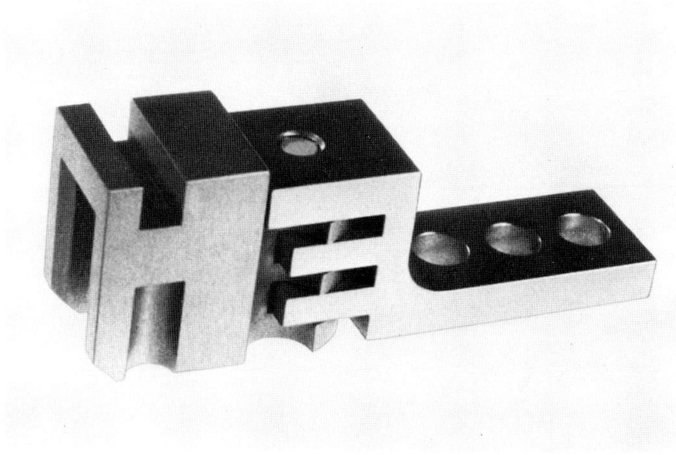

Fig. 128 Removable section of the Conex attachment. Note the parallel walls that provide a precise path of insertion.

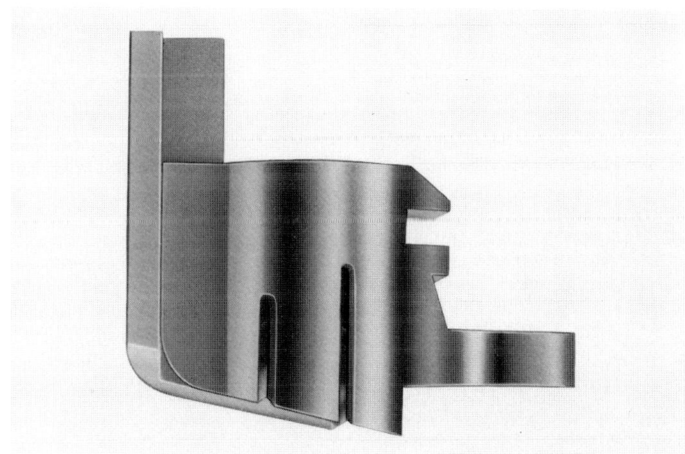

Fig. 129 The Dalbo extracoronal projection unit.

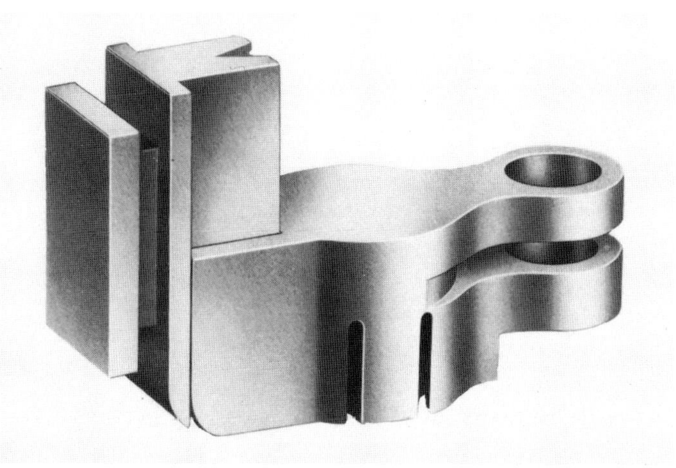

Fig. 130 Miniaturised version of the Dalbo extracoronal projection unit.

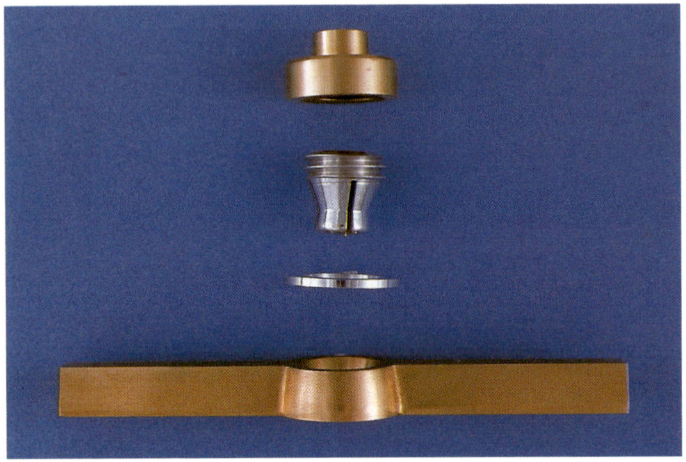

Fig. 131   The Ceka extracoronal attachment.

provide a rigid connection between the two sections of the prosthesis. Two types of intracoronal attachments are available:

1. Those whose retention is entirely frictional (Fig. 125).
2. Those whose retention is augmented by a mechanical lock (Fig. 126).

Semi-precision intracoronal attachments feature significant taper (Fig. 127). They may be cast from patterns or entirely laboratory produced. Unlike precision attachments, an additional retentive element is essential.

Extracoronal attachments

These attachments have part or all of their mechanism outside the crown of a tooth. Many of these units allow a certain amount of movement between the two sections of the prosthesis. Extracoronal attachments can be subdivided into the following groups:

1. Projection Units

The units are attached to the proximal surface of a crown. These groups can be divided in turn into:

a) Those that provide a rigid connection (Fig. 128).
b) Those that allow play between the components (Figs. 129 to 131).

2. Connectors

These units connect two sections of a removable prosthesis and allow a certain degree of play (Fig. 132).

3. Combined units

The attachments feature an extracoronally placed hinge-type unit connected to an intracoronal attachment.

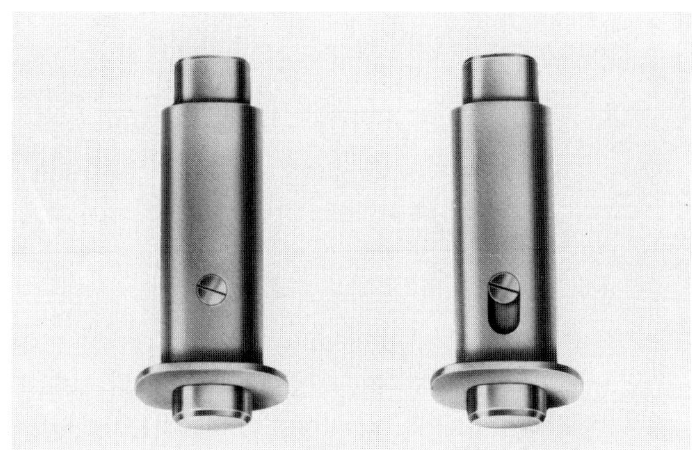

Fig. 132 Left: Rotation joint providing predetermined hinge movement. Right: Axial rotation joint providing restricted vertical travel together with predetermined hinge movement.

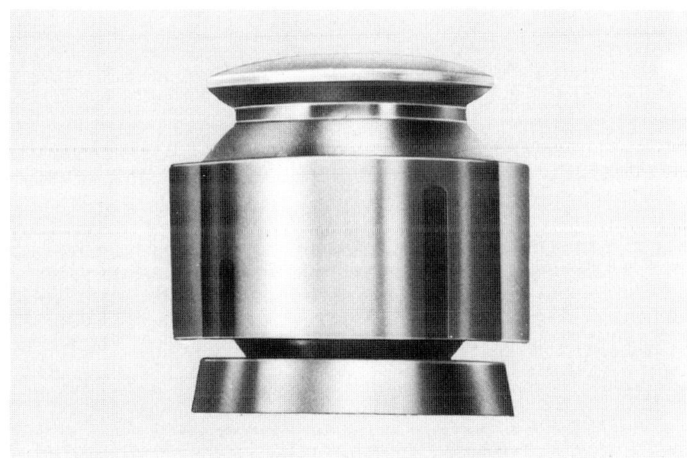

Fig. 133 The Dalbo stud unit. A small yet sturdy attachment particularly useful for joining a complete overdenture to root diaphragms.

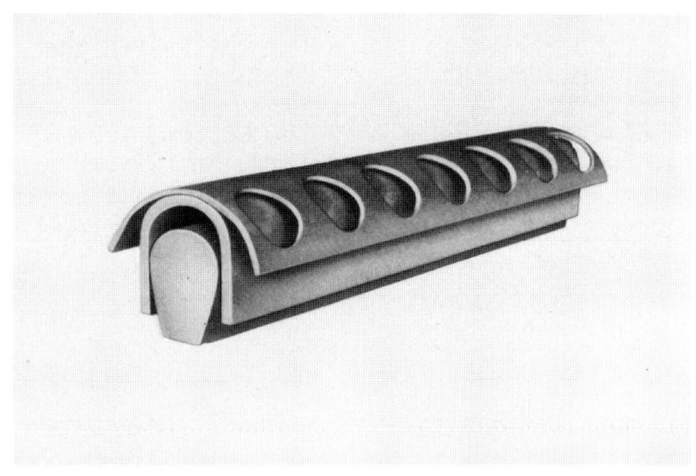

Fig. 134 The Dolder Bar Joint. A well-tested example of a single sleeve joint allowing vertical and rotational movements.

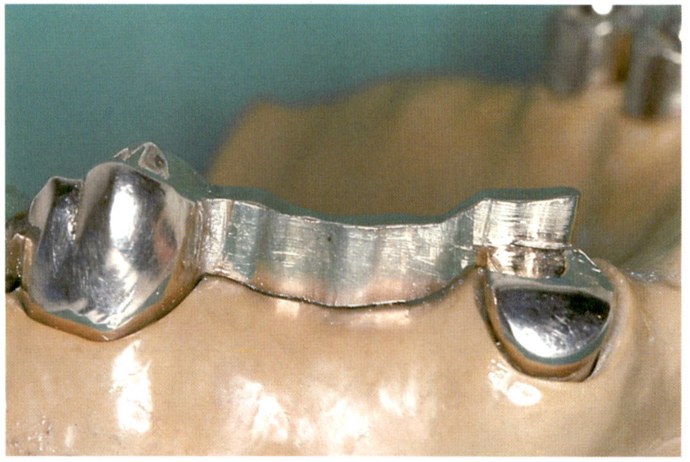

Fig. 135   A laboratory-produced example of a bar unit.

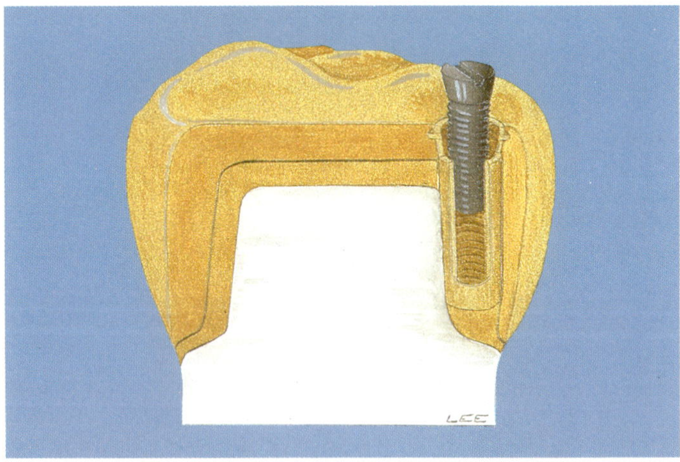

Fig. 136   By incorporating a precious metal threaded sleeve within the inner coping, the outer section can be retained with a screw.

Stud attachments

These attachments (Fig. 133) are so called because of the shape of the male units that are usually soldered to the diaphragm of a post crown. Some of these units provide a comparatively rigid connection; others allow movement between the two sections.

Bar attachments

Bar attachments consist of a bar spanning an edentulous area joining teeth or roots. The denture fits over the bar and is connected to it with one or more sleeves. Bar attachments fall into two categories:

1. Bar joints

These units (Fig. 134) allow play between the denture and the bar.

Fig. 137 (a) (b) Plunger unit employed to increase retention between the fixed and removable sections of a telescopic prosthesis.

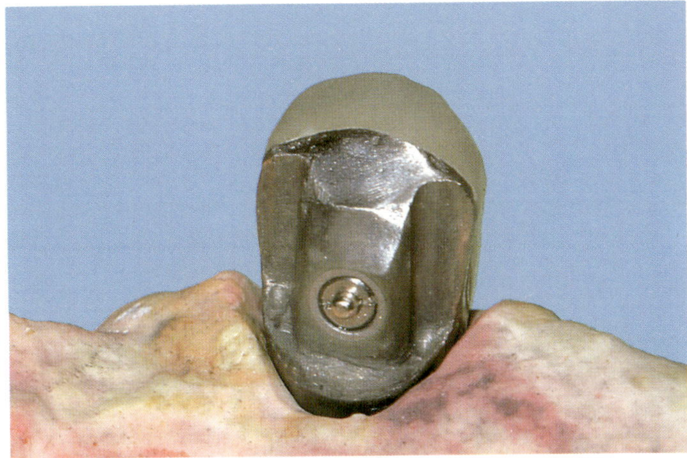

Figure 137 a

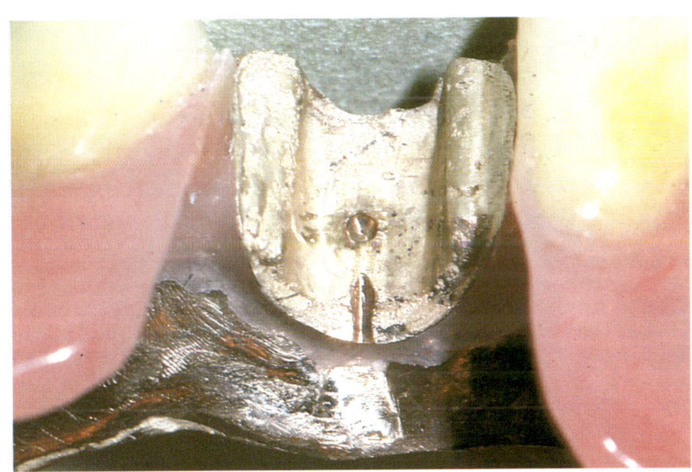

Figure 137 b

2. Bar units

With these attachments (Fig. 135) the sleeve/bar junction is rigid. Single or multiple sleeves may be used with either category.

1. Screw units

These devices (Fig. 136) are useful for securing and dismantling parts of a prosthesis in the mouth, when there is no common line of insertion of the whole. They are particularly useful for joining the two components of a telescopic crown.

Auxiliary Attachments

This miscellaneous group consists basically of:

2. Friction devices

Spring-loaded plungers are commonly employed to increase retention between

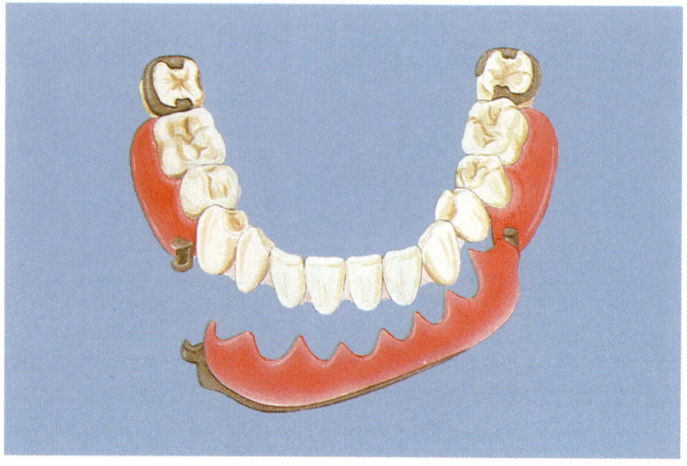

Fig. 138   A 'Swing-lock' prosthesis. The hinged labial flange allows proximal spaces to be used for retention.

the two sections of a telescopic prosthesis (Fig. 137 a, b).
Split posts can be used in conjunction with sectional dentures.

3. Bolts

Bolt units are used to connect the two parts of a sectional denture in the mouth. Each part of the denture is inserted separately and the patient locks them together with the bolt.

4. Hinged Flanges

This type of device (Fig. 138) allows mucosal undercuts and interdental spaces to be used for retentive purposes.
This volume covers the applications of intracoronal and extracoronal attachments. Stud attachments, bar attachments and auxiliary attachments are considered in Volume 2: Overdentures and Telescopic Prostheses.
Although components of prefabricated attachments are carefully matched, they are not all produced in identical metals. For example, sections of attachments to be joined to the fixed section of the prosthesis are available in platinised golds, compatible with abutments of similar alloys; the removable section of the attachment is likely to be made of a yellow gold. Apart from the vital difference in melting ranges, minor design differences are often to be found between components for use with yellow golds and those to be employed with bonded porcelain to gold techniques. Continued research with non-precious alloys holds promise of reduced component size in the future.

Chapter 6

Intracoronal Attachments

Intracoronal attachments consist of two parts: a slot and a flange. The flange is joined to one section of the prosthesis and the slot unit, embedded in a restoration, forms part of another section. In this way the two units can be joined in the mouth, the connection taking place within the contour of a tooth crown. Precision attachments have parallel-sided flanges; the flanges of semi-precision units are slightly tapered.

Towards the end of the last century, *Carr, Peeso, Parr, Alexander* and *Morgan* had all designed and used simple intracoronal attachments (Fig. 139).

Griswald had designed not only his own attachment, but also an ingenious paralleling device for alignment. In 1906, *Herman Chayes* designed the attachment which, with modification, is still in production today and carries his name (Fig. 140). His original idea was to position the attachment lingually, but subsequently a mesiodistal position was suggested.

Intracoronal attachments serve retentive and supportive functions, as do clasp units. The retention provided by the attachment mainly depends on the surface area of contact between the two parts. The bracing action is provided by the laterally facing surfaces of the attachment when used conventionally. In view of the excellent

Fig. 139 An attachment system designed by Alexander at the end of the 19th century. The male sections were joined to the crowns, the attachments were tapered and used with a buccolingual path of insertion for the prosthesis.

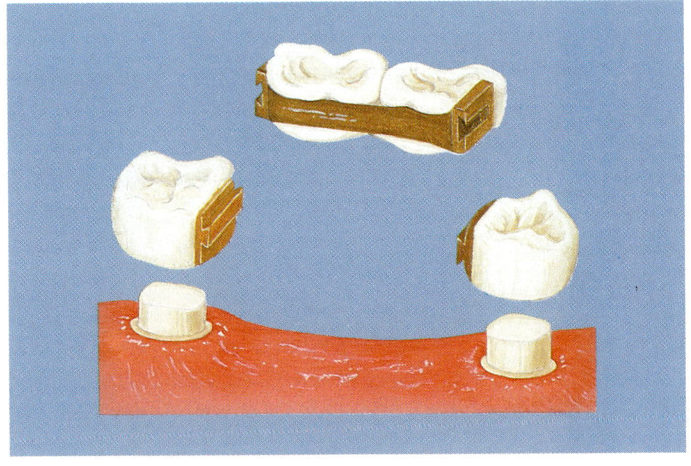

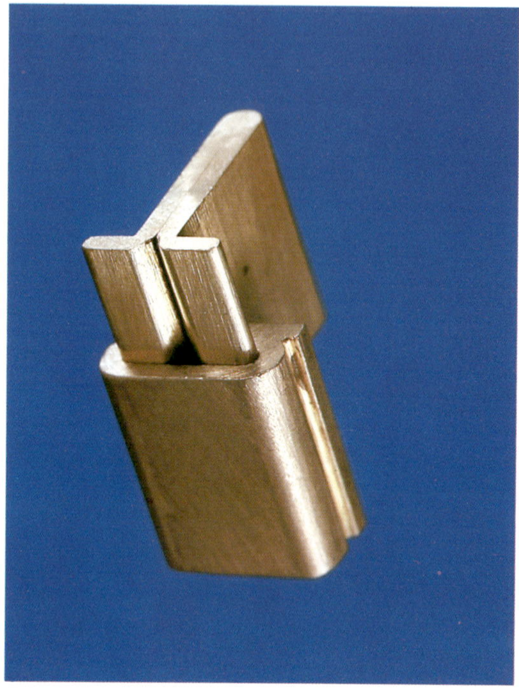

Fig. 140   The Chayes attachment, described in 1906. This T-shaped unit is still in production today.

retention and stability provided by intracoronal attachments, they have applications in both fixed and removable partial prostheses.

Since the retention provided by the attachment depends largely on contact between the two components, it is desirable to provide as much surface area as possible. The surface area available is a product of the cross-section of the male part and its length. The length of the attachment is governed by the height of the clinical crown of the tooth and is a most important factor in attachment retention and stability. The attachment cross-section is limited because it is necessary to recess the female part within the circumference of the tooth.

Failure to recess the female part of the attachment alters the tooth contour and leaves a permanent projection at the gingival margin of the restoration. The length of the attachment is then limited both by the gingival tissues and by the fact that it may intrude on the area where the tip of the opposing cusp occludes (Fig. 141).

Cross-sections of several attachment types are illustrated (Fig. 142) and it can be seen that the H-shaped flange of the modern attachment has great advantages over earlier T-shaped flanges. The external flange of the H-shaped unit virtually doubles the surface area and strengthens the attachment, without increasing the size of the female part. With some attachments, an external flange can be cast onto the

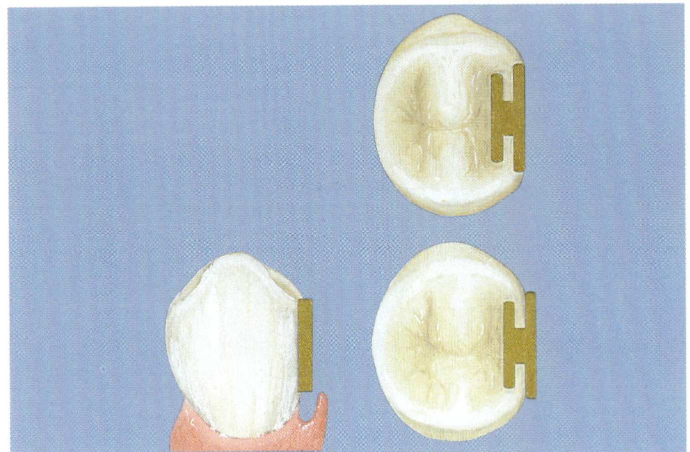

Fig. 141 The female part of the attachment should be recessed within the contour of the abutment crown (above). If this is not done, the contour of the tooth is completely altered and a permanent projection is left at the gingival margin.

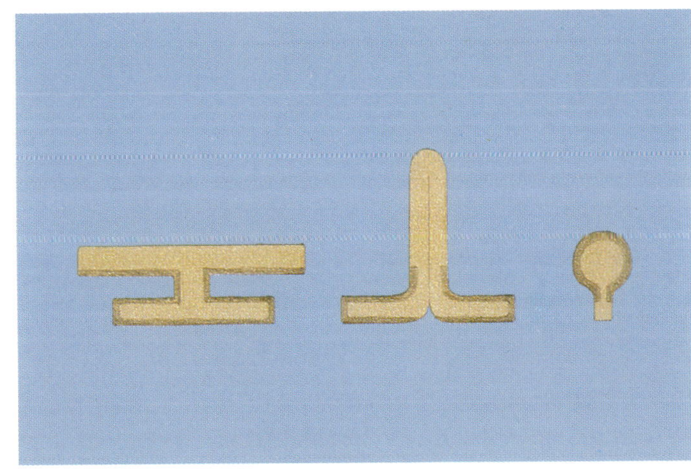

Fig. 142 Cross-sections of several types of attachment. The H-shaped flanges of the modern attachments are stronger and have nearly double the contact surface area of the earlier T-shaped flanges. Attachments with a circular cross-section are suitable only for joining two sections of a fixed prosthesis.

removable section. However, one cannot quite expect the accuracy of adaptation to match that of a precision engineered flange integral to the attachment.

Friction fit intracoronal attachments with adjustment potential

Constant insertion and removal of the prosthesis will cause the attachments to wear, so that some form of adjustment is desirable. While comparatively simple attachments, such as the Chayes unit, can be adjusted by opening the two halves with a razor blade or scalpel, the more complicated units require careful handling and strict adherence to the manufacturer's instructions. At one time, the male sections of some of the attachments were manufactured in two halves which were then soldered together. The soldered junction was comparatively weak and adjustment of the

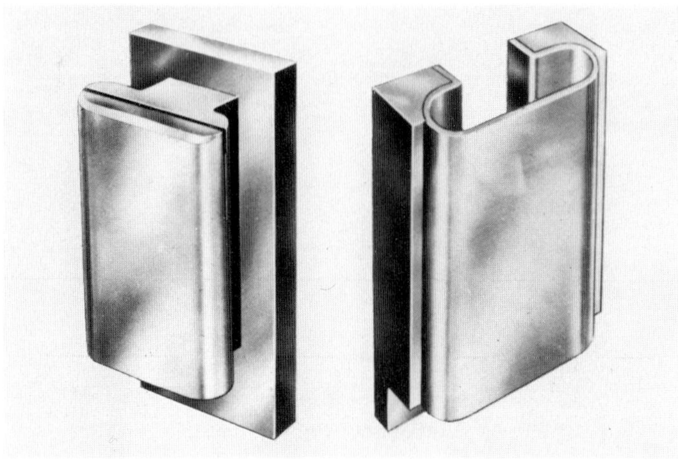

Fig. 143 The male and female parts of the Stern G/A attachment. These robust well-tried units are available in several sizes.

male part could lead to fracture. Numerous prefabricated attachments are produced by manufacturers in Europe and the USA. The choice of attachment is usually governed by its shape and size rather than any mechanical attribute claimed for it. Several examples of modern, well-tried attachments are illustrated (Fig. 142). The Stern G/A Unit (Fig. 143) is produced in the USA, the others in Europe.

The Crismani series of intracoronal attachments are available in two basic configurations. The narrower version (2.8 mm) features an adjustable central groove (Fig. 144). Refined over the years, this attachment now incorporates a chamfer and tapered gingival male section to facilitate insertion (Fig. 145). The unit is 7 mm tall, but can be shortened by up to 2 mm.

The McCollum attachment has now been redesigned for additional strength (Fig. 146 a, b, c). The adjustment split runs part way through the attachment from one side. Imagine a lower distal extension restora-

tion viewed from above. Since the splits should face laterally, it is necessary to produce left and right-sided attachments. The manufacturers have selected the lower restoration for their terminology. Rather confusing is the fact that when an upper denture is constructed, a left-sided attachment should be placed on the right side and vice versa if the slots are to face laterally.

The McCollum units are now among the most robust of those made. As with most intracoronal attachments, the units are available in metals compatible with bonded porcelain to gold techniques, as well as with conventional yellow golds. A combination is also produced in which the female element is to be employed with porcelain to gold, while the male is to be incorporated with yellow gold alloys.

The Ancra is a well-established intracoronal attachment. This unit features an 'H' shaped profile with external frictional flange, while the male unit incorporates

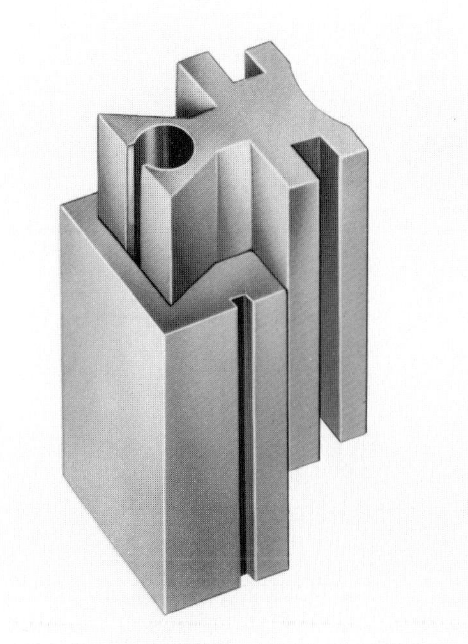

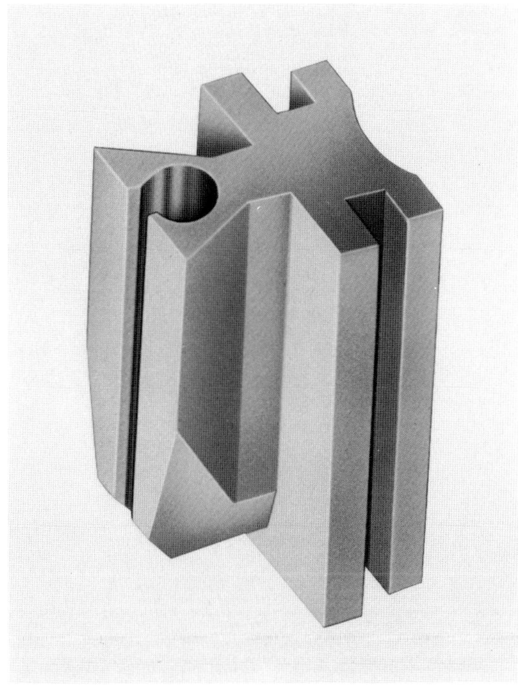

Figure 144

Figure 145

Fig. 144   The narrower of the two Crismani units features a central groove for adjustment.

Fig. 145   The male section of the Crismani unit. Note the chamfer and taper of the gingival section of the unit to facilitate insertion.

Figure 146 a to c

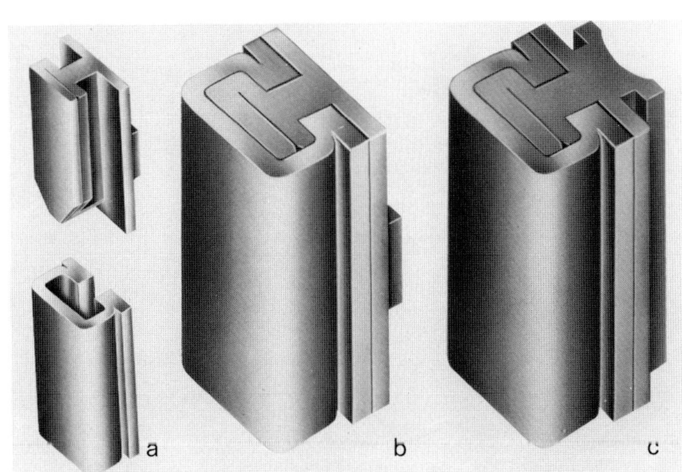

Fig. 146 (a)   The redesigned McCollum attachment. (b) The McCollum for use with conventional yellow golds. (c) The McCollum for use with bonded gold to porcelain techniques.

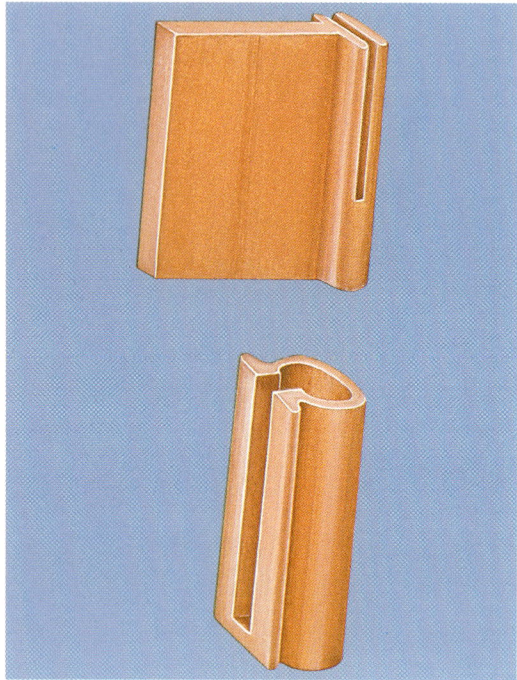

Fig. 147   The T-Geschiebe 123 intracoronal attachment.

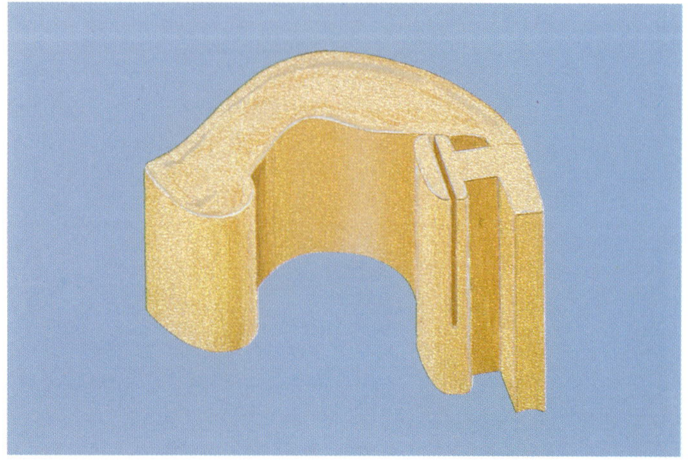

Fig. 148   Cast bracing arm and external frictional flange.

slots either side to allow for modification of retention. Two sizes of attachment are available and the female unit may be obtained in either high heat or conventional yellow gold alloys.

The T-Geschiebe 123 (Fig. 147) represents another approach to the problem. When used to retain removable prostheses, an external frictional flange is cast, together with a bracing arm (Fig. 148).

A new entrant to the field may herald a different approach to the concept of intracoronal attachments. The Biloc, by Cendres and Metaux, has a plastic pattern with the female element, that is burnt out with the wax model the abutment crown. The dimensions of the pattern are compatible with precious or non-precious alloys, but will be of particular interest to those using non-precious alloys.

The male element is prefabricated of a platinised gold alloy. The basic 'H' shape is modifed with the internal flange resembling two lobes with a small groove between them. The lateral facing surfaces and total areas of contact are far greater than those offered by a conventional intracoronal attachment and this may compensate for the reduced precision of fit between the two components. A bracing arm is recommended for this unit.

Two ingenious adjustment tools are produced to ensure continued useful service of the attachment. Minor adjustments should be particularly effective due to the curvature of the contacting areas.

Auxiliary retentive features

Since the shape and size of the tooth governs both the cross-section and length of an intracoronal attachment, there exists a definite limit to the retention available.

Auxiliary retentive features are incorporated in some attachments in an effort to provide more retention for a given contact area, although no extra stability is provided. A minimum of 4 mm vertical space is still usually necessary.

The wider Crismani units incorporate a wire clip to increase retention. Access to the clip is obtained by removing the screw in the male unit. Failure to tighten the screw correctly will prevent the male unit sliding into place. The female unit contains two depressions for the retaining wire and is 7.0 mm tall. No significant shortening should be carried out.

Other devices include a spring-loaded plunger within the male part, engaging a depression in the female element—rather like a simple cupboard door catch. The Schatzmann series (Figs. 149 a to f) are good examples of this type of unit. These attachments are robust and retentive, their applications being limited by their bulk.

The largest of the Schatzman series features a dismantling screw around the plunger (Fig. 149 a). As with any springloaded plunger system, access must be provided to allow the spring to be replaced. The male unit is manufactured in two configurations, one for soldering to the major connector, the other for burying in the acrylic resin of the denture base. Under normal circumstances it is preferable to solder an intracoronal attachment to the major connector. The female elements of the Schatzmann series include a retraction groove to engage the plunger within the male component (Fig. 149 b). The female elements are made of an alloy compatible with yellow golds, or another for use with bonded gold to porcelain techniques.

The smaller Schatzmann unit is about

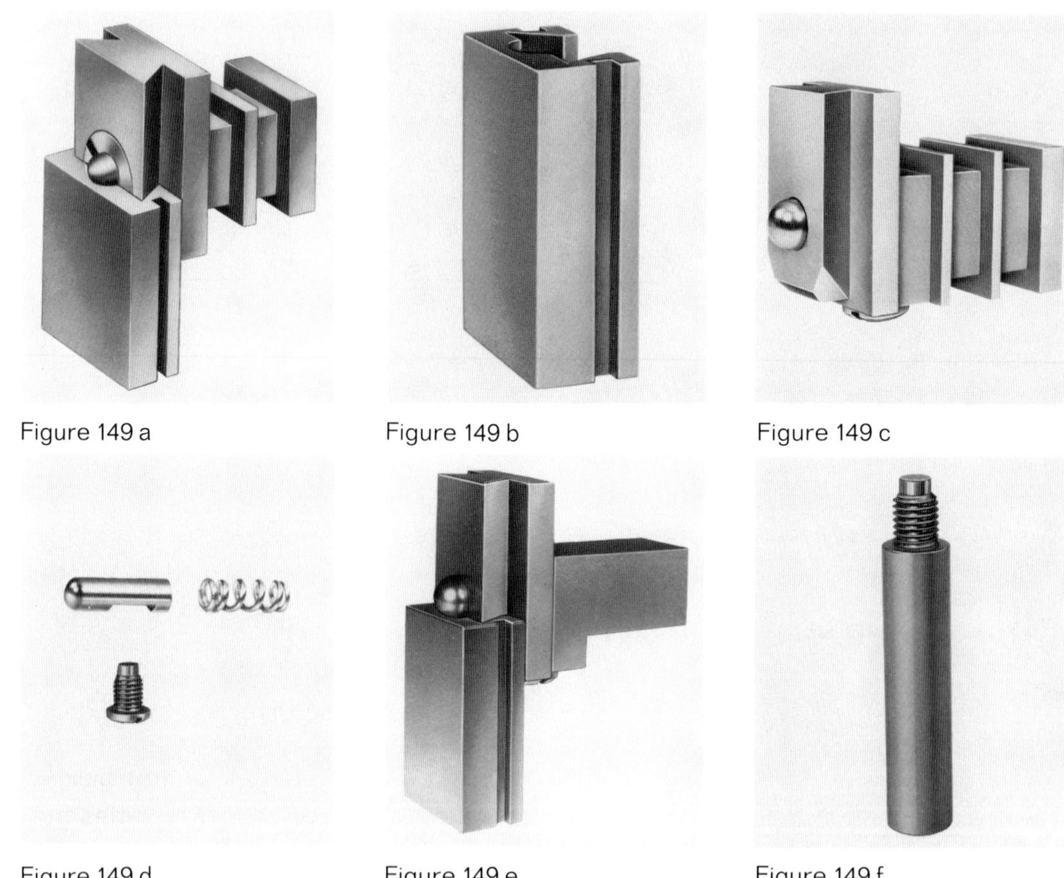

Figure 149 a

Figure 149 b

Figure 149 c

Figure 149 d

Figure 149 e

Figure 149 f

Fig. 149 (a)   The largest of the Schatzmann series features a dismantling screw around the springloaded plunger. This male unit is designed for burying within the acrylic resin of the denture base. (b) The Schatzmann female units are available in a choice of alloys for conventional yellow golds or bonded gold to porcelain techniques. Note the groove to retract the plunger on the male unit. (c) The smaller Schatzmann attachment. The width of the unit has been reduced by placing the dismantling screw under the attachment base. (d) The modified plunger of the smaller Schatzmann unit is held in place by the screw inserted through the base of the attachment. (e) The smaller Schatzmann attachment designed for soldering to the major connector. This arrangement is normally preferred. (f) Processing screw to prevent movement of this attachment during processing procedures.

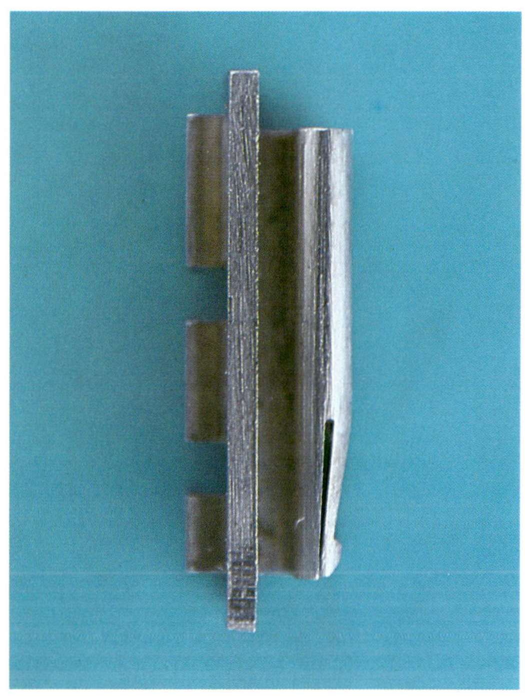

Fig. 150   The Stern gingival latch attachment.
The retention is adjusted by opening out the
base of the male unit with a special instrument.

0.7 mm narrower, a reduction in width achieved by modifying the plunger to allow it to be secured by a screw under the base of the attachment (Figs. 149 c to f). The design and construction of the partial denture must allow access to this vital screw component.

The Stern gingival latch attachment (Fig. 150) offers a novel method of additional retention. The base of the male unit is split and formed in the shape of a door latch. The result is to provide a lock as the male slide is engaged. Adjustments for retention are made with a purpose-built tool (Fig. 151).

Two sizes of unit are produced, standard and miniature. One of the factors limiting the extent to which the male unit can be shorted is the height of the split. On the standard unit the split is 2.5 mm high, on the miniature unit only 1.5 mm high. The manufacturers claim this allows the standard unit to be shortened to 3.6 mm and the miniature unit to 2.62 mm. From the point of view of the retention mechanism, this is obviously possible. However, the resistance to rotational forces is borne by the lateral surfaces of the attachments. Operators are therefore cautioned to think twice before reducing any intracoronal attachment below 4 mm if unacceptable movement is to be avoided at a later date.

Other modifications of the G/L system

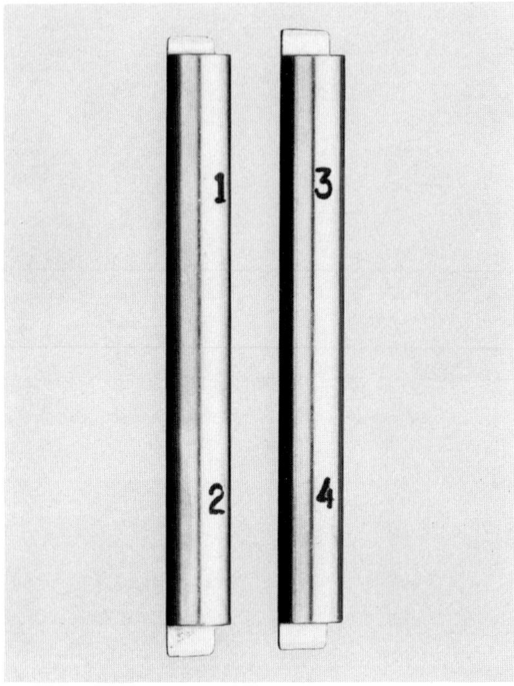

Fig. 151   The adjusting instrument for the Stern G/L attachment. The free ends are of varying thickness, and the male unit is adjusted by inserting the adjusting instruments in sequence until the retention desired is achieved.

include a unit with squared lateral surfaces, thereby allowing the buccolingual dimensions to be reduced. This unit, known as the Micro, is among the smallest of intracoronal attachments with auxiliary retention.

The 'dovetail' and ES1 versions are modifications of the tagging of the male unit. The dovetail design simplifies soldering and is useful when the attachment is used in a 'split-pontic' mode. The ES1 features a long extension plate that simplifies electro-soldering the male to the denture framework. Alternatively, the extension can be roughened to permit retention by the acrylic resin. Yet another innovation by Stern is represented by the Jacket Maintenance System. The male section of the attachment is covered by a nylon jacket and it is claimed that this virtually eliminates wear of either metal component. The jackets can be changed in a matter of moments and are available in three colours: yellow, red and black. The yellow jacket provides frictional retention only, the red jacket adds a light latch action, while the black jacket features a strong latch action. Operators and technicians are warned never to attempt to shorten the jacket by cutting it with a scalpel—discing is recommended. The manufacturers show their confidence in this new system by guaranteeing the male section against wear or breakage for the life of the patient.

Before choosing an attachment with auxiliary retentive devices, the following factors should be considered:

1. Bulk.
2. Adjustment.
3. Retention mechanism.
4. Trimming the attachment.
5. Plaque control.

Bulk

Any retentive device requiring a larger female element is defeating its own purpose. The purpose of the device is to increase the retention available from a given box size. If a larger box is necessary, a larger attachment would give better results; it would not only give more retention because of the greater contact area, but it would also be stronger and provide greater stability to horizontal and rotational loads. The best retention devices are the simple ones, and generally their female elements are practically identical with a simple intracoronal attachment, except for a small recess. It should be remembered that these devices usually increase the retention, but seldom the bracing action, of the attachment.

The plunger or spring mechanism has to be incorporated within the male element. In a well-designed attachment the retention mechanism should not affect the cross-sectional size of the part engaging the female element.

Adjustment

The adjustment of any retentive device must be straightforward. Many retention devices are spring-activated and, since it will be necessary to replace the springs at 6-monthly or yearly intervals, easy access to the spring should be provided.

Retention mechanism

Most attachment breakages occur while they are being adjusted. Incorrect heat treatment during construction of the prosthesis may play a part, as may incorrect adjustment by the dental surgeon. However, it is also important to select a sturdy attachment and reduce even further the chances of accidental breakages. Any springs incorporated in the mechanism should be protected from impaction of food.

Trimming the attachment

It is sometimes necessary to shorten an attachment to accommodate it within a tooth. The retention device should work at least halfway down the attachment. If it engages near the occlusal surface it will be damaged as soon as the attachment is shortened.

Plaque control

The retentive mechanism should be straightforward to clean without nooks and crannies to complicate plaque removal.

Friction fit intracoronal attachments without adjustment potential

Lack of adjustment potential renders this type of unit unsuitable for removable prostheses, as repeated insertion and removal will cause the attachment to wear. They are, however, useful for joining a series of crowns without a common path of insertion. Round profiles are useful where anterior teeth are concerned (Fig. 152),

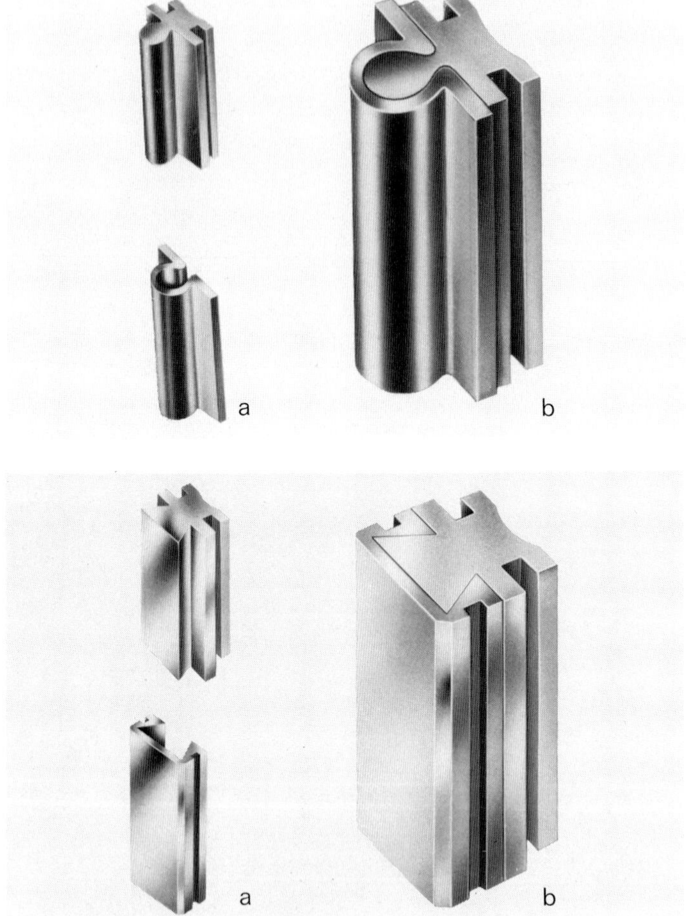

Fig. 152 Two useful attachments for connecting anterior crowns.

Fig. 153 (a) The Beyeler Attachment for use in posterior quadrants. (b) The Beyeler Attachment assembled.

whereas the Beyeler attachment offers more contact surface area in the posterior quadrants (Fig. 153 a, b). Note that both units feature an external frictional flange.

Applications of intracoronal attachments

Intracoronal attachments are among the most commonly used of all prefabricated attachments. A minimum of 4 mm vertical space is normally required, and preferably 5 mm. Furthermore, almost as much buccolingual space is needed, while pulpal and anatomical considerations must allow the female section to be accommodated within the crown contour. Careful analysis of diagnostic casts is indicated, as mistakes with space requirements can be extremely expensive to correct at later stages. The small tolerances of the attachments dictate

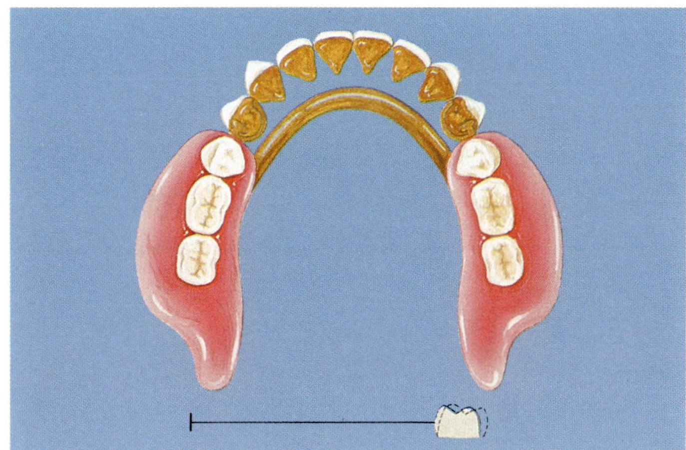

Fig. 154   A bilateral prosthesis is able to resist horizontal loads between the teeth and mucosa of both sides, while rotational loads applied to one side are resisted by the retainers of the opposite side acting with the mechanical advantage of the width of the arch.

precise clinical techniques and technical skill. Frequently overlooked is that they also require a degree of manual dexterity on the part of the patient. Intracoronal attachments are easily damaged by clumsy or careless patients. With these provisos, their many valuable applications can be considered under two headings: retainers and connectors.

Retainers

Intracoronal attachments are effective and almost invisible retainers for bilateral and unilateral prostheses.

Connectors

Sections of a fixed prosthesis may be joined with intracoronal attachments. This possibility can be useful where:

1. Prostheses do not share a common path of insertion yet can be connected rigidly in the mouth.
2. The operator prefers to limit the length of individual castings while making a large span fixed prosthesis.
3. The prognosis of a distal abutment is dubious. Connecting the posterior segment with an attachment allows its subsequent removal without damage to the main restoration. The attachment slot can be used for later construction of an attachment-retained denture.

Removable partial dentures for bounded spaces

Intracoronal attachments may be used to retain unilateral and bilateral dentures. For the purposes of description, the two types of restoration, the bilateral and unilateral denture, will be discussed separately.

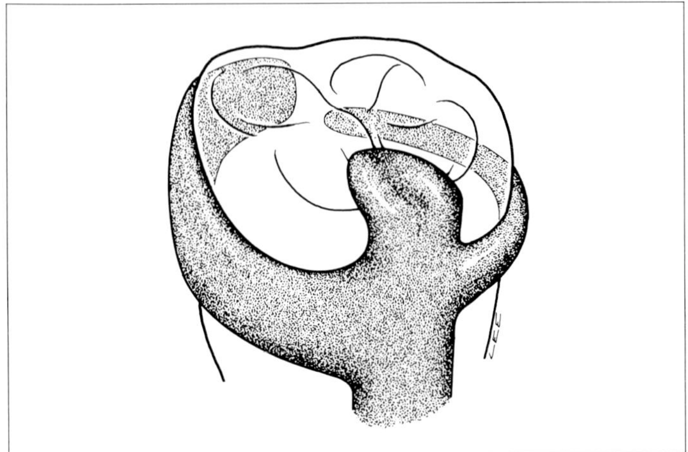

Fig. 155 An intracoronal attachment serves the function of a retaining arm, occlusal rest and bracing arm.

The bilateral denture

The major connector provides cross-arch support that contributes to the stability of the prosthesis. Horizontal displacing forces are resisted by the retainers of the opposite side, acting with a considerable mechanical advantage (Fig. 154).

When used for this type of prosthesis, an intracoronal attachment serves the functions of a clasp arm, occlusal rest and bracing arm (Fig. 155). The relative merits of the two types of retainer should therefore be considered. The intracoronal attachment has the following advantages over the clasp retainer:

1. Appearance.
2. Retention unaffected by crown contour.
3. Reduced bulk.
4. Stability.
5. Elimination of food stagnation.
6. Stresses on abutment teeth minimised.

Appearance

Since there is no need for buccal or labial clasp arms, the appearance is far better. This factor becomes particularly important in anterior parts of the mouth.

Retention unaffected by crown contour

The intracoronal attachment provides excellent retention, irrespective of the crown contour: a clasp arm can only provide retention if its free end is able to engage an area undercut to the path of insertion of the denture. The clinical crowns of canines and premolars in young patients may be virtually free of undercut, while aesthetic problems may preclude positioning a clasp arm to engage what little undercut may be present.

Reduced bulk

Since an intracoronal attachment fits within the contour of a tooth crown yet serves the functions of an occlusal rest, clasp arm

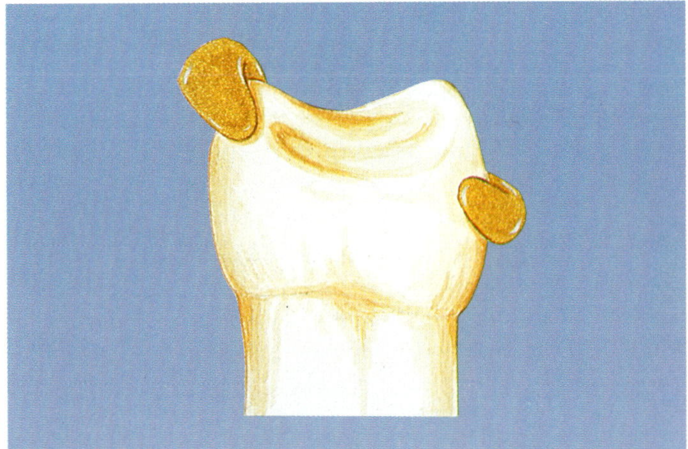

Fig. 156　When a clasp-retained partial denture is inserted, the clasps have to be deformed before they engage the undercut. If this occurs before the bracing arm engages the tooth, lateral tilting loads will be applied.

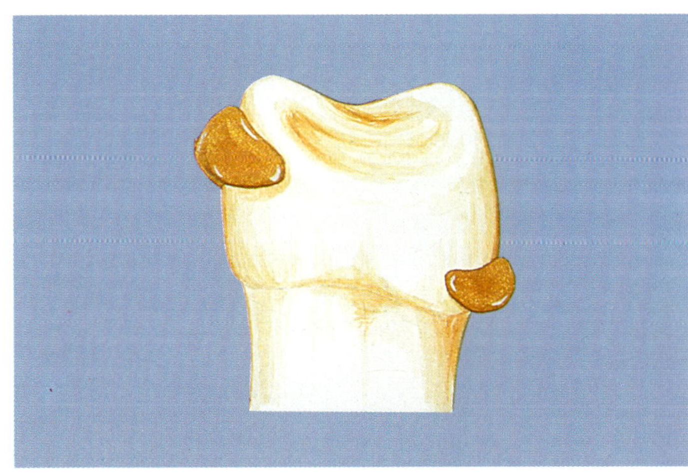

Fig. 157　In theory, tilting of the abutment teeth could be caused by a badly made clasp retainer, as the bracing arm is seldom at the same height as the clasp arm.

and bracing arm, there is a considerable reduction in the bulk of the prosthesis.

Stability

Intracoronal attachments provide good resistance to horizontally inclined or rotational displacing forces. This stability can be augmented by a palatal bracing arm constructed to fit within the contour of a tooth. In comparison, rigid bracing arms of a partial denture would be bulky.

Elimination of food stagnation

Complex designs of clasps, especially those used on posterior teeth, may lead to food stagnation, gingival irritation and caries. The elimination of this potential source of trouble is a major advantage.

Stresses on abutment teeth minimised

When a clasp-retained partial denture is inserted, the clasps have to be deformed until they engage the undercut (Fig. 156). During deformation they apply lateral loads to the clasped teeth, whereas an attachment should slide into place without this lateral stress. Provided the clasp has been correctly designed and constructed, the advantage possessed by an attachment in this respect is theoretical rather than real.

Some authorities feel that a clasp may cause rotation of the teeth, since it is not always possible to apply a 'reciprocal' at the same level as the clasp (Fig. 157). The term 'reciprocal' is misleading, since the clasp should be passive while at rest and should only become active when the denture is displaced. Convincing clinical evidence of this type of mishap has not been presented, but there is no possibility of it occurring if an intracoronal attachment has been used.

To summarise, intracoronal attachments can be used to provide a well-retained and stable partial denture with the minimum of bulk and with no clasp arms to mar appearance. However, the use of these attachments has some drawbacks, and these should be considered as well:

1. *Extensive preparation of abutment teeth required.* Intracoronal attachments require extensive preparation of all the abutment teeth and their neighbours. This is probably their greatest disadvantage. Most clasp-retained partial dentures require only reshaping of the occlusal surfaces or recontouring of proximal surfaces.

2. *Cost and time.* It takes considerable chairside time to carry out the procedures involved in making an appliance with intracoronal attachments, and even more laboratory time. This extra expenditure of time and materials must be reflected in the cost; the cost of the actual attachments themselves is comparatively small.

3. *Crown length and pulp size.* Intracoronal attachments require a minimum of 4 mm vertical space. Since they need to be recessed within the crown contour, extensive preparation of the abutment tooth is required. Where buccolingual room is restricted, or the pulps are large, there may be inadequate space available for the attachment. Occasionally, a cantilevered pontic can be employed, but the occlusal load and its distribution then requires considerable attention.

4. *Difficulty.* Constructing an attachment-retained denture requires no skills other than those employed in the fields of fixed and removable partial prostheses; however, it does show up small errors and requires careful planning of the treatment.

Intracoronal attachments are by no means substitutes for all conventional clasp units. If employed carefully they can provide a prosthesis combining many of the advantages of a fixed and of a removable prosthesis.

The unilateral denture

A unilateral denture can be made when the teeth on either side of the space can be made into sufficiently strong abutments. The problem then resolves itself into one of anchoring the prosthesis to the teeth.

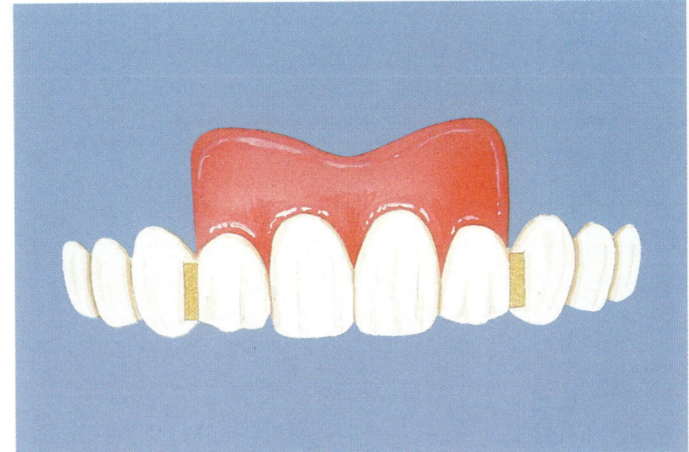

Fig. 158 Where bone loss needs to be replaced with artificial mucosa, intracoronal attachments allow the construction of a small, rigid, and well-retained prosthesis.

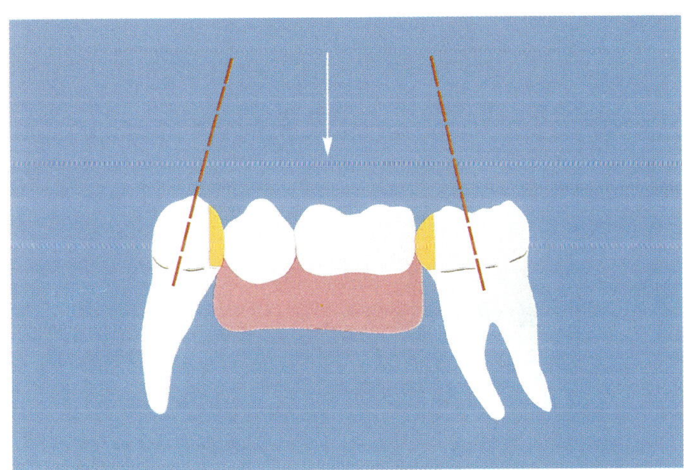

Fig. 159 An attachment-retained prosthesis consists of three basic units: a removable section and two groups of abutments either side.

The unilateral clasp-retained 'side-plate' partial denture requires undercut on both lingual and buccal aspects of the teeth. The retention and stability of this type of prosthesis frequently cannot resist the displacing forces to which it will be subjected, so that the hazard of the patient inhaling or swallowing the denture must be taken into account. If a clasp-retained denture is to be made, it usually requires support from more than one quadrant of the mouth; a major connector should therefore be incorporated.

The fixed prosthesis is usually the restoration of choice for restoring small gaps. However, where a flange is necessary for appearance or support, a removable prosthesis has much to offer. It is here that intracoronal attachments are useful, allowing the construction of a small, rigid and well-retained prosthesis removable by the patient (Fig. 158).

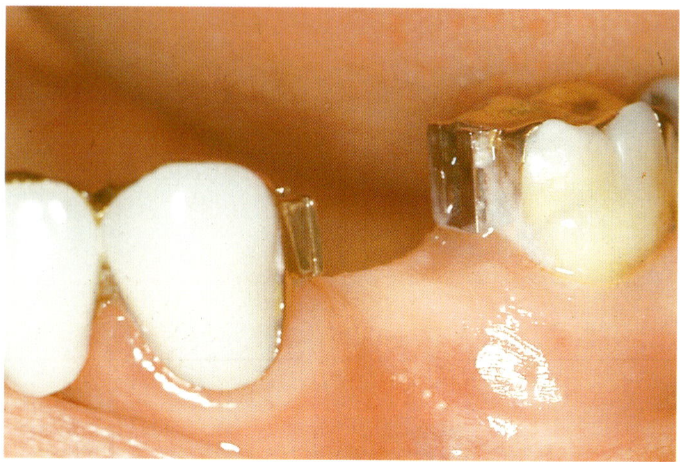

Fig. 160 An example of poor treatment planning. The prosthesis was loose due to lack of retention from the short anterior attachment. Furthermore, the projection of the attachment led to considerable gingival damage. (Mirror view.)

Although the attachment-retained prosthesis has a superficial resemblance to the fixed prosthesis, the principles involved in the construction differ. A fixed bridge is one solid structure and requires all the abutment preparations to be mutually aligned. It may be necessary to devitalise teeth and use telescopic crown procedures, but once inserted it locks all the abutments together and has only to resist the occlusal loads applied to the structure.

An apparently similar attachment-retained prosthesis consists of three basic units: a removable section, and the two groups of abutments on either side (Fig. 159). While the attachments must be aligned with precision, the paths of insertion of the two groups of crowns and that of the removable prosthesis may differ. A slight divergence between the various paths of insertion can be helpful, in fact, for the abutment crowns have to resist not only the occlusal forces, but the considerable displacing forces exerted when the prosthesis is removed. The retention available for the prosthesis is governed in the end by the retention of the abutment preparations, while the size of the attachments is determined by the size of the boxes that can be cut into the abutments adjacent to the gap.

Once the prosthesis is made removable, the mucosal coverage can be treated as a partial denture flange. The flange may contribute to the support of the prosthesis and can be rebased should further resorption occur. The ability to remove the prosthesis naturally simplifies plaque control.

The main problem posed by intracoronal attachments in the anterior quadrant of the mouth is that of finding space for the female section within the contour of the abutment teeth. Devitalisation may help, but not always. For example, some lateral incisors cannot accommodate the bulk of an intracoronal attachment even when devitalised. An intracoronal attachment may be placed closer to the centre of a non-vital tooth, but if the crown has insufficient buc-

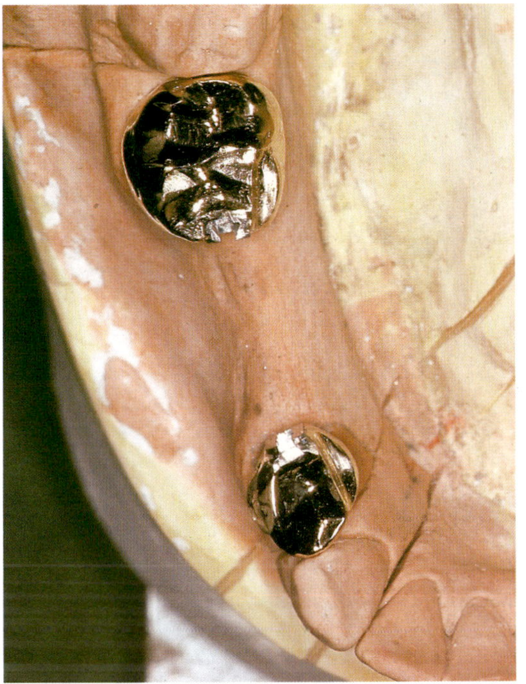

Fig. 161   The abutment restorations remade. Note lingual steps in the crowns, prepared for bracing arms of the removable section.

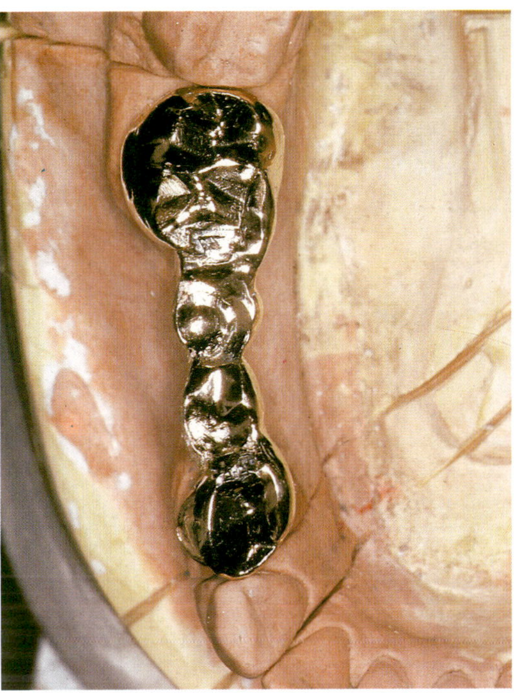

Fig. 162   Metal framework of the removable section in place.

colingual space the attachment still cannot be employed. Overcontouring crowns, or leaving the female section projecting, results in several problems (Fig. 160). The appearance will be poor, and the attachment may be shortened to such an extent that the retention may then be unsatisfactory. The projection at the gingival margin, together with the poor gingival contour, is likely to lead to periodontal damage.

Where adequate crown bulk exists, intracoronal attachments are neat and effective retainers. They are usually simpler to employ with older patients whose clinical crowns are longer and whose pulps are smaller.

Posteriorly, it is easier to find room for the attachments. As with anterior restorations, the great advantage of the attachment-retained prosthesis rests with the fact that the removable part can be treated as a partial denture. Wide mucosal coverage is, therefore, possible; it has considerable hygiene advantages, and facings on artificial teeth can be replaced in the laboratory. On the other hand, the splinting action between the two groups of abutments is never quite as effective as that exerted by a one-piece restoration.

Unilateral attachment-retained prostheses may be employed to restore many types of gaps (Fig. 161 to 163). However, there must

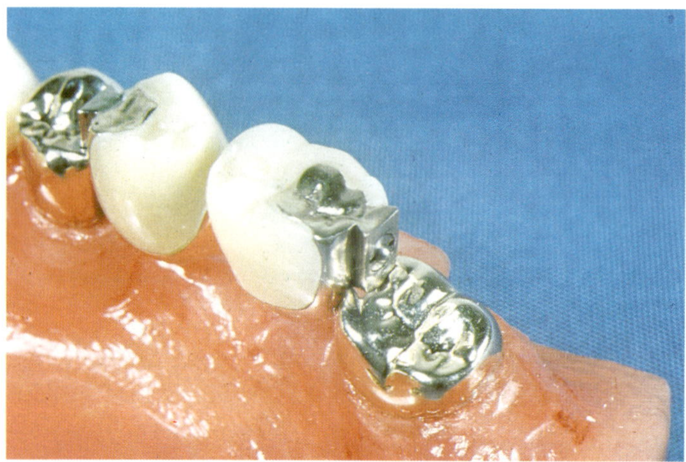

Fig. 163 (a) (b)   Two examples of unilateral attachment-retained prostheses.

Figure 163 a

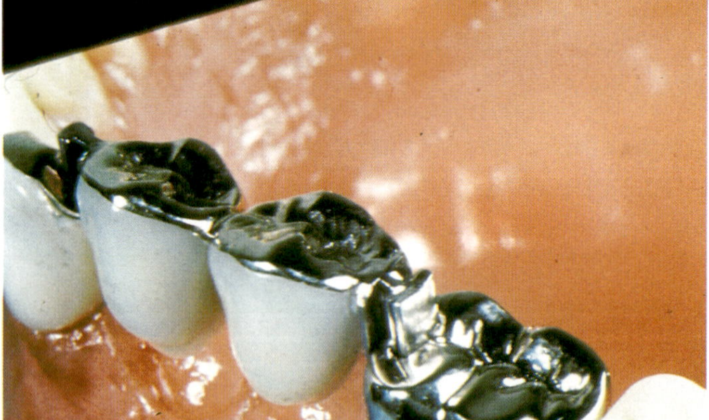

Figure 163 b

be a definite reason for making a restoration removable, and every advantage then taken of this facility.

Removable distal extension partial dentures

The relative merits of intracoronal attachments and clasp arms as retainers have already been discussed. The excellent retention and stability provided by the path of insertion of the attachment is particularly valuable in the case of distal extension prostheses. Intracoronal attachments provide a neat and rigid junction between

Fig. 164 (a) (b) A laboratory produced semi-precision retaining device that features a lingual arm.

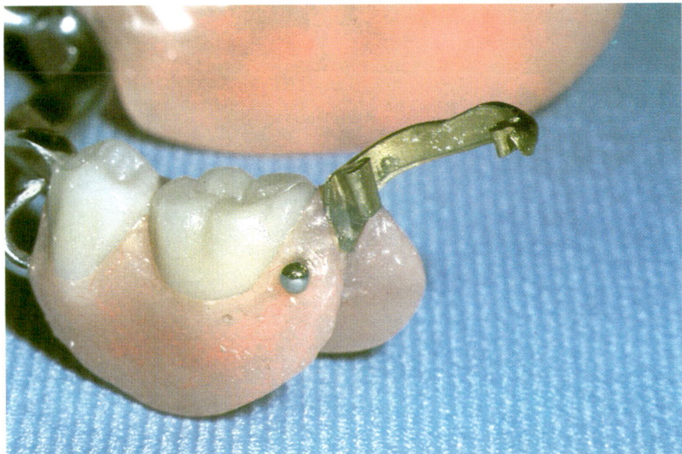

Figure 164 a

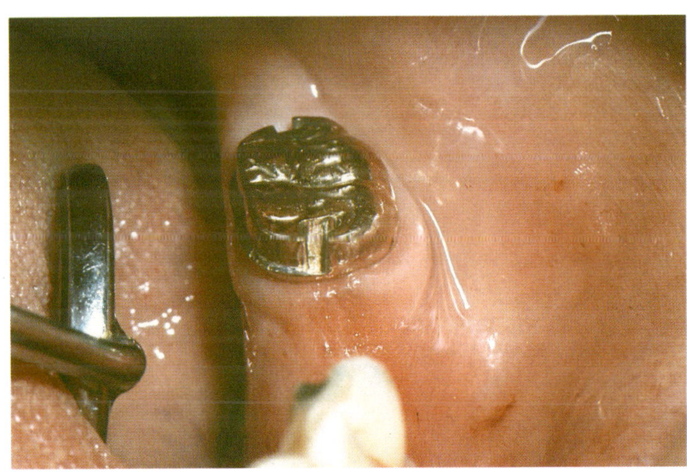

Figure 164 b

the denture and abutment crowns. They are the attachment of choice whenever they can be used. It is essential, however, that the design and construction of the denture reduces to a minimum forces applied to the attachment and to the abutment teeth.

No matter how carefully the denture is designed, intracoronal attachments used to retain distal extension dentures are subjected to considerable forces. Strong attachments should be selected and used in conjunction with lingual bracing arms (Fig. 164 a, b).

The lingual bracing arm reduces the loads to which the attachment is subjected, thereby minimising wear. Where possible the arm should be the same height as the attachment and carried around to the opposite proximal space (Fig. 165). This arm not only adds to the stability of the prosthesis, but also provides the patient with a

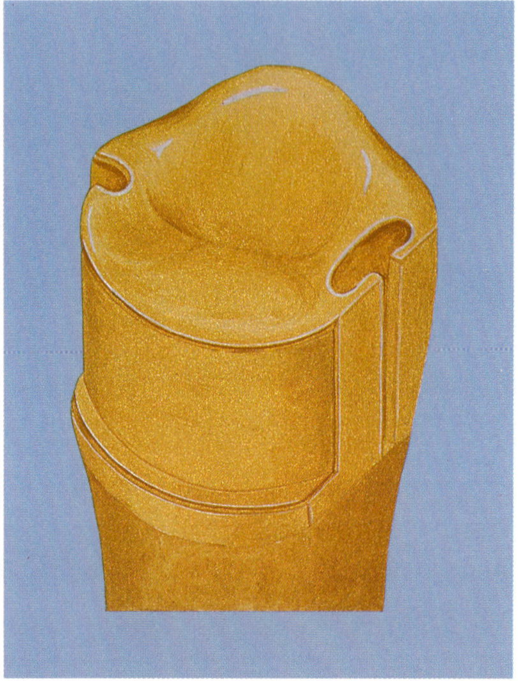

Fig. 165   The lingual bracing arm should be the same height as the attachment and carried around to the opposite proximal space.

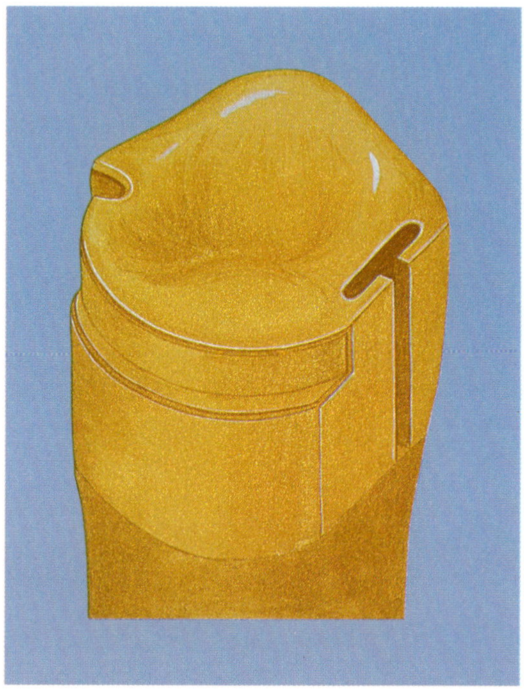

Fig. 166   Lingual space requirements can be reduced by making the step near to the occlusal surface and carrying a skirt of metal to the full depth of the attachment.

handling point to aid removal and insertion of the denture. Additional lingual tooth reduction is necessary to accomodate this arm. Where lingual space is restricted, the step can be placed near the occlusal surface and a narrow skirt of metal carried down the lingual surface of the crown (Fig. 166).

Distal extension prostheses require a minimum of two splinted abutment teeth on either side. Where there are seven or fewer anterior teeth remaining, it is necessary to splint them all together to form one rigid abutment.

Prostheses for bilateral distal extension spaces

Intracoronal attachments may be used to provide a well-retained and stable prosthesis without visible buccal or labial re-

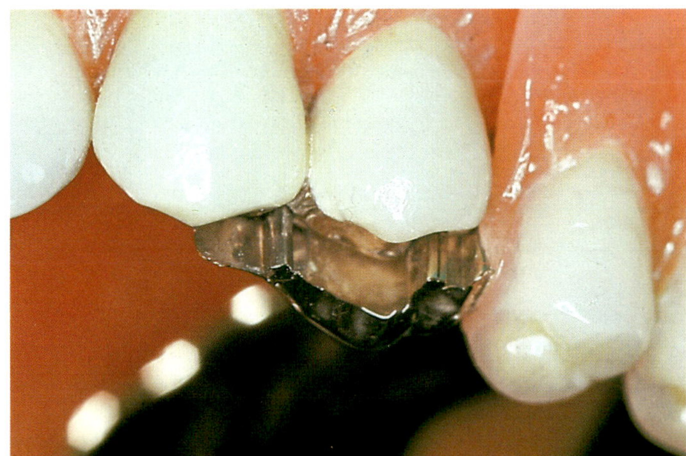

Fig. 167 An attachment-retained denture being inserted.

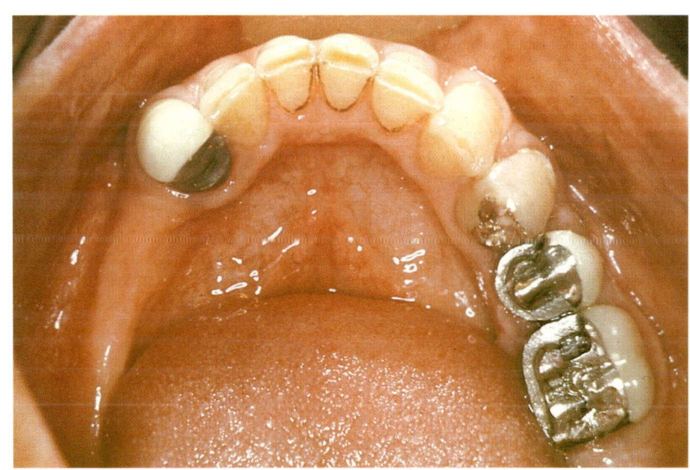

Fig. 168 Overcontouring resulting from failure to prepare the abutments in accordance with the attachment space requirements.

tainers. They are particularly useful where only several anterior teeth remain as clasp retainers might be ineffective and unsightly in these situations. The additional space normally available in upper teeth makes them more useful intracoronal abutments (Fig. 167). Devitalising canines, or other teeth for that matter, may allow the attachment to be placed closer to the centre of the tooth but will be of no avail if there is inadequate labiolingual space. While intra-coronal attachments can be employed to retain many different types of bilateral distal extension prostheses, the limiting factor must always be the provision of adequate abutments with sufficient vertical and buccolingual space (Fig. 168).

Where there is insufficient room within the most distal abutment for the attachment, an artificial tooth can be cantilevered from it to carry the attachment (Fig. 169). This arrangement has considerable advan-

161

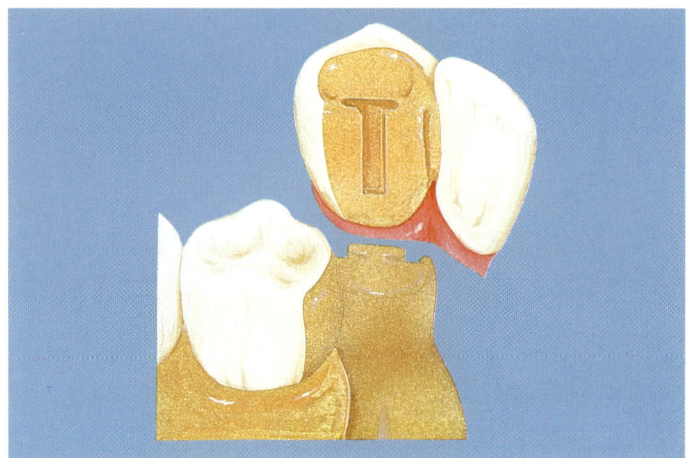

Fig. 169   Where there is insufficient space for an attachment within an abutment tooth, an artificial tooth can be cantilevered from the splinted abutment.

tages, for the attachment does not interfere with the contour of the abutment crowns, no box preparation is required in the abutment teeth and the maximum length and size of attachment can be used. For these reasons, many experienced operators prefer the method, especially as there can be no question of the denture attachment damaging the gingival papilla of the abutment tooth.

The cantilevered extension can result in considerable torques falling upon the abutments so that the total load and its distribution requires careful assessment. The hazards of damaging forces applied to the abutments are increased if the prosthesis is opposed by natural teeth.

The loads applied by the denture to the teeth are transmitted through the attachments now positioned at right angles to the way in which many were designed to function. Most prefabricated attachments work perfectly well in this position, but it is wise practice to protect their lateral surfaces with a component of the denture framework.

Prostheses for unilateral distal extension spaces

A distal extension prosthesis requires support from both sides of the jaw, even if the gap to be restored is only on one side. In view of the extensive tooth preparation required for attachment prostheses, the relative merits of a clasp-retained denture should be considered. An attachment-retained denture to replace the gaps shown in Figure 170 would require crown preparations on a minimum of four teeth and probably more. It is doubtful, in this instance, if the retention and stability achieved for the prosthesis would be significantly greater than that for a correctly designed clasp-retained denture.

On the other hand, advantage can be taken of attachments when extensive restoration of the abutments is necessary. Where there is a space on the opposite side, the denture can gain support from an attachment placed buccolingually in a fixed prosthesis restoring the gap (Fig. 171).

The advantages of restoring the jaw in this

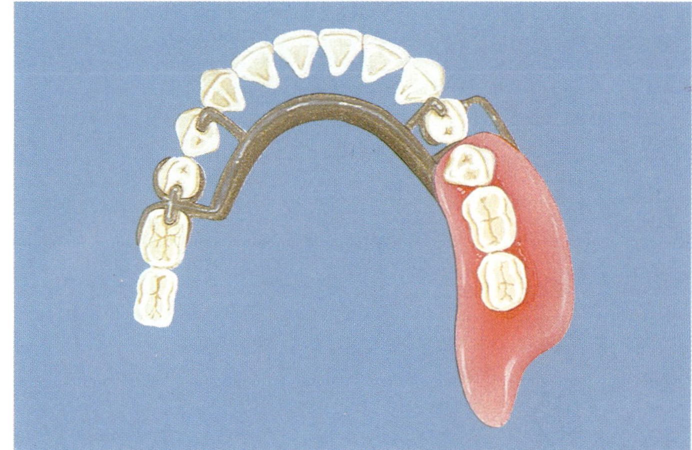

Fig. 170 A clasp-retained denture may be preferable for some unilateral spaces. The extensive tooth preparation required for an attachment-retained prosthesis may not be offset by its marginal advantages in retention and stability.

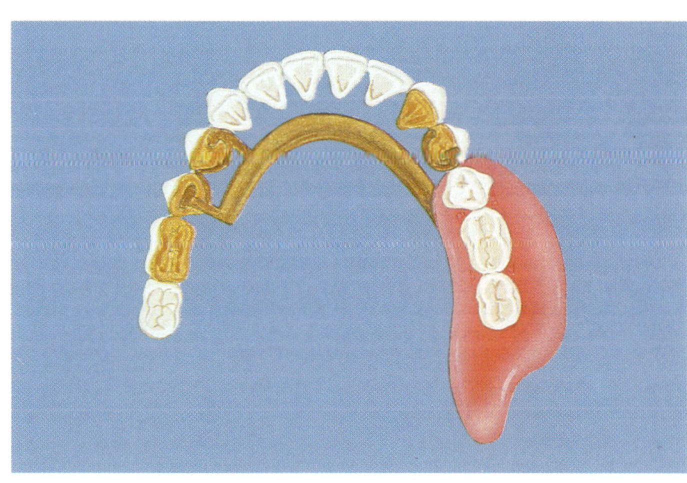

Fig. 171 Where there is a space on the opposite side to the distal extension base, the denture can gain support from an attachment placed buccolingually in a bridge restoring the gap.

way, compared with the alternative method of replacing the spaces either side with the denture, are discussed in Chapter 4. The fixed prosthesis unites the mesial and distal abutments, allowing the positioning of a generous sized attachment in the pontic (Figs. 172 and 173). Only two attachments need to be aligned, and box or wide shoulder preparations are necessary on the side to be restored with the fixed restoration.

The attachment and associated bracing components forms an extremely neat and effective retainer (Figs. 174 and 175). Since intracoronal attachments cannot be rocked or rotated out of place, removal of the denture could be extremely difficult as there is so little purchase available. An additional handling point should be provided, preferably in line with the attachment (Figs. 176 to 178).

It might be tempting to shorten the major

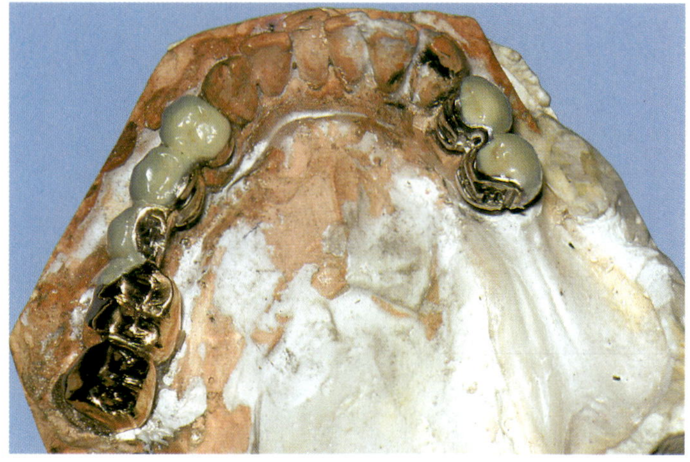

Fig. 172 Buccolingual positioning of the attachment in the pontic allows the use of a generous sized attachment and simplifies alignment of the retainers.

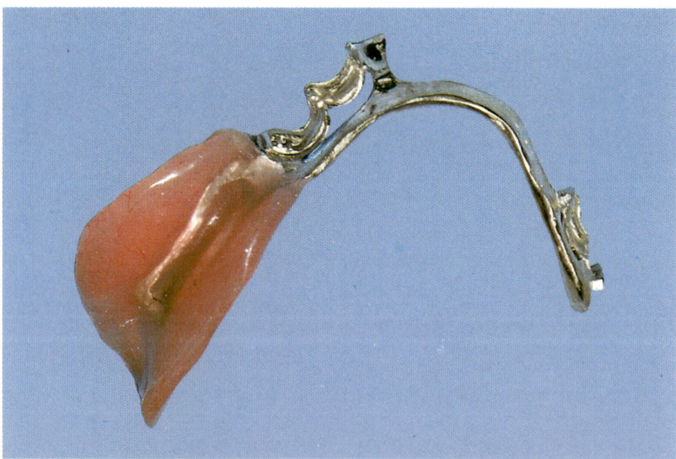

Fig. 173 The removable section of the prosthesis. Note the attachment and additional bracing component.

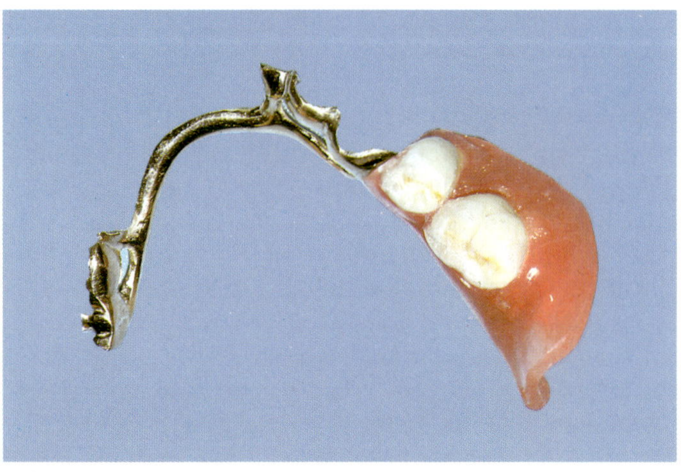

Fig. 174 Occlusal view of the denture. The bracing components act as handling points to aid removal and insertion of the prosthesis.

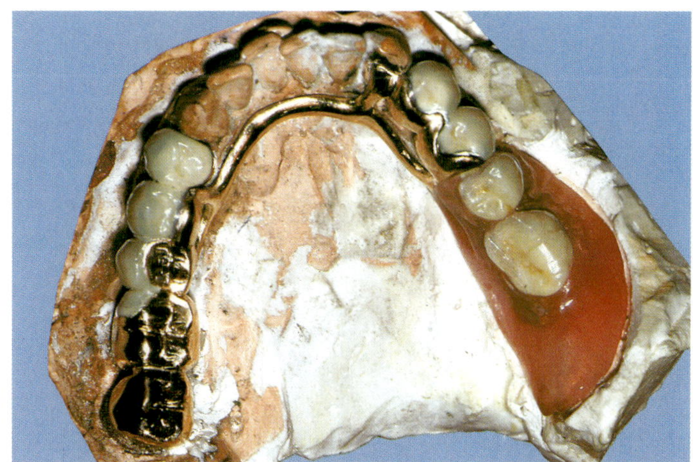

Fig. 175 The assembled prosthesis on the master cast.

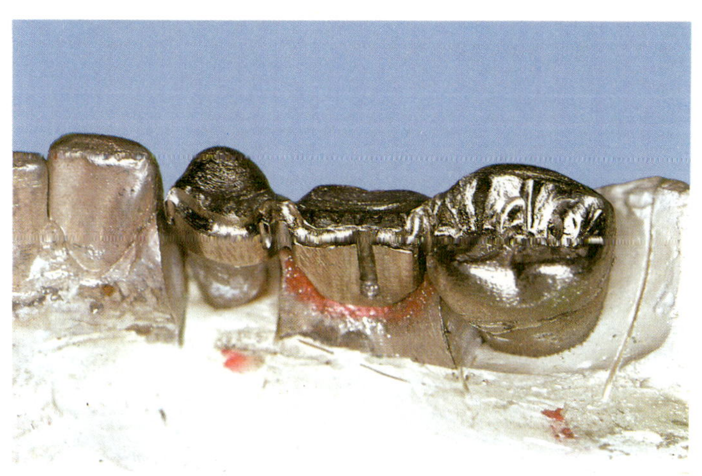

Fig. 176 Unpolished casting showing positioning of the attachment in the pontic together with the provision of additional bracing components.

connector by joining it to the mesial section of the bracing components rather than to the attachment itself. Unfortunately, this results in an increased buccolingual bulk of the restoration while the handling aid for the patient is malaligned with the attachment (Fig. 179).

Lower anterior teeth seldom possess adequate labiolingual space for intracoronal attachments. In order to accommodate such a unit, even a non-vital lower canine or premolar may need to be overcontoured (Fig. 180). This arrangement is obviously far from satisfactory. Where sufficient abutments and vertical space are present, a cantilevered extension may be used, otherwise another retaining system should be selected.

Where no space exists on the opposite side of the jaw, the denture may be joined to the teeth of that side by means of telescopic crowns (Figs. 181 to 184). Some form

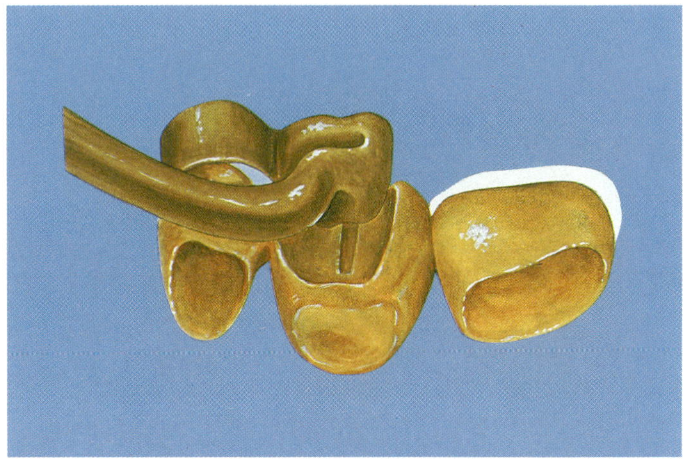

Fig. 177 Lingual view to show depression above the attachment to facilitate withdrawal along its path of insertion.

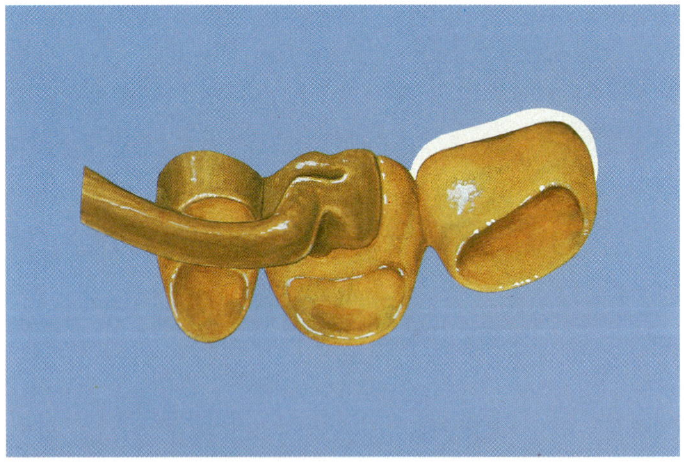

Fig. 178 Attachment seated.

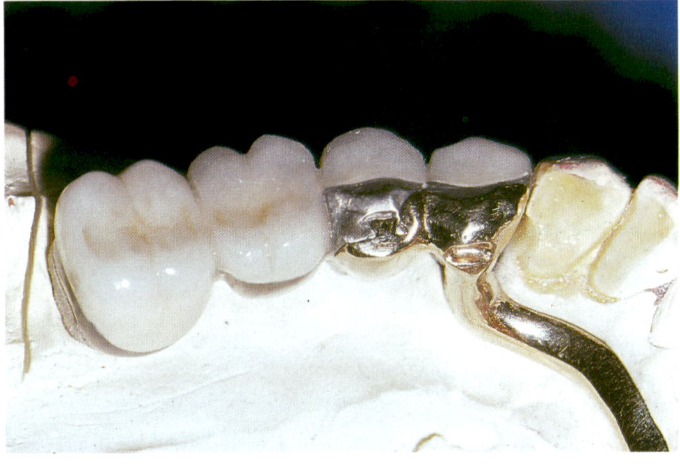

Fig. 179 Joining the major connector to the bracing components, rather than to the attachment, increases the buccolingual bulk of the restoration and places the handling aid out of alignment with the attachment.

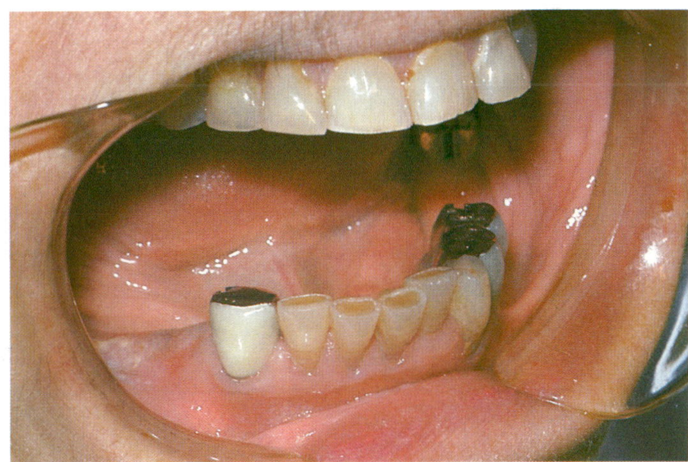

Fig. 180 Lower canines and premolars seldom possess adequate buccolingual space for intracoronal retainers without grossly distorting their contours.

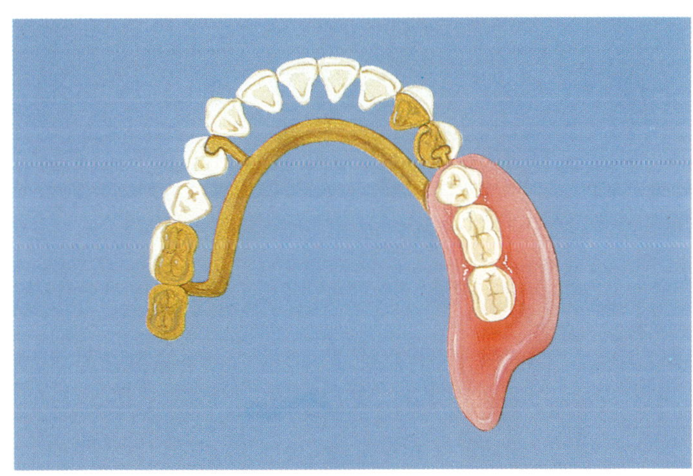

Fig. 181 Where no space exists on the opposite side of the jaw to the distal extension space, telescopic crowns may be employed to join the denture to these teeth.

of indirect retainer should be incorporated where possible. Intracoronal attachments placed between the teeth are seldom satisfactory as they encroach upon the gingivae, while clasps placed around the teeth and used in conjunction with attachments on the other side of the jaw frequently lead to unfavourable load distribution and damage.

The principles involved in the construction of a distal extension denture are the same, be it retained by clasps or by an attachment system. The clinical application of these principles may differ slightly and they are described in the relevant sections.

Connectors

Intracoronal attachments can be employed to join sections of a fixed prosthesis.

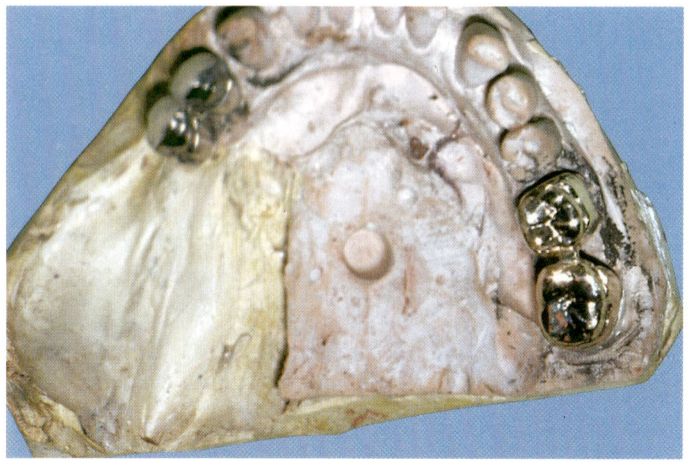

Fig. 182 Master cast showing fixed sections of the prosthesis.

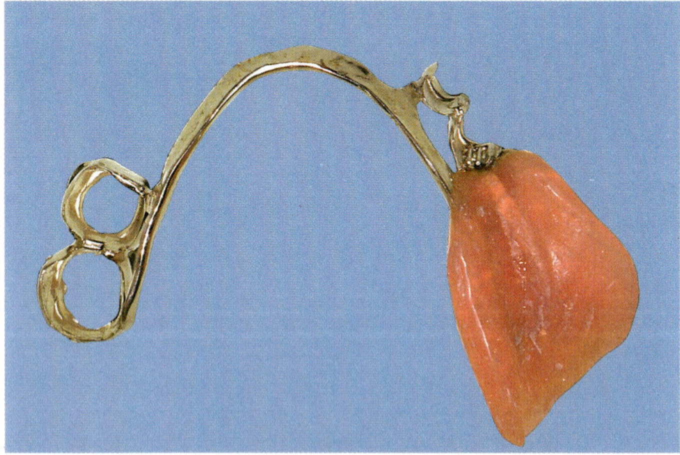

Fig. 183 The removable section of the prosthesis.

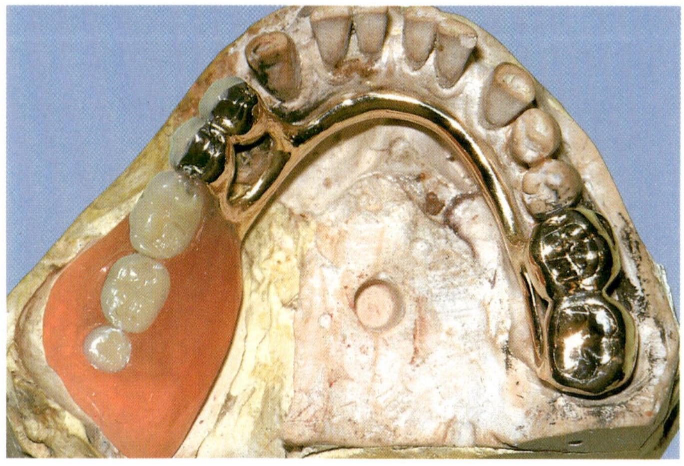

Fig. 184 The assembled restoration on the master cast.

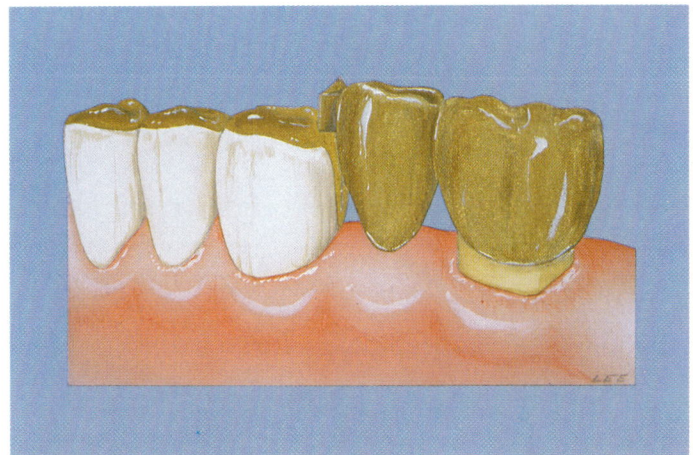

Fig. 185 Intracoronal attachment used to join crowns without a common path of insertion.

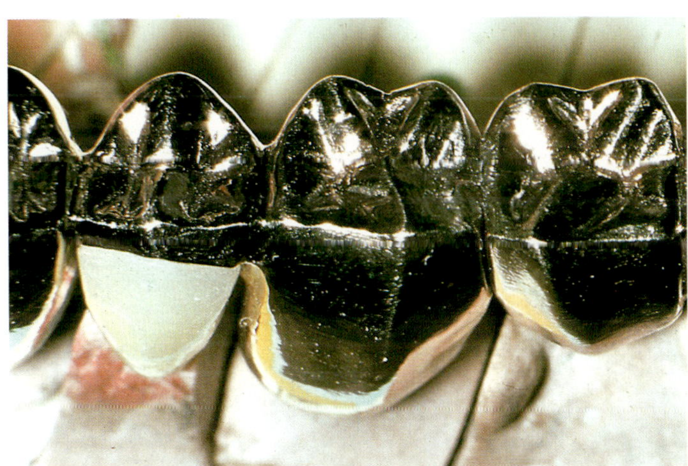

Fig. 186 Attachment in place.

A distinction must be made between instances where the operator employs attachments to limit the length of individual castings, or connect abutments without a common path of insertion, and those in which he may be faced with constructing a partial denture at a later date.

Where the restoration is to remain fixed, the attachments will not be subjected to the constant wear and tear of removal and insertion. Comparatively small units can be selected, as subsequent adjustments will be unnecessary. If there is a possibility of replacing a distal section with a partial denture, provision should be made for an attachment of adequate strength together with a bracing arm.

Suppose a misalignment of abutments on the master cast is discovered in the laboratory. Splitting the casting and connecting the two sections in the mouth with an attachment might save the day. But where is

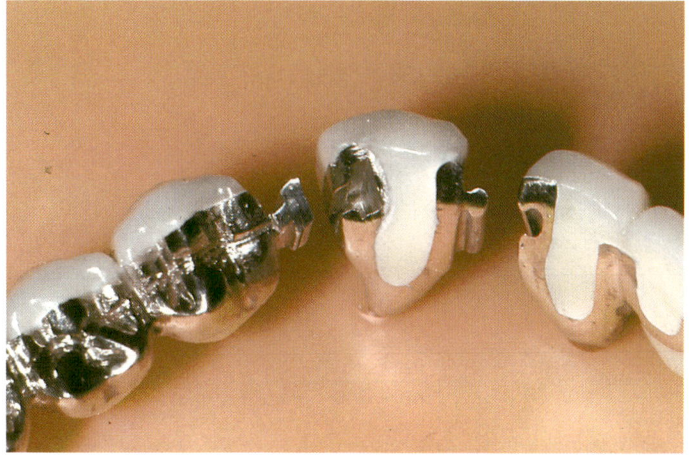

Fig. 187 Intracoronal attachments employed to split a large bonded porcelain to gold restoration into small sections.

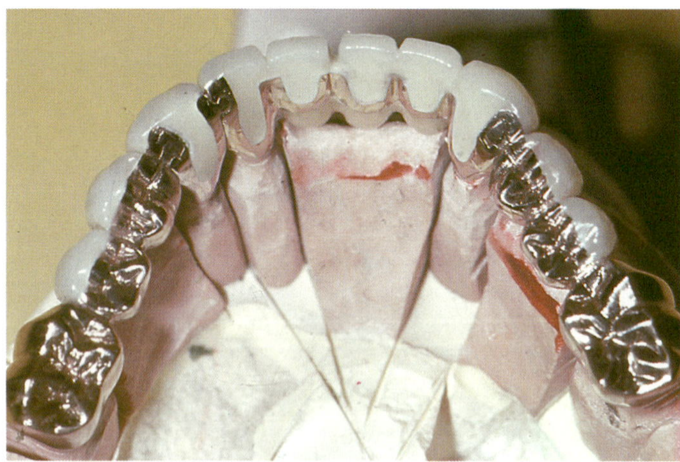

Fig. 188 Prosthesis assembled on the master cast.

the attachment to be placed? Long clinical crowns and good fortune might provide adequate space. Otherwise one is faced with repreparing several of the teeth and a new impression. It is obviously far better to plan the restoration on diagnostic casts, assess the alignment of teeth and design the preparation to include sufficient vertical and adjacent proximal space for the attachment, the neck of which will cross this proximal area. There must be adequate room for plaque control. Where teeth are missing, it is possible to place the connection in a pontic.

If attachments are employed, the crown preparations can be aligned in groups, and these groups of crowns then joined with intracoronal attachments. Ideally, the attachments should be sited distally in teeth. The groups of crowns are inserted separately and interlock in the mouth with intracoronal attachments (Figs. 185 and 186).

170

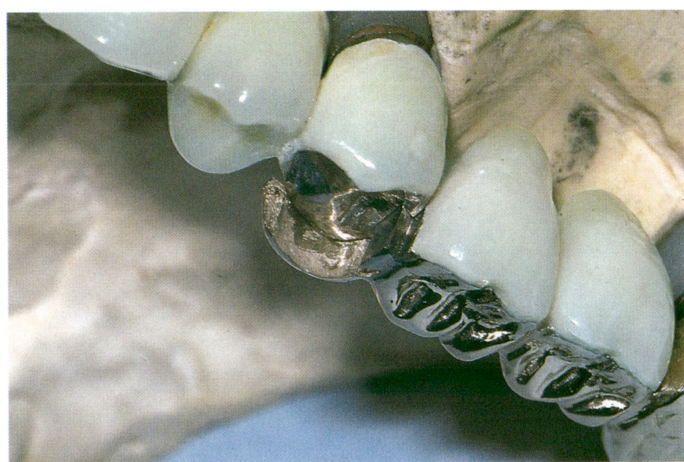

Fig. 189 Intracoronal attachment connecting two sections of the prosthesis. Parallel-sided units of adequate size must be employed to prevent play.

Assembling the prosthesis in this manner may avoid devitalisation of several teeth. It allows a large prosthesis to be assembled from comparatively small castings, preferred by some when porcelain fused to gold is employed (Figs. 187 and 188). Others claim that there is some physiological advantage in constructions of this nature. While this point is questionable, there is little doubt that it minimises the effects of casting distortion during the firing of the porcelain.

Figure 189 shows an example of an intracoronal attachment used to join two sections of a prosthesis. Placement of the attachment requires some care if the proximal space is not to be restricted. To prevent play between the connected sections, a parallel-sided unit of adequate dimensions must be selected. Where space permits, a bracing arm should be incorporated as well. Figures 190 and 191 show the principle applied to a lower prosthesis where malalignment of the teeth dictated the use of four attachments.

While it is obviously possible to design and construct one's own connecting attachment in the laboratory, it is easier to employ prefabricated units where space permits. Recently introduced plastic blanks, such as the Plasta unit, are useful. Both male and female components are made of combustible plastic and each is incorporated in the wax-up of its respective group of crowns.

When the prognosis of a bridge abutment is dubious, the segment of the prosthesis carried by this abutment can be joined to the main part of the structure with intracoronal attachments. Provision should be made for a bracing arm. Should the abutment be lost subsequently, it can be replaced with an attachment-retained denture. When considering the possibility of a future bilateral denture, the attachments each side must not only be sturdy, but they must be aligned with each other. Cantilevered pontics, at least on one side, can be used in some of these situations (Figs. 192 and 193).

There are many other situations where this flexible treatment planning can be useful.

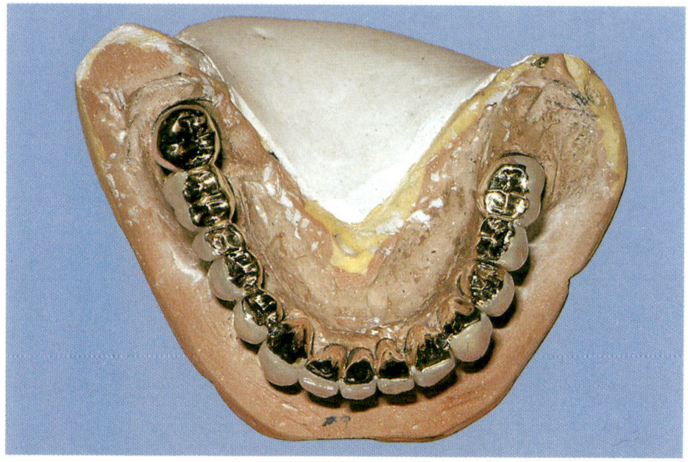

Fig. 190 A lower restoration made in four connected sections due to malalignment of the abutments.

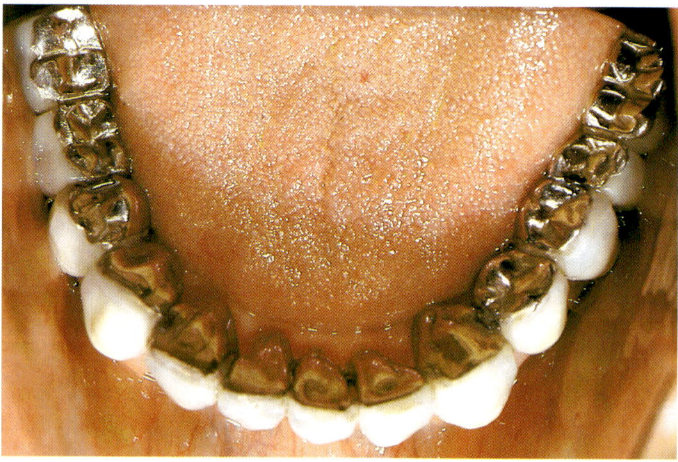

Fig. 191 Prosthesis in the mouth 9 years later.

Although the male section can be easily removed from the female unit, the female unit cannot be removed with the male section in place. This is because the female slot has a base and is only open at the occlusal surface. It is, therefore, vital to ensure that the prosthesis and restorations are planned so that the male part of the attachment is joined to the section of the prosthesis carried by the dubious abutment.

No matter how rigid intracoronal attachments may appear to be, a small degree of play is inevitable, particularly after they have been used a while. The length of span must be considered when connecting it to another section of a prosthesis. Take for example a first molar distally displaced and connect it with a fixed prosthesis to an attachment distal in the canine. After a period of months the patient is likely to complain that the prosthesis moves slightly and, on

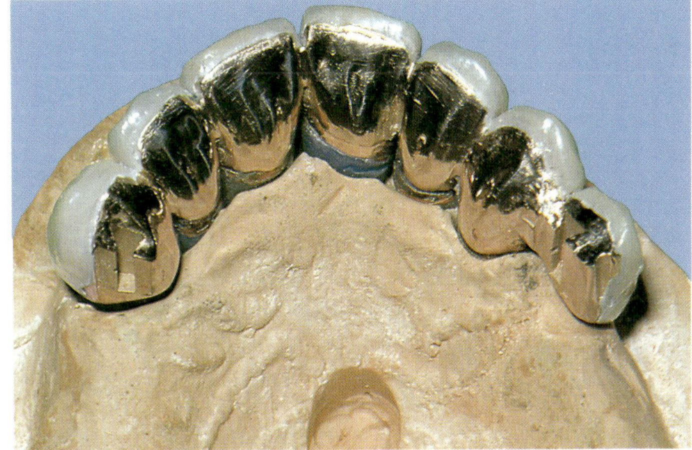

Fig. 192 The anterior teeth are splinted and joined to the posterior sections with intracoronal attachments. Following loss of the molars, a bilateral distal extension denture retained by attachments can be constructed.

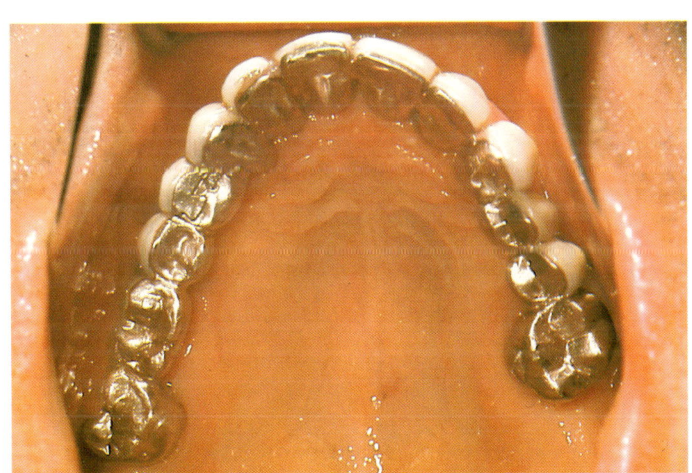

Fig. 193 Restoration in the mouth 10 years later.

examination, a minute degree of play will be found. For the sake of argument, assume the span of the prosthesis to be 30 mm, just 1 degree of play in the attachment will allow movement of 0.5 mm of the distal section. In practice, the reverse appears to be the case with the pontics effectively cantilevered from the molar until the minute play is taken up. Incorporating a bracing arm will prevent this complication. Alternatively, the attachment can be placed distally, or buccolingually, in a cantilevered pontic thereby reducing the length of span of the distal section.

Intracoronal attachments therefore allow a considerable flexibility in treatment planning. Demanding upon both operator and technician, they cannot be employed haphazardly. Nevertheless, their popularity shows just how many are prepared to take the time and trouble to ensure they are employed in a correct manner.

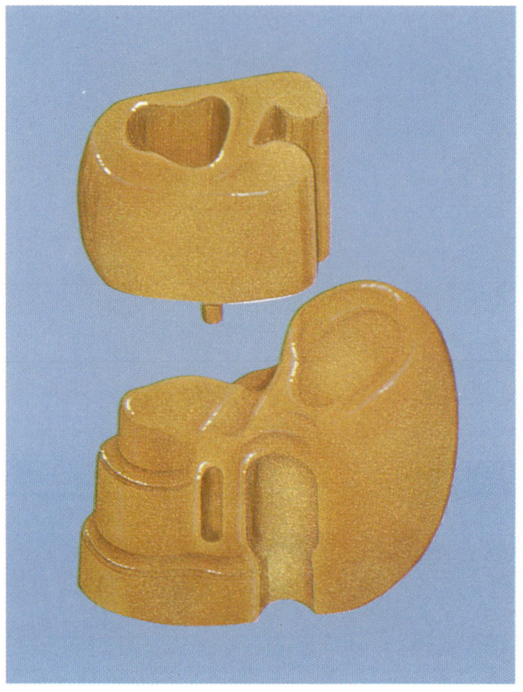

Fig. 194   Simplified diagram of Channel Shoulder Pin (CSP) System. This design provides excellent retention and stability.

The channel shoulder pin system

If a design study were undertaken to improve the retention and stability of a conventional intracoronal attachment and lingual bracing arm, it would probably result in the development of something resembling the Channel Shoulder Pin system (CSP). This technique was originally developed by Steiger and is admirably described in his book (*Steiger* and *Boitel* 1959). This design gives a remarkably firm bracing action and resistance to rotational displacing forces. The removable section is retained primarily by a series of parallel-sided pins, secondarily by the vertical surfaces of the unit, and is guided into place by retention grooves (Figs. 194 to 197). The

clinical procedures place special emphasis on impression techniques, methods of location and jaw relation records, for not only must the two sections interlock with precision, but the occlusal surfaces must be accurate. The difficulty of making occlusal adjustments to the sections of the crown covered by the removable part of the attachment should be borne in mind. Both parts of the attachment have to be produced in the laboratory and the processes are exacting. Unlike most attachment work, a rigid surveyor will not suffice for these techniques, which require precise milling facilities as well. Examples of two popular models of milling machines, combined with surveyors, are illustrated in Figures 198 and 199. While the CSP system

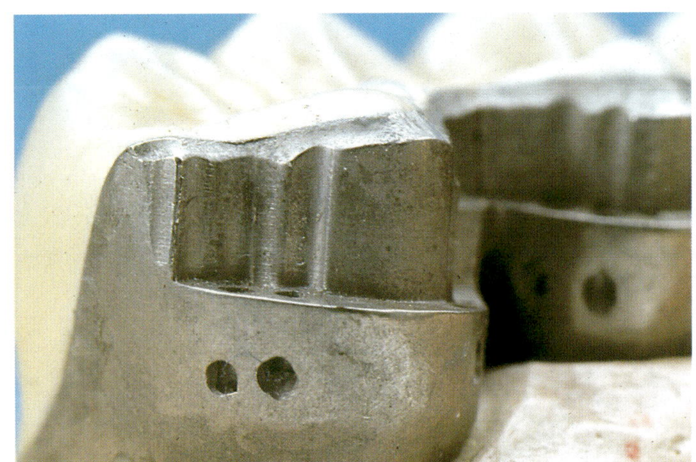

Fig. 195 Lingual view of CSP type units showing drainage channels.

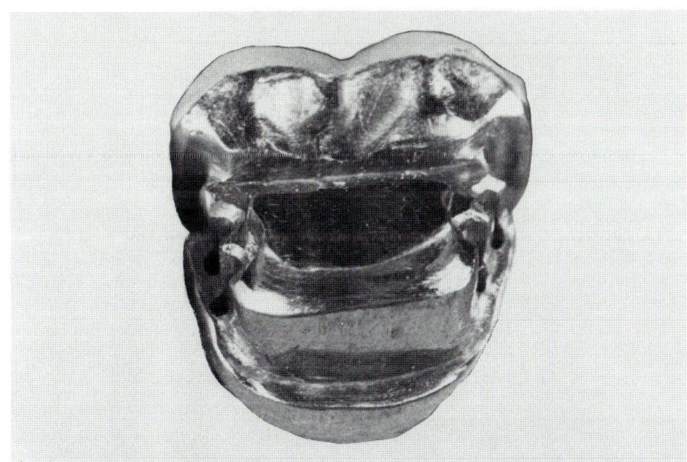

Fig. 196 The cemented section of the attachment. Note the large areas for contact in both the horizontal and vertical plane.

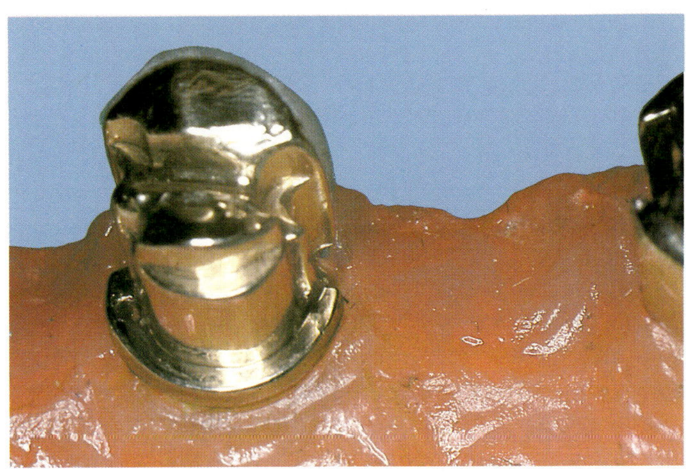

Fig. 197 Another example of the CSP principle.

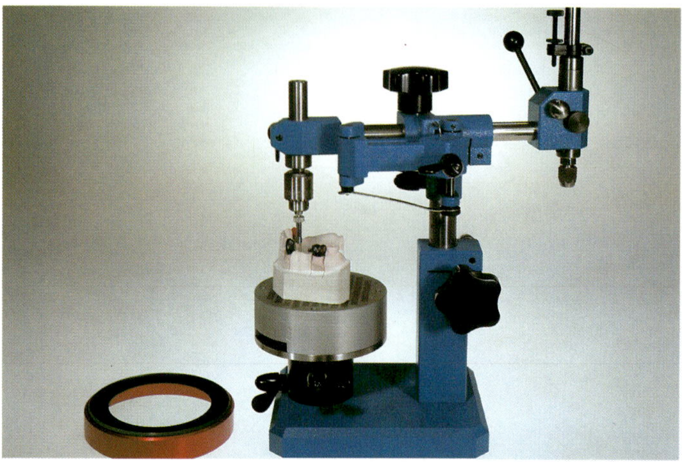

Fig. 198 (a) The Bachmann Parallelometer. (b) The Bachmann instrument prepared for use as a milling device.

Figure 198 a

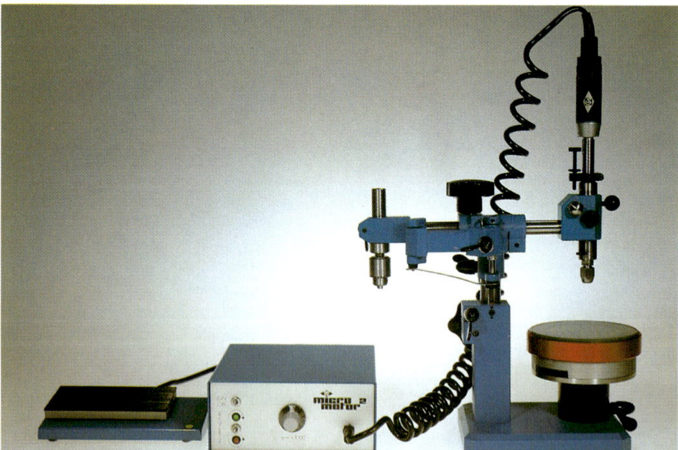

Figure 198 b

gives excellent results, it can only be recommended when both operator and technician have had experience with other types of attachment.

The multiple parallel-sided pins, together with the other frictional surfaces used in this technique, have a much greater surface area than an intracoronal attachment of equivalent length. The CSP system, or modifications of it, can therefore be used, albeit with some difficulty, where lack of vertical space would preclude the use of other types of attachment. Figures 200 to 203 show examples of a modified CSP principle where the vertical space available for an attachment was particularly limited.

The Channel Shoulder Pin system works equally well for lower restorations and Figures 204 to 207 show examples.

A major problem of maintenance is a bent pin, for the actual culprit has to be identified

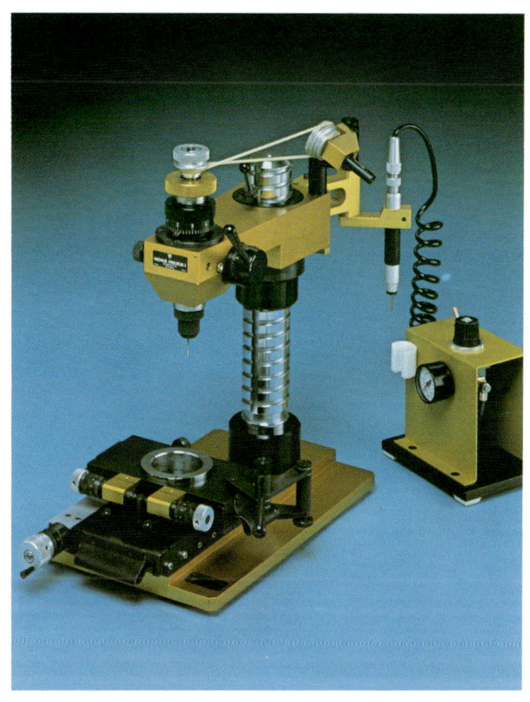

Fig. 199   The MP 2000 Parallelometer.

and straightened or removed before the restoration can be placed in the mouth. It is apparent that this retainer is not suitable for clumsy patients or those with a tendency to make their own adjustments! A broken pin is easier to repair. A small hole is drilled through the gold over the pin in question and a new one inserted through the seated denture into the hole in the crown. The pin is then connected with resin, preferably Duralay, and the denture removed from the mouth and handed to the laboratory.

Due to the problem of construction, many operators have devised their own simplified versions of the CSP system. Where there is adequate crown height, one can dispense with the pins and rely on the para-llel surfaces, grooves and shoulders to give stability and retention. Once the principles of the CSP design and construction have been mastered, the operator is free to design his own retainer according to the needs and space available for each retainer. There is certainly no merit in complexity for complexity's sake.

A far simpler laboratory-produced attachment is shown in Figure 208 a, b. The outer layer slides over the inner section and is supported by a shoulder running around the gingival portion of the inner layer. Parallel retention grooves add to the frictional surface and, although the efficiency of the device cannot match that of the CSP type of assembly, it is considerably easier to produce.

177

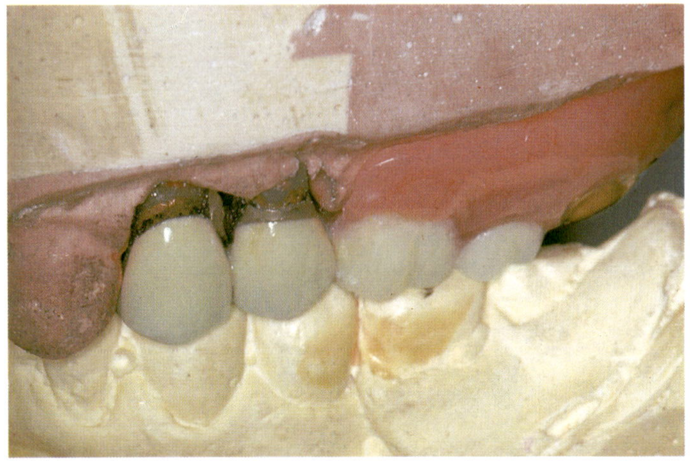

Fig. 200 The CSP system, or a modification of it, is particularly useful where lack of vertical space precludes the use of other attachments.

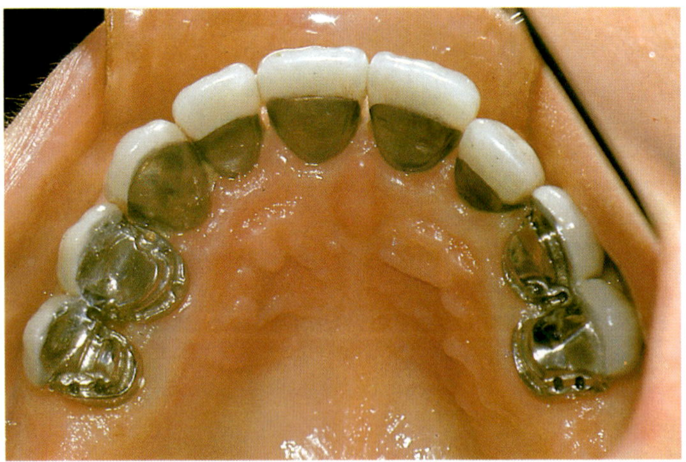

Fig. 201 Occlusal view of the restoration.

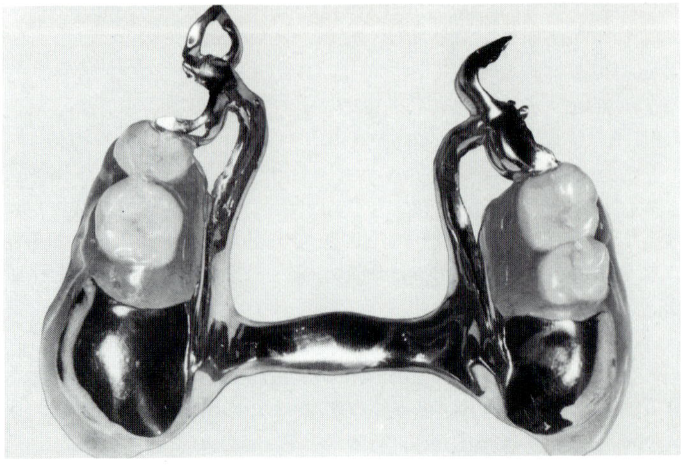

Fig. 202 Occlusal surface of a denture retained by a modified CSP technique. The modification was dictated by lack of space and the position of the opposing cusps.

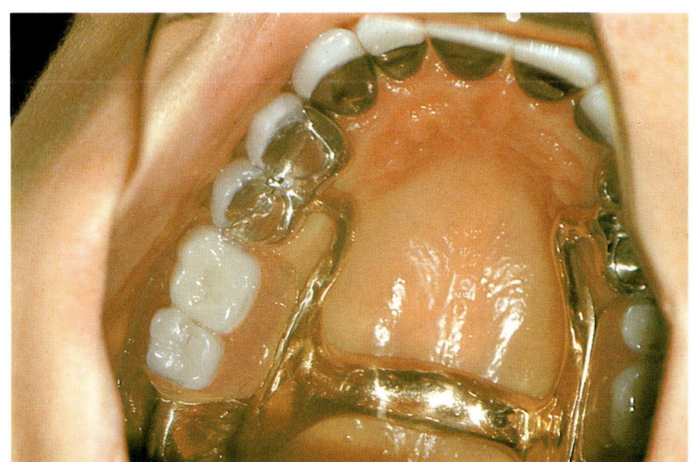

Fig. 203 The restoration in the mouth.

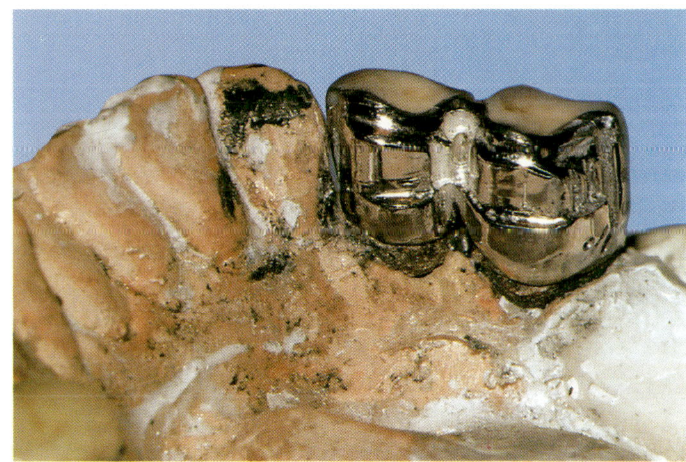

Fig. 204 The Channel Shoulder Pin (CSP) on two lower premolars. Note the vents to allow the removal of debris from the retention holes. The guiding groove is clearly visible.

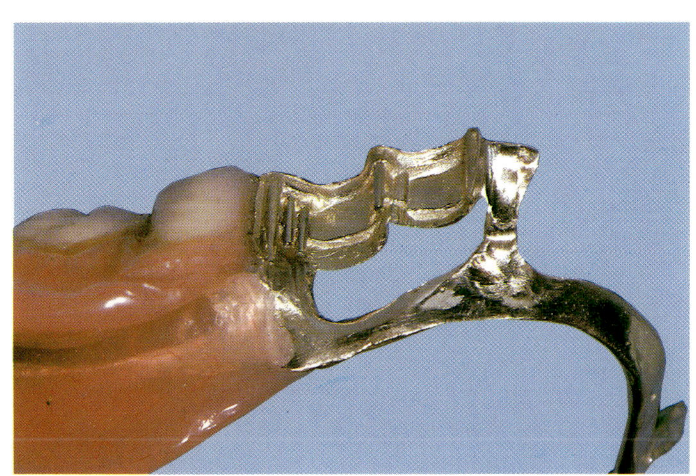

Fig. 205 Removable section of the prosthesis showing the long, slightly tapered, guides and the shorter parallel-sided retaining pins.

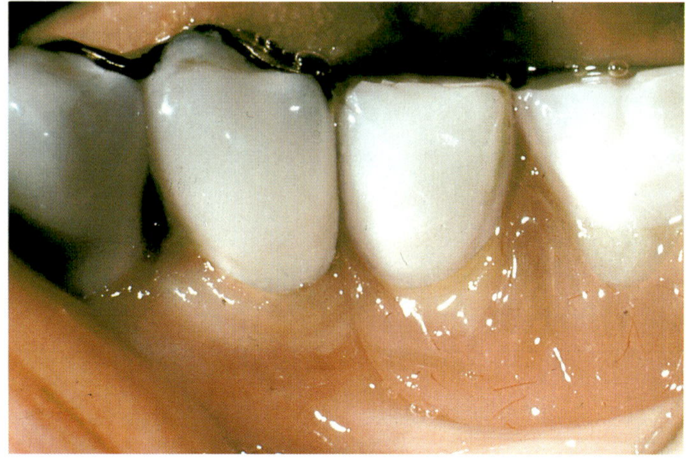

Fig. 206 Mirror view of the restoration in the mouth.

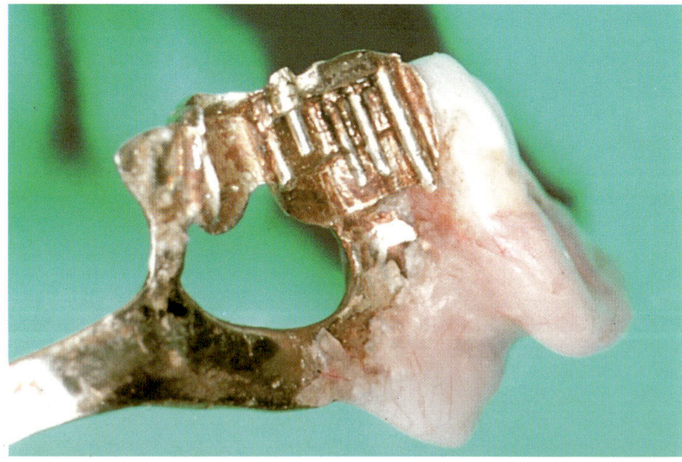

Fig. 207 CSP unit after 9 years service.

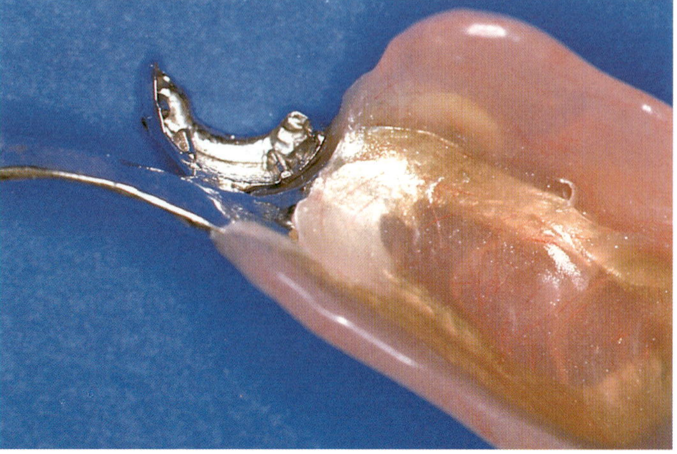

Fig. 208 (a) (b) A greatly simplified laboratory-produced attachment which works well, provided there is sufficient vertical space available.

Figure 208 a

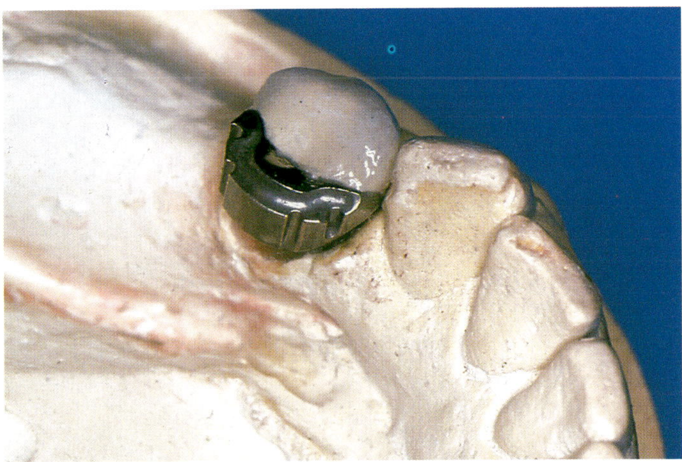

Figure 208 b

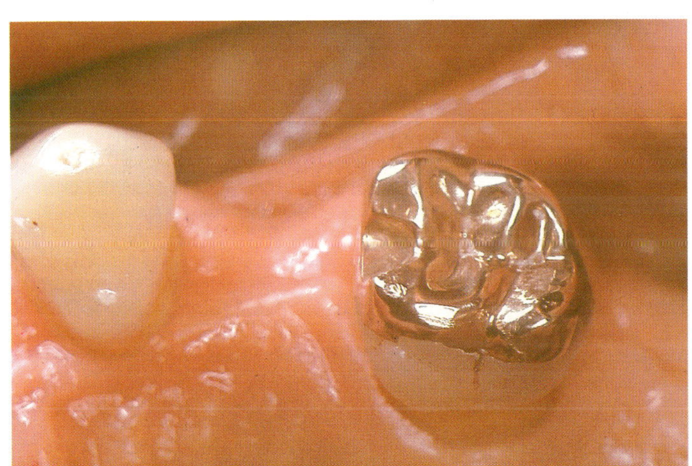

Fig. 209 A simple occlusal rest seat. Note the prepared guide plane.

The semi-precision rest

A semi-precision rest can be considered as an intracoronal attachment with tapered sides. Like a precision attachment it provides occlusal support, but the bracing action may be less and it cannot be relied upon by itself to produce adequate retention.

When an abutment tooth is to be crowned, guide planes can be incorporated on the proximal surface. Furthermore, the rest seat can be deepened and contoured to the operator's requirements (Fig. 209). As the rest seat is deepened, the ability to transmit lateral forces is increased until the bracing action may be considerable. In these circumstances, it is possible to dispense with a bracing arm and to construct a unit consisting of a rest and a retaining arm (Figs. 210 a, b and 211).

While the components of a semi-precision

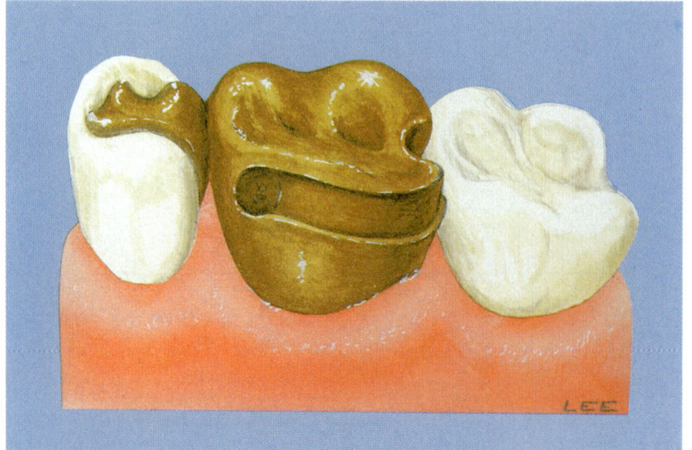

Fig. 210 (a) A deepened rest seat with a lingual step prepared for a retaining arm. Note the depression at the mesial section of this step. (b) Diagram to show the design of the removable component. Note the ball-shaped end of the lingual retaining arm.

Figure 210 a

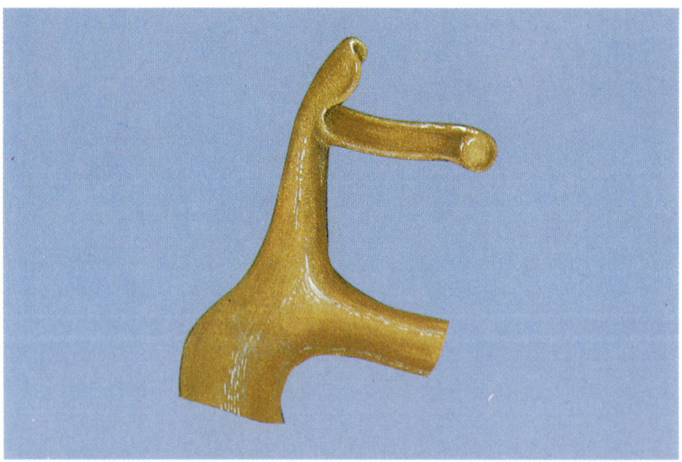

Figure 210 b

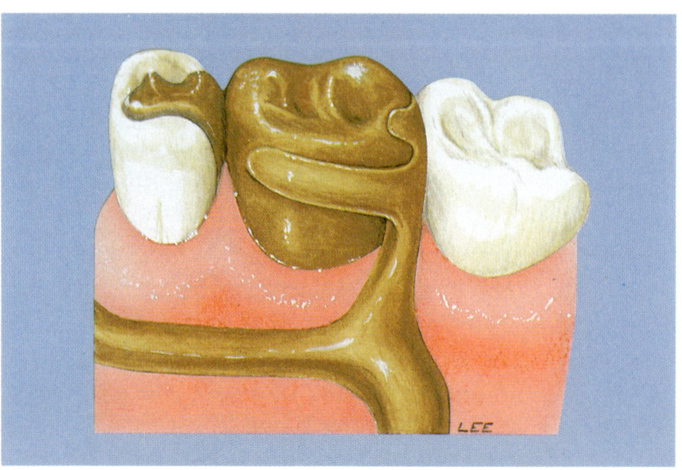

Fig. 211 The removable prosthesis in place.

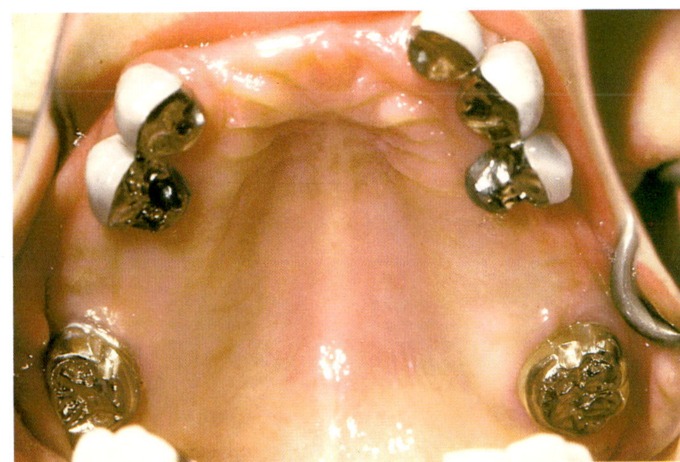

Fig. 212 Crowns incorporating semi-precision retainers.

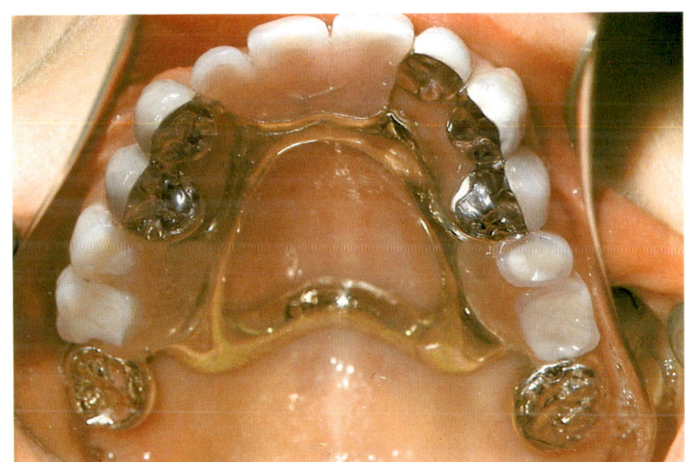

Fig. 213 Removable section in place.

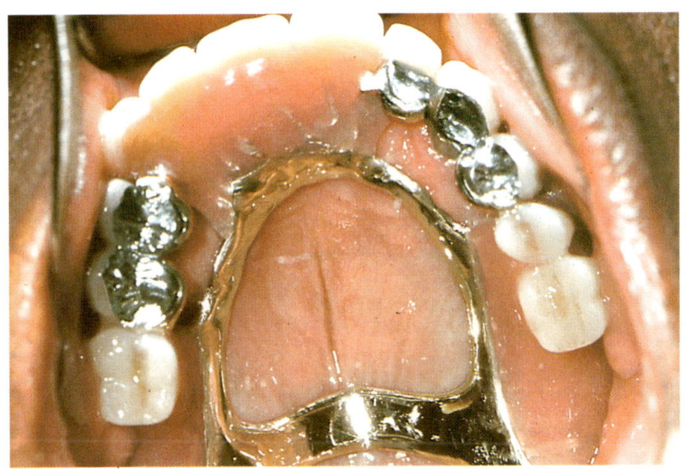

Fig. 214 Another example of a prosthesis retained by semi-precision attachments. Note absence of buccal retainers.

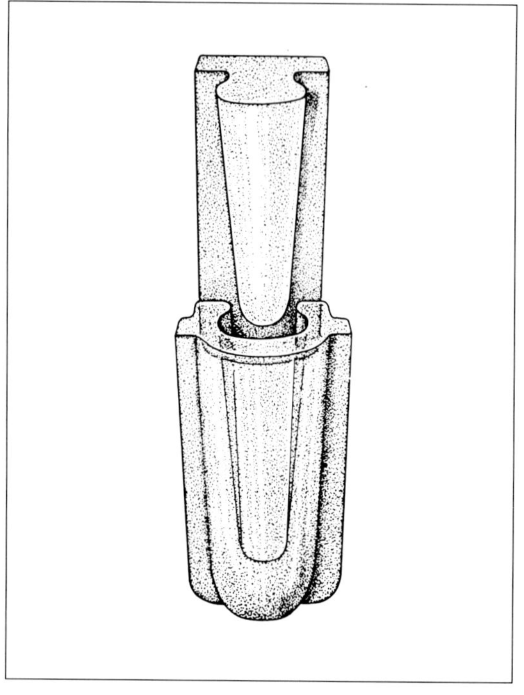

Fig. 215   The Stern resin pattern for a semi-precision attachment.

rest system resemble those of an intracoronal attachment and bracing arm, their roles are reversed. Unlike the precision attachment, it is the arm of the semi-precision unit that provides the retention, and the rest component the bracing action. In practice, of course, the functions are by no means separated. There are operators who prefer to make comparatively rigid bracing arms with semi-precision rests. The results are perfectly satisfactory, although adjustments are difficult and the restoration unnecessarily complex. Semi-precision retainers are comparatively neat and simple to employ. They are usually more economical than their precision counterparts, yet allow the construction of an effective, good-looking restoration without buccal arms to mar the appearance (Figs. 212 to 214).

Semi-precision rests may be carved in wax with the aid of a surveyor and then produced in the laboratory. Alternatively, preformed resin patterns may be purchased that are incorporated in the waxed-up crown and subsequently burnt out with the wax (Fig. 215). The male section of the unit is normally cast as part of the framework of the removable prosthesis. A lingual arm is essential (Figs. 216 and 217). These attachments can also be placed buccolingually in a pontic, like other intracoronal attachments (Fig. 218).

The design and positioning of the occlusal rest influence the functions it will serve. *Blatterfein* (1969) has suggested that the

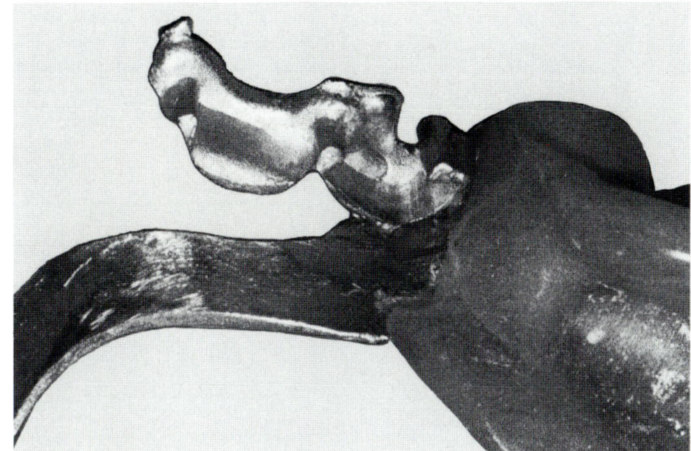

Fig. 216 Stern semi-precision attachment with lingual bracing arm.

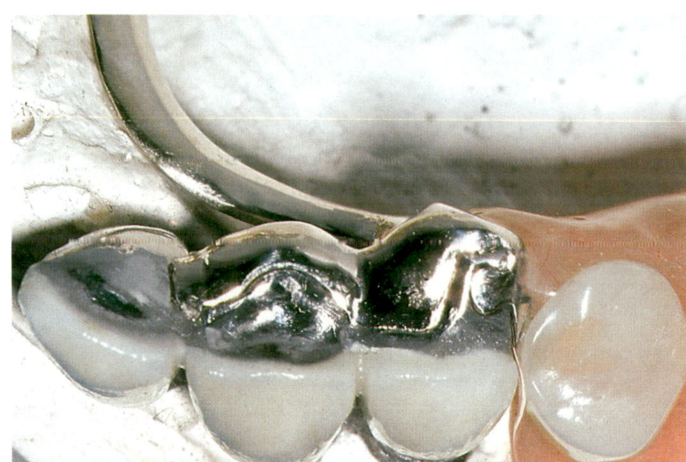

Fig. 217 The prosthesis in position.

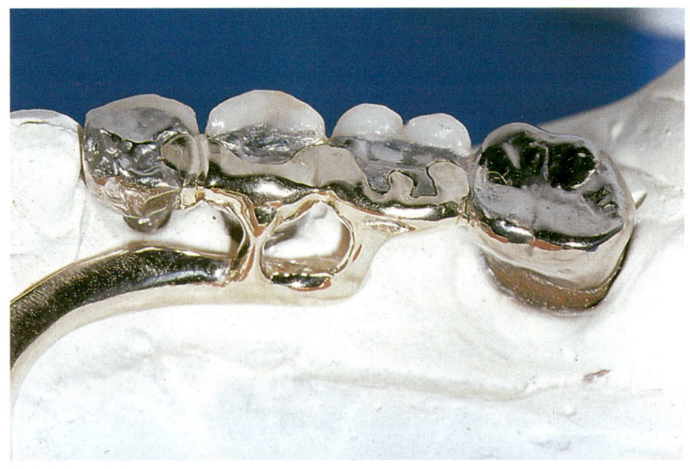

Fig. 218 Stern semi-precision retainer placed buccolingually in a pontic with associated bracing components.

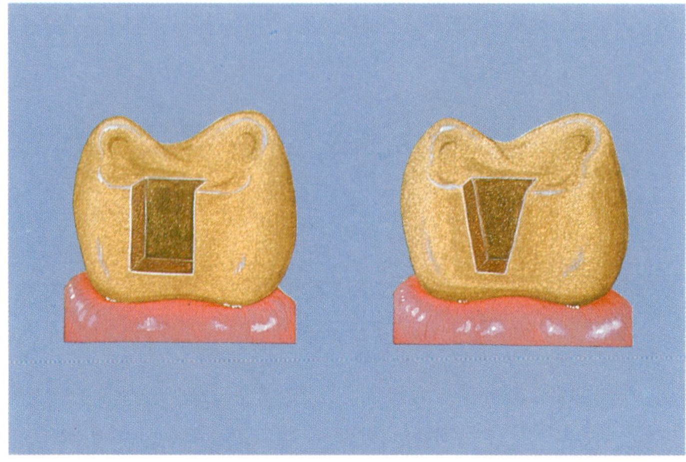

Fig. 219 Depth and taper of the rest seats influence the retention and bracing action obtained. Convergence of more than 5° significantly reduces the retention obtainable from the lateral walls of the box.

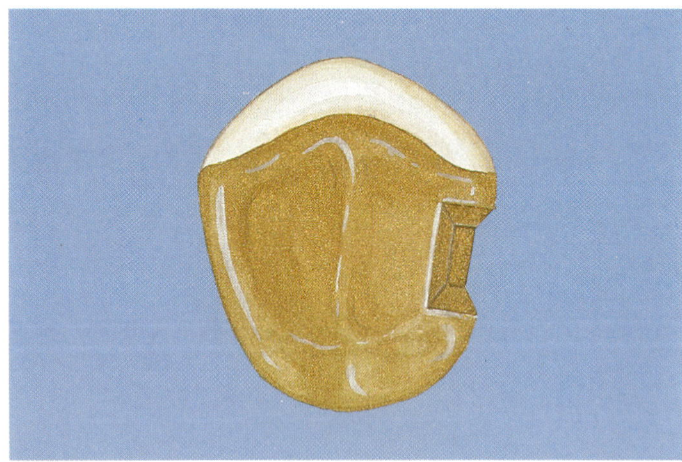

Fig. 220 The occlusal outline is basically rectangular. For strength and ease of manufacture a neck width of not less than 3 mm is recommended.

design be considered from four aspects: proximal form, occlusal form, gingival floor form, and proximal surface placement.

The depth and taper of the rest seats are important considerations of the proximal form (Fig. 219). If some measure of retention together with bracing action is required, the rest seat depth should not be less than 3 mm and the convergence of the lateral walls should not exceed 5°. Increasing the angle of convergence of the walls facilitates insertion and removal of the prosthesis, but decreases the bracing and retentive action of the unit. These properties are rapidly reduced as the rest seat depth increases.

The occlusal outline is basically rectangular (Fig. 220). For strength and ease of manufacture, a neck width of not appreciably less than 3 mm is recommended, unless a prefabricated unit is employed. A rectangular shape does not resist dis-

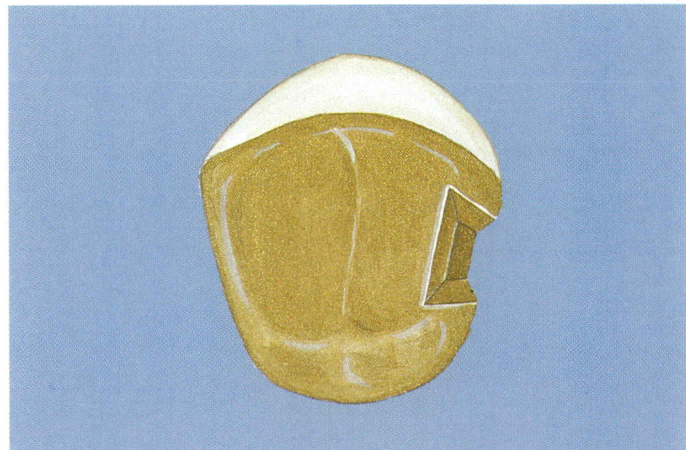

Fig. 221 Dovetail designs resist movement of the denture away from the tooth. They are desirable features of the preformed patterns, but complicate the construction of laboratory-produced units.

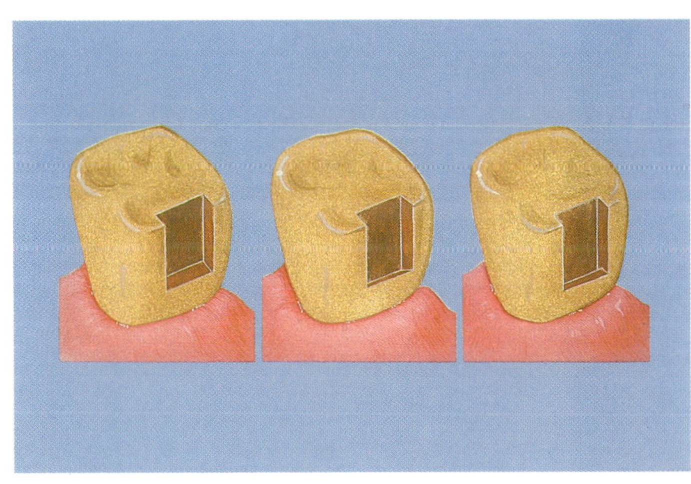

Fig. 222 A flat gingival floor is normally recommended. Inclined or channelled floors may improve the resistance to displacement, but are difficult to produce and clean.

placement of the prosthesis away from the abutment tooth (Fig. 221). When semi-precision rests are placed either side of a bounded space, this problem is of no significance. Where distal extension prostheses are concerned it does mean that a rigid component of the framework must resist this movement. Relying on a flexible lingual retainer to resist distal displacement would be foolhardy.

A preformed pattern with inclined walls has apparent advantages for distal extension prostheses. Circular or dovetail forms may be used.

Inclined and channelled floors provide additional resistance to displacement. However, it must be appreciated that they complicate construction and cleaning (Fig. 222).

Retention is provided by the lingual arm, usually engaging a dimple on the lingual surface of the crown. The free end of the

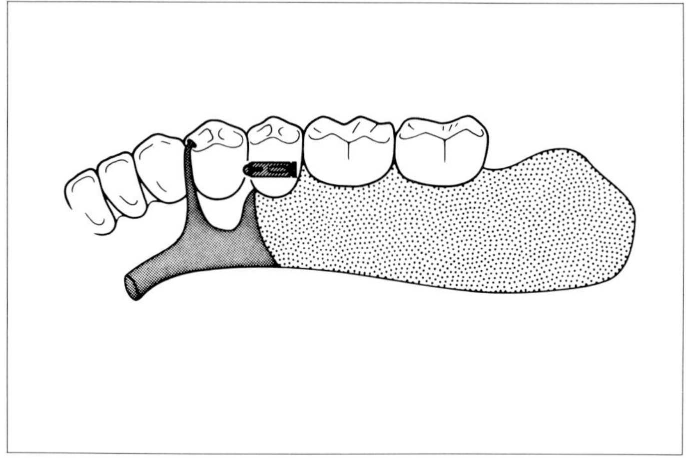

Fig. 223 The Tach-E-Z Unit. A commercially-produced spring-loaded plunger used in conjunction with a mesially placed semi-precision rest.

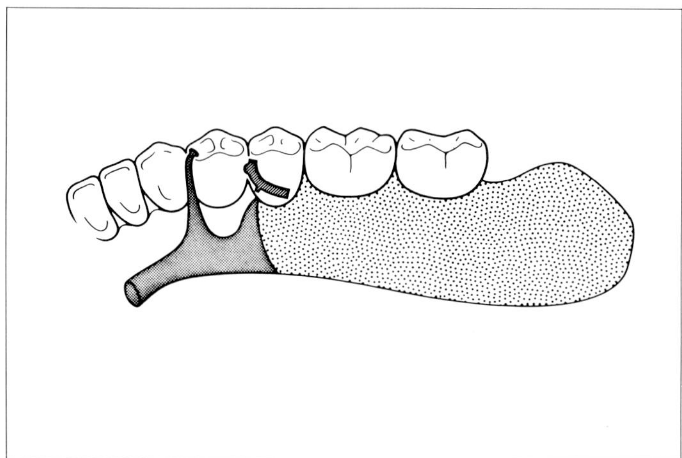

Fig. 224 The C and L Unit. This commercially-produced spring clip provides additional retention to a mesially placed occlusal rest.

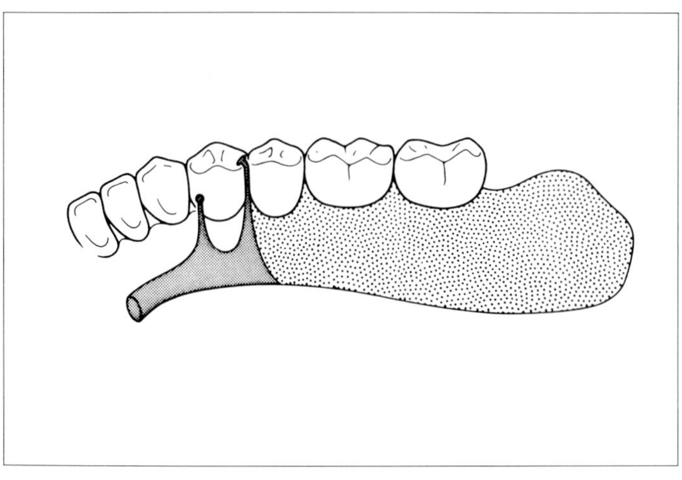

Fig. 225 A laboratory-produced retaining system employing a distally placed semi-precision rest and a lingual retaining arm engaging a dimple in the crown.

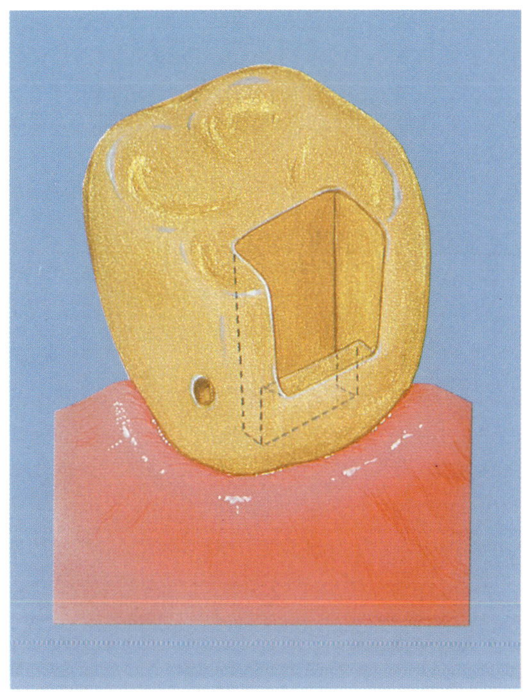

Fig. 226 The Thompson dowel. A well-tried laboratory-produced unit that enjoys popularity after more than four decades of use.

arm must therefore be flexible, although the arm will be rigid near its origin. The arm then contributes to the stability of the prosthesis and helps prevent wear of the rest.

Prefabricated retentive devices such as the Tach-E-Z and C and L system (Figs. 223 and 224) are available. A neat laboratory-produced system can also be employed (Fig. 225), but lacks the stability afforded by the lingual arm. As a result, it may need frequent adjustment to maintain retention.

The Thompson dowel semi-precision intracoronal retainer is an excellent example of a unit that enjoys popularity after more than four decades of use (Fig. 226). *Koper* (1973) and *McLeod* (1977) have analysed the unit in some detail. Apart from support

and bracing, a small degree of hinge potential is provided. Movement in the opposite direction is prevented by components acting as indirect retainers, such as the distal wall of the gingival well below the shelf and the occlusal part of the axial wall above the shelf. Retention is provided by a minor connector engaging a dimple on the lingual aspect of the crown. *Koper, Knowles* and *McLeod* have pointed out that *Thompson* was not entirely correct in assuming that the axis of hinge movement was the midwell area of the dowel. It is more likely to be in line with the inner shelf line of the retaining abutment. However, there is another point that should be considered. The design of this unit goes back to the days when considerable hinge movement was felt desirable. For this reason, the retaining dimple was placed in line with the dowel, or rest seat. Had this not been done, the retaining arm would have jumped out of its dimple each time load was applied to the denture base.

Placing the dimple in line with the rest seat introduces a complication. How do you obtain a flexible arm that runs into the dimple adjacent to the rest seat? The normal solution was to employ a split lingual connector. This type of connector, particularly in lower restorations, has proved awkward to produce, difficult to clean and prone to fracture.

Nowadays a well-made denture should have only the slightest tendency to move under load, and so there appears little drawback to placing the dimple away from the rest. The dimple can be engaged by a simple flexible arm originating from the rest. Construction and subsequent maintenance is greatly simplified, but does depend upon the production of a correctly made denture base.

Becker and others (1978) point out that the precursor to the Thompson dowel semi-precision attachment system was designed by *Clark* in 1938. *Clark* had a lingual retentive arm engaging a mesial lingual undercut, but *Thompson* later modified *Clark's* attachment system by placing the retention undercut directly on the fulcrum line. One drawback to the *Thompson* dowel concept is simply the cost of constructing a partial denture framework in gold. This can be overcome by using a chrome-cobalt major connector to which the gold alloy dowel rests are soldered. Primary retention is obtained by using stainless steel ball clasps to engage the retention dimples. The entire framework can, in fact, be cast in chrome-cobalt. Another

limitation to the Thompson dowel system is the difficulty of hand carving the dowel rest seats.

Dr *Alex Koper* writes:

Components and dimensions of the Thompson dowel retainer

'The receptacle (female) portion of the Thompson dowel retainer consists of two parts (Fig. 227). The superior part is called the tapering recess, and the inferior section is called the well. The tapering recess opens occlusogingivally (Fig. 228 a). The lingual wall of the tapering recess parallels the lingual wall of the tapering recess of the opposite side of the arch and its buccal wall flares enough to eliminate mechanical lock during function. Minimum measurements are 2.5 mm buccolingually and 3 to 3.5 mm occlusogingivally. The tapering recess extends gingivally to become the well which is oval-shaped buccolingually at the bottom and continuous with the axial, buccal and lingual walls (Fig. 228 b).

Minimum measurements for the well are about 2 mm buccolingually, 1.5 mm mesiodistally, and 1.5 to 2 mm in depth. At least 0.5 mm more depth is added for the well on a maxillary tooth because additional retention is necessary for an upper partial denture. For an upper tooth, the well should never be less than 2 mm in depth. The well is bounded proximally by the shelf with a minimum width of 1 mm.

The axial wall of the receptacle of this retainer extends from the occlusal surface of the tooth to the bottom of the well for a minimum height of 4 to 5 mm. The metal on the axial wall should be a minimal thickness of 0.4 to 0.5 mm (Fig. 228 c).

The dimensions indicated for the receptacle are minimal ones and if a tooth cannot contain them, it is too small for use as a dowel rest retainer. This condition is rarely encountered. This retainer may be adapted for use in long, short or wide crowned teeth. Dimensional variability is an important feature of this retainer.

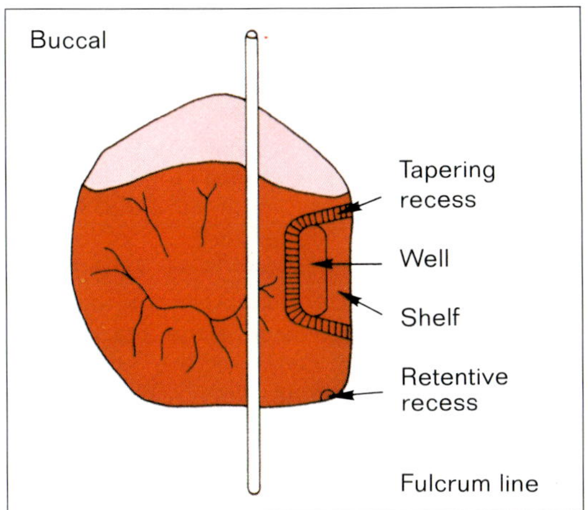

Fig. 227   An occlusal view of the receptacle of the semi-precision retainer.

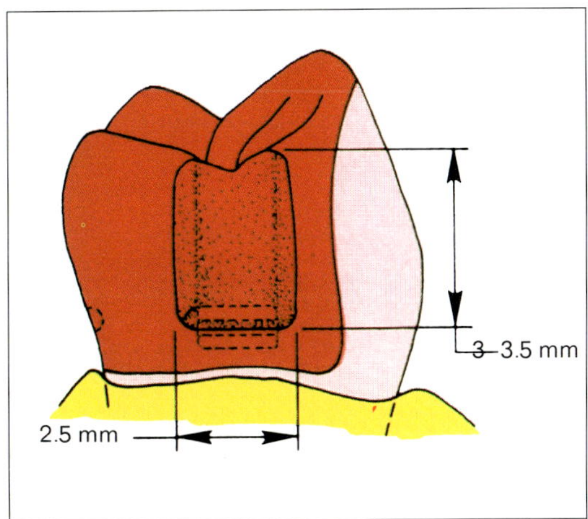

Figure 228 a

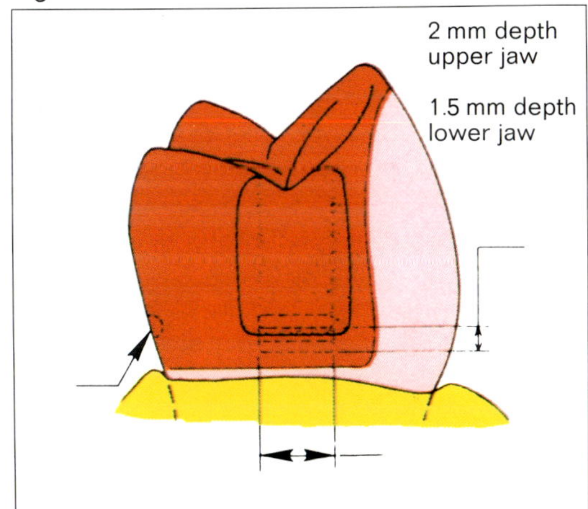

Figure 228 b

Figure 228 c

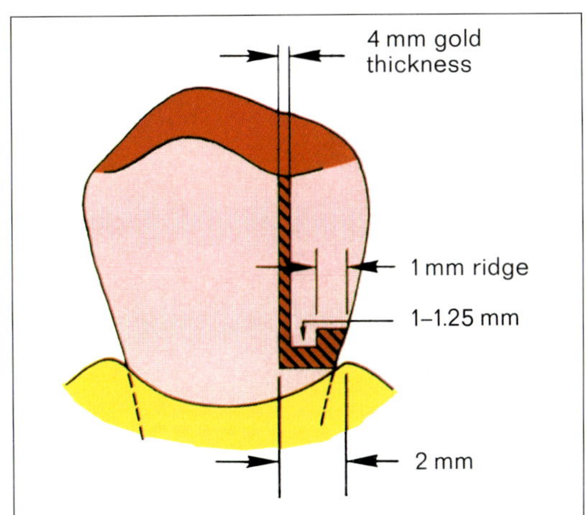

Fig. 228 (a) (b) (c)   The minimum dimensions for the receptacle should be as large as the retaining tooth allows.

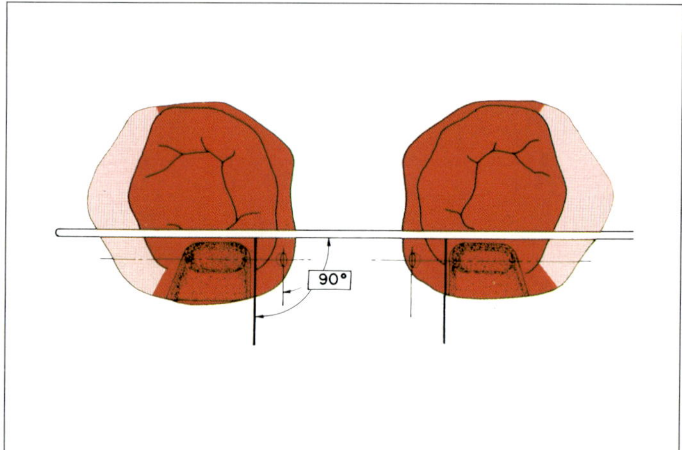

Fig. 229 The retainers on opposite sides of the dental arch are designed so that the lingual walls of the tapering recesses and wells parallel one another with just enough taper to allow for placement without binding. The lingual surfaces of the retaining teeth taper slightly toward the occlusal surface and are squared in the distolingual area opposite the shelf and well to allow for proper placement of the retentive recess.

Components should be as large as the retaining tooth permits. For example, a short but wide lower molar may have a tapering recess and well of minimum height, but the buccolingual width may be 4 to 5 mm.

The tapering recesses and wells on both retainers should be placed so that their axial walls are parallel to the fulcrum line with their lingual walls at right angles to the fulcrum line. This angulation gives proper direction to the vertical forces acting on the extension bases (Fig. 229). The retainers do not always open to the edentulous ridges. Their placement is determined by the positions of the teeth in the arch (Figs. 230 a, b and 231).

The retentive recess is located on the lingual surface of the tooth at the level of the shelf and in a line continuous with its inside edge (Fig. 232). The recess is usually one-half the depth of a No. 4 or 5 round bur and its margins are carefully polished to eliminate sharpness.

The attachment (male counterpart) is cast to fit the receptacle (female counterpart) and is continuous with the edentulous frame of the removable partial denture. The part of the attachment that fits in the well of the retaining tooth is known as the dowel (Fig. 233).

An extension of the major connector, a lingual spring-retaining arm, contains a boss which fits into the retentive recess described above. This flexible arm is located adjacent to the lingual surface of the retaining tooth and often has an extension to the mesial or distal which has no retentive features but which serves as a guiding arm to orient placement of the removable partial denture. Most dentists who describe the retaining arm mention that the retention is supplied by this lingual spring lock, while *Thompson* (1949, 1957) mentioned that *"The retentive feature of this attachment is not dependent solely on the snapped clasp but on the friction and locking effect of the dowel when the end of the saddle is displaced occlusally"*.

Positioning the retentive recesses opposite the shelf areas affords retention even during vertical loading of the extension base. The retentive recesses must be placed parallel with the fulcrum line which intersects both wells. Locating the retentive recesses off the fulcrum line is a common error.

A short removable arm is also placed inconspicuously on the buccal surface of the retaining tooth and this aids in the removal of the denture. This arm has no retentive or stabilizing features and may be removed when the patient gains familiarity with the restoration.

Fig. 230 (a) (b) The fulcrum line determines the position of the retainers in the abutment teeth.

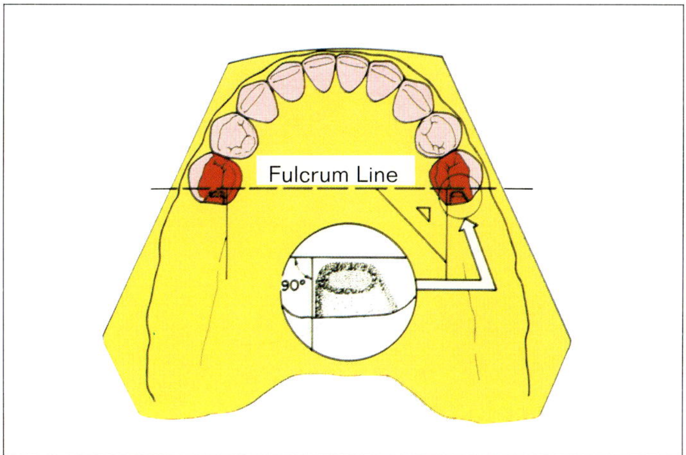

Figure 230 a

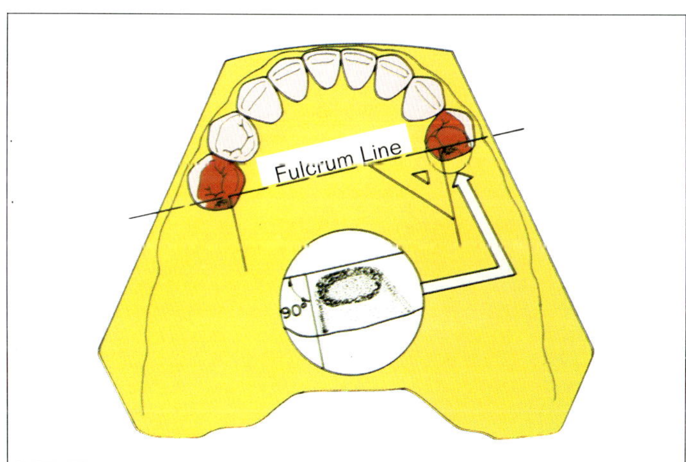

Figure 230 b

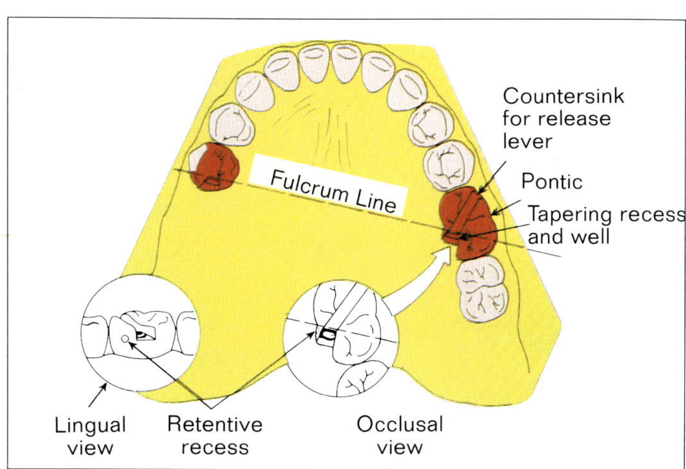

Fig. 231 The retaining recess is often placed in a pontic.

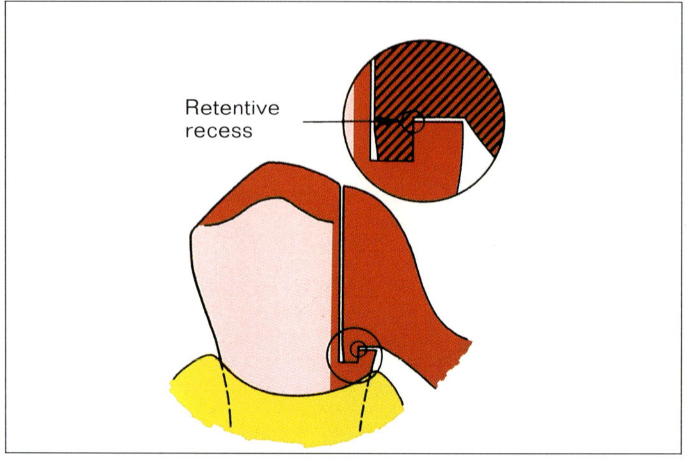

Fig. 232 The retentive recess is one-half the depth of a No. 4 or 5 round bur.

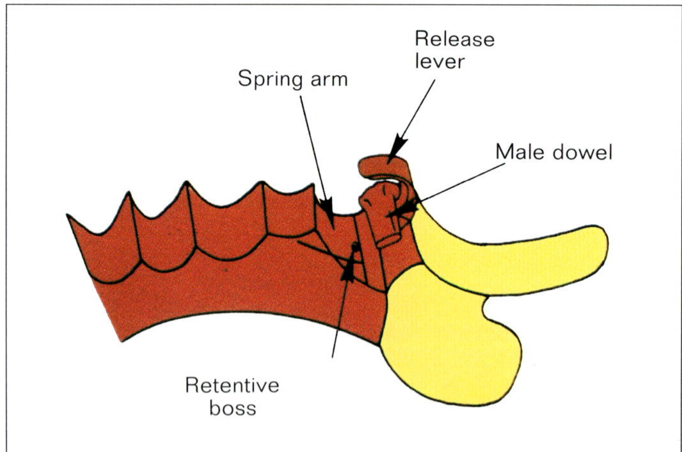

Fig. 233 The attachment of the intracoronal retainer is a part of the framework of the removable partial denture.

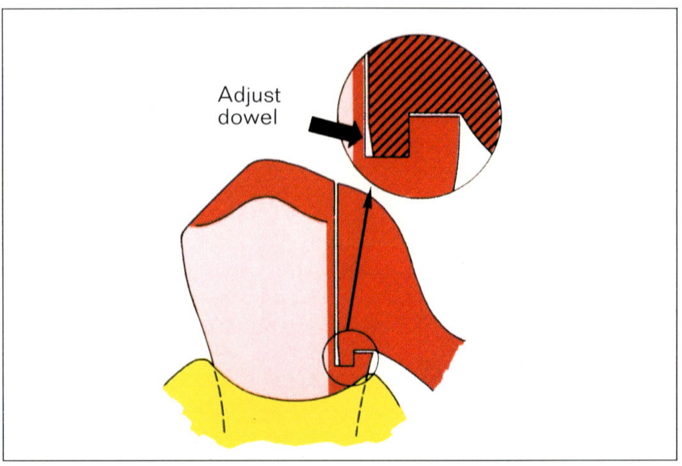

Fig. 234 The dowels are trimmed less than 0.5 mm to allow movement of the denture bases as they displace the tissues during function.

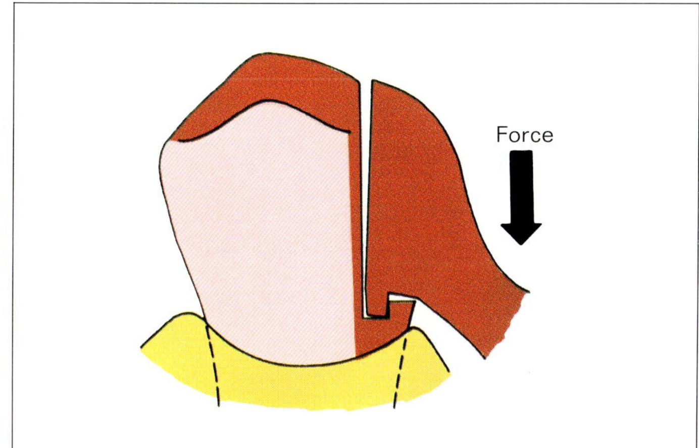

Fig. 235   Note that the occlusal portion of the dowel moves slightly posteriorly when the denture base moves towards the mucosa during function.

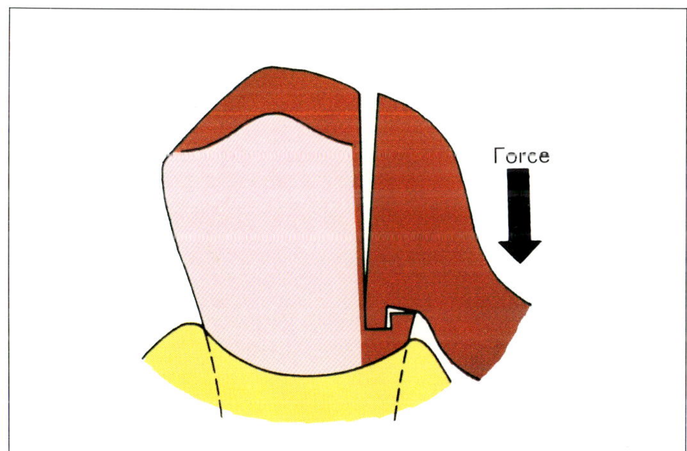

Fig. 236   Note that the shoulder of the receptacle contacts the dowel during maximum displacement of the distal extension denture base.

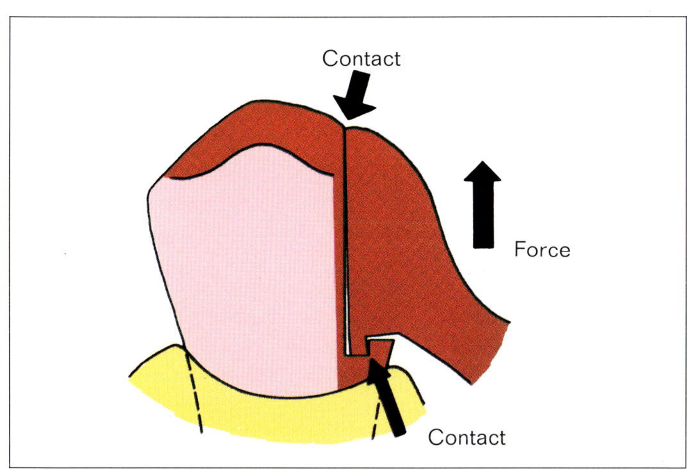

Fig. 237   The distal corner of the well must be a right angle to retain the dowel when forces pull the extension bases away from the tissues.

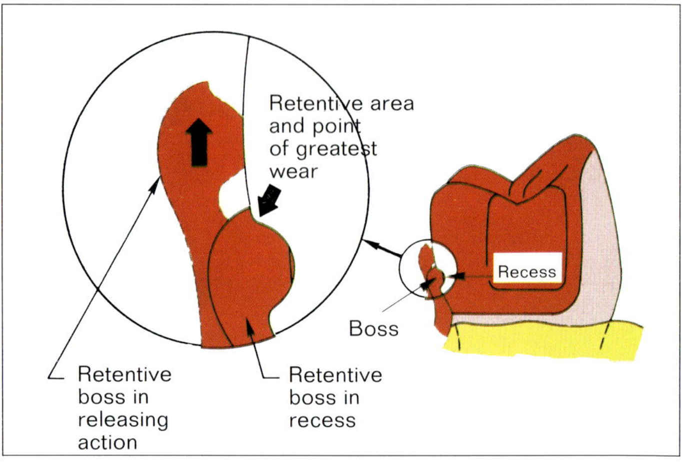

Fig. 238 The lingual retentive boss fits into the recess to provide retention for the removable partial denture.

Dynamics of function of the Thompson Dowel Retainer

Vertical support for the removable partial denture is provided by the base of the dowel as it rests in the well. Bracing is provided by the lingual walls in the retaining teeth and the seating of the dowels within the wells. Cross-arch support is also achieved by the parallel dowels in the abutment teeth on opposite sides of the dental arch (Figs. 229; 230 a, b; 231).

In distal or mesial extension removable partial dentures, pressure on the tissue-borne denture base utilizes a stress-breaking function of the retainer. The dowels are trimmed slightly in the well portion of their axial surfaces so they may tip distally in the wells and minimise torque to the abutment teeth (Fig. 234). Where the connector bearing the dowel approaches the abutment shelf, a space of 2 mm must be available to allow the dowel to rotate. As the bottom of the dowel moves slightly toward the axial abutment wall, the occlusal portion of the dowel opens slightly (Fig. 235).

The shoulder should relieve the bottom of the dowel as the distal extension denture base moves tissueward (Fig. 236). The dowel should be so designed that it does not contact the shoulder until maximum distal displacement of the denture base occurs. This movement of the attachment within the contours of the tooth, with loading close to its bony support, allows the abutment to function with a minimum of torque.

When forces pull the distal extension denture bases away from the tissues, indirect retention is achieved by the occlusal portion of the dowel as it contacts the axio-occlusal line angle in the abutment tooth (Fig. 237). The dowel moves distally at the bottom of the well and affords additional indirect retention.

Extracoronal retention is achieved when the spring-loaded lingual retaining arm seats the boss in the retentive recess (Fig. 238). The convex surface of the boss that fits into the recess is flattened slightly to minimise the movement of the spring arm. Retention occurs at the junction of the boss with the occlusal half of the retentive recess. During removal of the partial denture, the boss springs out of the recess.

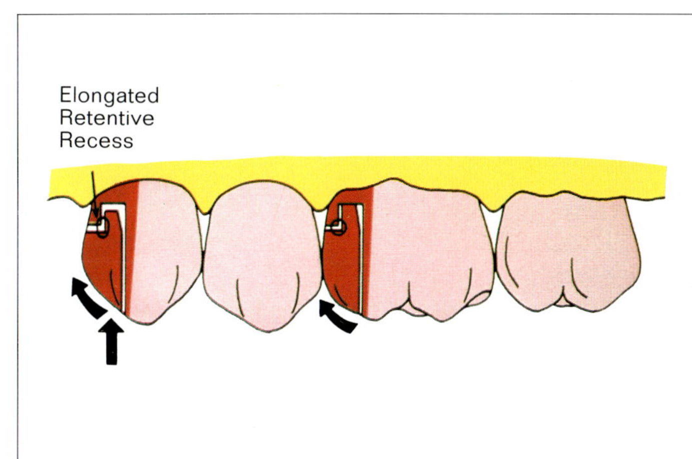

Fig. 239   The elongated retentive recess is not always necessary if there is parallelism of sliding dowels on both sides of the edentulous space.

The Sliding Dowel

Situations exist where it is necessary to allow the extension denture base to move a limited amount as the resilient tissue is displaced under stress, and yet not allow the removable partial denture to move occlusally. This is often important in a mesial extension type of removable partial denture where insufficient anterior teeth remain to support the functional load. The sliding dowel allows some vertical movement on the resilient tissues before the dowel contacts the floor of the well (Fig. 239). The recess and well are not tapered, but constructed with nearly parallel walls. The male part of the attachment is trimmed to produce the desired amount of vertical movement. If a retentive recess is used on the lingual surface of the crown, the recess is elongated gingivally to equal the amount of adjustment to the dowel. In most instances, recesses are not placed on these crowns, as it is better to place the retainers on the major retaining teeth farther back in the mouth. The sliding dowel assists indirect retention and, by limiting the amount of tissueward movement in the anterior region, maintains the proper functional relationship while providing occlusal support'.

Unlike many intracoronal attachments, the Thompson dowel does not provide a positive lock. In order to overcome problems that would arise when an altered cast impression technique is employed, an incisal hook is usually added to the framework. This incisal hook is particularly useful for orientating the removable partial denture framework on the master cast and for processing acrylic resin. It is subsequently removed following denture construction. Rebasing problems, however, are another matter and these should be considered along with extracoronal attachments that have similar problems.

There is, of course, no limit to the design and shape of retainers that can be produced in the laboratory to suit individual problems. Their versatility must be one of their greatest assets.

Semi-precision rests are simpler and more economical to employ than precision attachments. They require the preparation of few abutment teeth and allow the operator to design the unit for a particular situation.

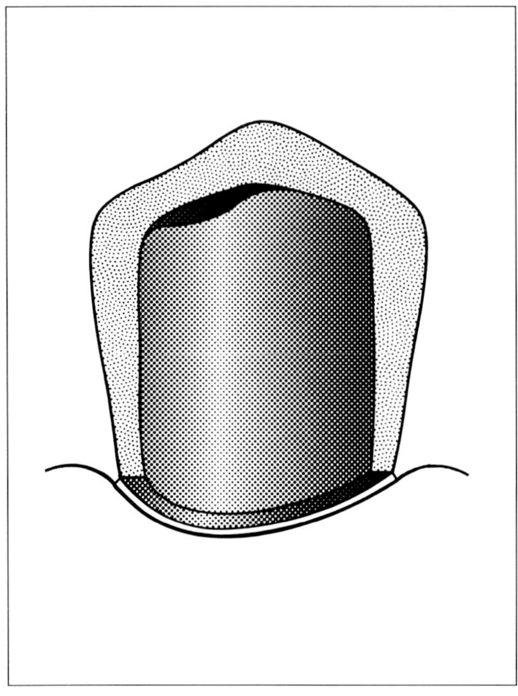

Fig. 240 A shoulder preparation results in considerable removal of tooth substance, but provides the technician with greater latitude for alignment of the attachment.

A partial or full coverage restoration is normally required in conjunction with a shoulder preparation. The full width of the shoulder should be carried through the proximal surfaces and carried onto both lingual and buccal surfaces. The semi-precision rest is neat, effective and versatile. It should be considered for use where neither the clasp nor the attachment retainer is entirely suitable.

Abutment preparations

The key to success lies in careful treatment planning. For this, all the diagnostic aids possible must be available, including full-mouth radiographs and mounted diagnostic casts. In difficult situations, the diagnostic casts may be duplicated and the duplicate set used for practise of the preparations. It takes little time and can be a valuable aid in showing up difficulties ahead. The plaster preparations may also be used as a basis upon which the temporary crowns can be made.

Recommended abutment preparations are basically full crowns modified to accommodate the female part of the attachment. This modification may take the shape of a wide shoulder carried through the proximal surface and onto the lingual surface of the tooth. Alternatively, a box may be cut in the crown preparation to accommodate the attachment. The shoulder provides the technician with greater latitude for posi-

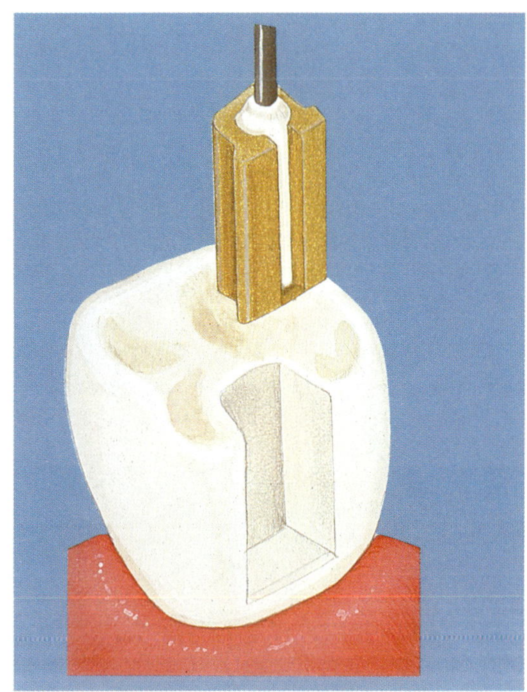

Fig. 241   Until experience is gained, the attachment can be measured against the box preparation. It is easier to judge the depth of the box by cutting it before the crown is prepared.

tioning the attachment, but results in more tooth substance removal (Fig. 240). Either way, one must be sure that adequate space has been made for the attachment if one is to avoid demoralising and time-consuming repreparation when the work has reached an advanced state. One simple method is to take the female attachment, join it to a short piece of wire with compound or plasticine, and measure it against the space that has been prepared for it. Up to 0.5 mm clearance is required for the surrounding gold (Fig. 241). When a lingual or palatal bracing arm is to be incorporated within the abutment crown, more tooth substance must be removed from these surfaces, otherwise the final crown will be bulky.

Thompson dowel retainers

Dr *Alex Koper* writes:

'All fundamentals of accurate diagnostic procedures and careful planning must be observed. Such factors as the parallelism of the retaining teeth and the position and size of the pulps of the teeth must be considered. If, after careful planning, preparations must be extended into the pulp chambers of vital teeth, prophylactic endodontic therapy is indicated. The alternative might be preparations with box forms that are too shallow, resulting in over-contoured abutment teeth which may be more detrimental to the health of the teeth than loss of vital pulps.

After the retaining teeth have been selected and a path of insertion has been determined, the preparation of the retainers should be planned from properly mounted casts. Positioning box forms of adequate dimension at right angles to the fulcrum line is one of the basic considerations in the preparation of abutment teeth. A device which has value in locating and preparing the box forms is a simple template made on the diagnostic casts when the box form areas have been identified (Figs. 242 and 243). This plastic template fits over each abutment tooth. The box form is prepared according to the outline supplied by the template. The remainder of the preparation is planned according to the dictates of occlusion and other considerations such as aesthetics, caries, parallelism and the path of insertion (Figs. 243 and 244).

Only two retaining teeth, that is, two dowel retainers, should be planned for each removable restoration. The retainers should be on opposite sides of the dental arch and if the design is properly planned will provide adequate retention. Additional dowels, without retentive recesses, may be used in certain situations, such as the sliding dowel, but retaining dowels, with their extracoronal retentive boss and recess retainers, must be limited to two teeth on extension removable partial dentures for proper function.

Design of abutments varies with the needs of the patient. Abutments must be three-quarter crowns, full crowns, or full or partial veneer crowns. The crown must be made of a metal of the same hardness as the type IV gold used in the framework of the removable partial denture. A retaining tooth partially veneered with porcelain must be made of metal of similar hardness and the wells and tapering and retentive recesses must be metal, not porcelain.

The occlusal edge of the retentive recess on the abutment tooth is subjected to wear by the convex boss of the retentive arm as it slips in and out. The shelf and other housings for the dowel will also wear unless they are made of a metal of similar hardness and resistance to abrasion as the dowel, The choice of abutment teeth is important in planning the design of these removable partial dentures. In a bilateral distal extension situation, the choice of abut-

ments is the most distal tooth adjacent to the edentulous space. In a unilateral distal extension partial denture, the tooth adjacent to the edentulous space is always used. The other retainer should be located as far distally on the other side of the dental arch as possible, but not necessarily on the most distal tooth. Much depends upon the position and strength of these teeth. Often the side opposite the edentulous space needs a fixed partial denture and the retaining recess and dowel may be placed in a pontic. The choice of the retaining teeth for Kennedy Class IV type of removable partial dentures, where the edentulous space is in the anterior region, is as far back as the first or second molars.

This dowel-retained removable partial denture offers an opportunity to replace anterior teeth where it is not possible to prepare teeth for fixed partial dentures. The missing anterior teeth may be restored with excellent retention without requiring preparations on the teeth adjacent to the edentulous space.'

Impression materials

For those brought up on reversible hydrocolloids there is no other impression material. Certainly, the combination of stone dies and reversible hydrocolloid gives an accuracy that cannot be surpassed. Where attachments with bracing arms are to be employed, many technicians prefer a plated cast. Polyethers have grown in popularity for use where tissue undercuts are small. The high stiffness of polyether materials, coupled with their medium tear energy, makes them difficult to remove from the mouth. The spacing of trays should be slightly greater than those employed for silicones or polysulphides. *Craig* (1977) has pointed out that this stiffness also dictates care when removing

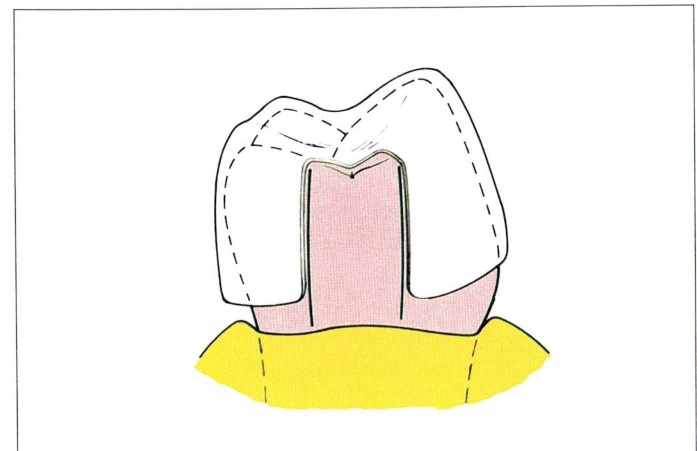

Fig. 242 The acrylic resin template provides an outline for the box form. This is followed when preparing the tooth.

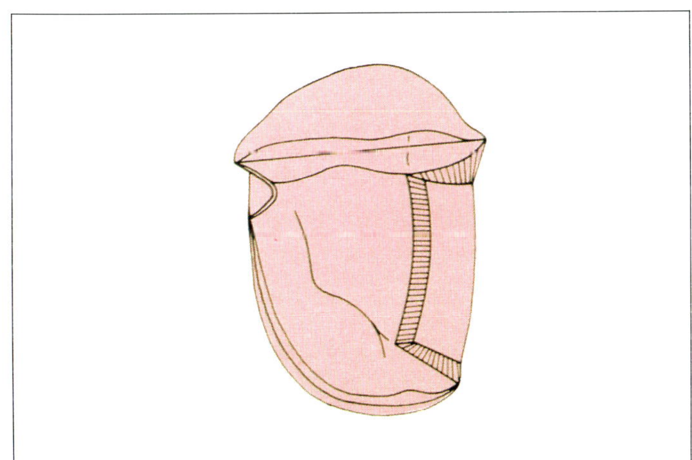

Fig. 243 A typical preparation is modified to accommodate the box form.

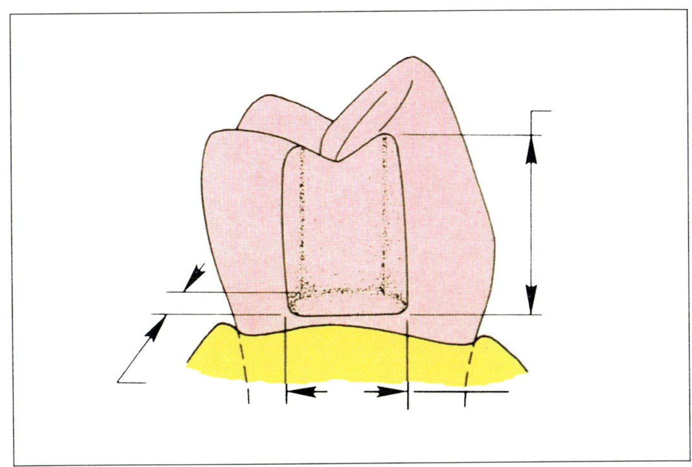

Fig. 244 A proper box form assures intracoronal placement of the retainer, a fundamental which should not be overlooked in preparing the retaining tooth.

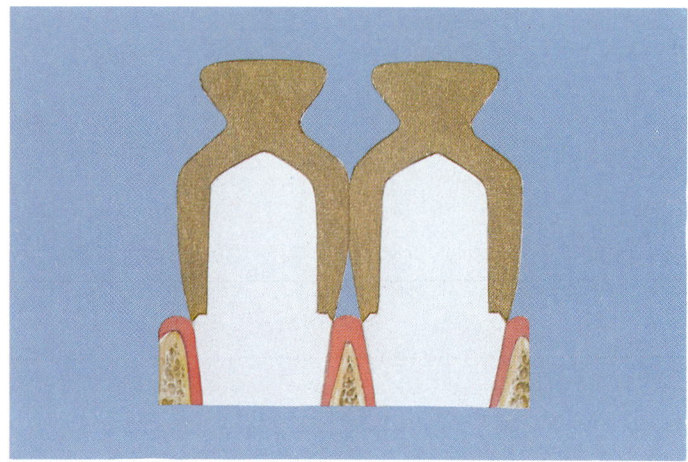

Fig. 245 Cast metal transfer copings should have small holes cut near the incisal edges to ensure correct seating. Copings on adjacent teeth should be checked to ensure they do not interfere with each other's seating.

gypsum products from the impression. The accuracy of polyether is among the highest of all elastomeric impression materials, but its dimensional accuracy is only good if the impression is kept dry. Silver-plated polyether impressions are more accurate than other materials (0.005 % compared with 0.056 % for polysulphide rubber), a useful property to bear in mind when plated casts are required.

Mercaptan rubbers are easier to remove from the mouth and can be silver-plated. Polyether and mercaptan rubbers require a closely adapted rigid acrylic resin tray. Flexing of poorly made trays under load is one of the most common causes of subsequent problems with castings.

With all elastomeric materials, problems appear to resolve around providing healthy gingival tissues, correct placement of margins and adequate retraction.

Frowned upon by many as out of date, the copper ring technique is capable of producing excellent results. It is still used by at least one of the world's authorities on fixed prosthodontics. Having obtained individual impressions of each preparation, the problem is then one of location. Metal transfer copings are recommended, although Duralay resin copings can be used with care (Fig. 245). Copings must have windows to ensure correct seating and adjacent copings connected in the mouth with resin. Plaster is still the most reliable overall locating impression, it is rigid and tends to absorb the slight moisture occasionally overlooked on copings.

Having made facebow and jaw relationship recordings, the master cast can be mounted on the articulator and the metal framework tested for accuracy. Intracoronal attachments are precise testers of impression accuracy. In fixed restorations, errors of location show up in two ways. The prosthesis may not slide into place, or it may do so by disturbing the seating of one of the crowns. Either way the fault must be found, the casting sectioned with a disc and a plaster or polyether locating impression made. Where the error is due to an inaccurate die, the casting of the preparation concerned must be removed, the remainder of the metalwork placed in the mouth, and an overall impression of the preparation made. The metalwork is removed with the impression. Polysulphides and mercaptan rubbers are best for this method.

When a removable partial denture is retained by intracoronal attachments, the impression procedure is modified. The initial impression procedure is identical to that of a fixed prosthesis, but the female attachments are subsequently aligned and included in the casting. Having checked the accuracy of the abutment castings, the denture framework can be made. There is one frequent problem however. In sectioning the cast to produce the dies, the region corresponding to the denture-bearing area is often damaged, and a new impression is required. To accomplish this, construct a rigid acrylic resin tray, spaced over the castings but closely adapted over the denture-bearing area. Place the castings in the mouth, ensure they are dry, and make an overall impression in which the castings are removed. Polyether impressions are excellent for this step. The cast can then be rearticulated and the denture framework made.

For distal extension prostheses, an altered cast technique is preferred. Impression techniques for these situations are considered in further detail in Chapter 4.

The denture framework is made and the denture base area covered with closely adapted acrylic resin bases. The abutment crowns are placed in the mouth, the adaptation of the framework assessed and the borders of the bases examined. The framework is now removed and a zinc-oxide impression paste or fluid wax* placed in the acrylic resin bases before the framework is reseated. No seating load must be applied to the occlusal aspects of the bases —only to the metal components of the framework. Remove the denture, together with abutment crowns, to preserve intact details of the distal gingivae. The master cast is now sectioned to remove the areas corresponding with the edentulous ridge. This allows the crowns and connected denture to be placed on the remains of the cast. Stone can now be poured into the impression surface of the denture base to reconstitute the cast. Intracoronal attachments are particularly useful in this manner because of their precise location and lack of movement potential. Where the abutments represent most or all of the remaining teeth in the arch, a modified approach is recommended. The abutment crown and denture framework are removed in an overall alginate impression. The dies are placed in their respective crowns and a new master cast poured.

Inserting the restoration

Large restorations are best inserted with a temporary non-setting cement for a period of several days. This period of trial insertion allows the restoration to be removed and polished after any subsequent corrections to the occlusal surfaces have been made. It also allows inspection of the plaque control of proximal spaces and

---

* Korecta Wax, D & R Miner Dental, 14 Lavina Court, Orinda, California 94563, USA.

these spaces can be modified if necessary. This trial period might also allow for slight tooth movement to compensate for any minute migrations that might have occurred while the prosthesis was being constructed.

The precise location necessary for intracoronal attachments can be disturbed by the layer of cement between crown and preparation; it would be disastrous to spoil the whole restoration at this late stage by such an error. To prevent this mishap, no crown or group of crowns should be cemented unless all the other components are placed in the mouth before the cement has hardened. Following removal of excess cement, patients with removable prostheses can be sent away for 24 hours, with instructions not to remove their dentures.

At the next visit, the occlusion and articulation are checked. The adaptation of the denture base to the mucosa is checked with disclosing paste. If an error has occurred in this respect the denture will need to be rebased immediately.

With the aid of a large mirror the patient is shown how to remove the prosthesis and to reinsert it. A demonstration model or diagram is useful to explain the term 'path of insertion'. Above all, the danger of applying force to the prosthesis must be stressed. With a bilateral prosthesis, considerable leverage can be exerted if only one side is moved.

Cleaning instructions should reinforce not only plaque control, but also denture hygiene. The female units may be cleaned with an 'interspace' toothbrush that is also useful for cleaning around the male attachment.

Once the patient can manipulate his pros-

thesis he may be seen one week later, and subsequently in one month for the final post-insertion checks and post-treatment radiographs. Regular 6-monthly examinations should then suffice.

Adjustment of retention

Clumsy adjustment of intracoronal attachments is the one clinical procedure that is most likely to result in breakage. It must be carried out very carefully and in small stages according to the detailed instructions given by manufacturers.

With a precise path of insertion and large contact areas, only the smallest adjustments are required to produce a surprising difference in retention. Attachments such as the Stern G/L with auxiliary retentive features require special adjustment instruments. For most of the European attachments, spring replacements or retaining clip adjustments may be necessary. A screwdriver of the correct size should be available. With the correct instrument, adjustment takes only a few moments, without it the attempt may not only fail but damage the attachment as well.

Intracoronal attachments with small slots, like the Stern G/A and McCollum units, can be adjusted with an annealed razor blade. The razor blade is simply inserted into the slot, thereby opening it very slightly.

Other types of attachment, such as the Chayes and smallest Crismani, can be adjusted with a small jeweller's screwdriver.

Over a period of years there seems to be a tendency for the female sections of the

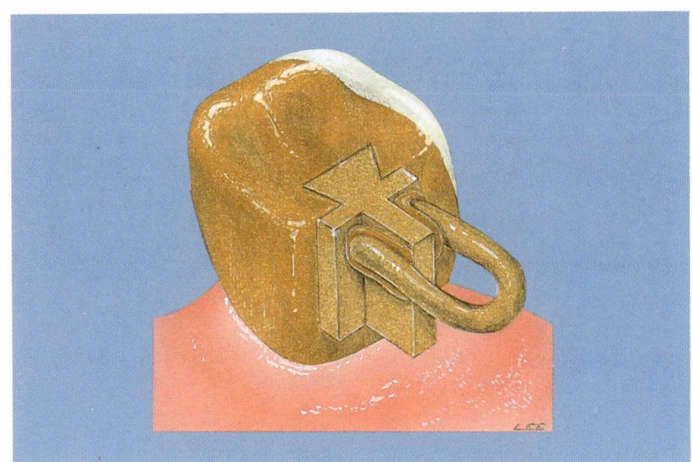

Fig. 246 Tagging soldered to the male section of the intra-coronal attachment to facilitate its withdrawal in the impression.

attachments to open slightly; this type of wear or distortion occurs more rapidly with patients who tend to use excessive force when inserting their prosthesis. A lingual bracing arm reduces this type of wear and also lessens the effect of such wear as it occurs. Oversize male attachments, available for some of the Stern range of units, are useful for repairing this type of damage.

Remaking a removable prosthesis

Remaking a removable prosthesis retained by intracoronal attachments presents one particular problem—that of reproducing the slots of the female section of the attachments.

The most reliable method involves placing the male attachments in the mouth to engage the corresponding female slots. Additional tagging is soldered to these male units (Fig. 246) enabling them to be removed in an overall impression. Where possible, the tagging of the two male units should be joined by wire and united to it with self-polymerising acrylic resin. Plaster used to be the most popular localising material, but its use required extremely careful waxing out of proximal spaces and other undercut areas. Furthermore, the impression obtained was seldom satisfactory for partial denture construction. Polyether materials, such as Impregum, are more straightforward to employ and provide best results if used in a carefully adapted acrylic resin tray. Waxing out of proximal spaces is still important, while the tagging and connecting elements must be scrupulously dried before the impression material is inserted. Before casting the impression, matching female units are inserted over the male sections of the attachments. In this way the new master cast incorporates the actual female sections of the attachments.

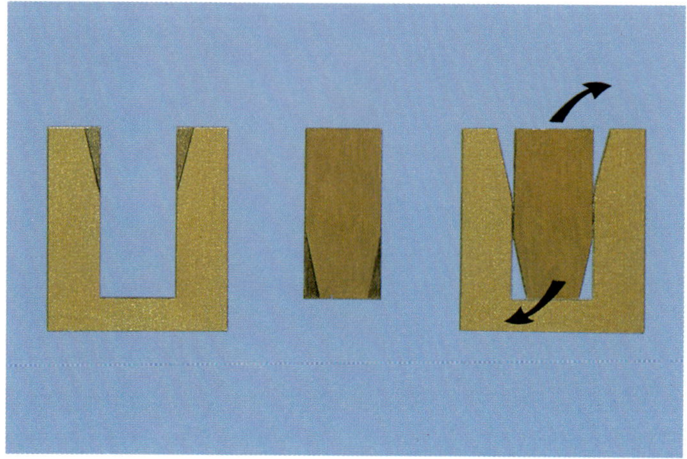

Fig. 247 The pattern of wear is usually more pronounced at the gingival portion of the male section and the occlusal third of the female section. This wear may result not only in loss of retention, but also in loss of bracing action.

Technical considerations

Most manufacturers provide detailed technical advice on the use of their attachments. The operator should be familiar with some of the factors involved as several technical aspects influence the design of the restoration.

An intracoronal attachment provides a removable prosthesis with direct retention, resistance to dislodgement along the path of insertion, and also first-class resistance to horizontal and rotational displacing forces. The direct retention is provided by the entire surface of contact together with a mechanical retentive device, if this is incorporated. The lateral aspects of the attachment play an important part in its resistance to horizontal and rotational displacing forces. These lateral aspects are usually small and in many attachments they cannot be adjusted once worn. An attachment with a spring-loaded tensioning device may have its retention increased by substituting a spring with greater tension.

However, this does not directly affect its ability to resist horizontal and rotational displacing forces, so that while the prosthesis might stay in place, it might still feel slack to the patient. This example may overstate the case because increasing the retention of an attachment is not without effect on its bracing action, but it does show the importance of designing the prosthesis to protect the lateral surfaces of the attachments. The pattern of wear is seldom even, and is usually more noticeable at the gingival portion of the male unit and the occlusal third of the female slot (Fig. 247). Where patients have been clumsy, the female slot may in fact be distorted.

Distortion of the female section may also be seen in a mesiodistal direction, but is usually limited to the area adjacent to the occlusal surface (Fig. 248).

Most attachment wear occurs when a prosthesis is being inserted and removed. Wear of attachments can and does take place while they are in position, but it appears that the amount of wear that takes place is comparatively small. Attachments serving the functions of connectors between two fixed prostheses wear far less than those anchoring a removable prosthesis to its abutments.

A patient may insert and remove the prosthesis several times a day, so that the attachments may wear over a period of years. Few patients can consistently slide their prostheses in and out of place without a few false start. Each time they make a mistake the appliance will jam and must go back to its original position before a fresh attempt is made. It takes little imagination to visualise the effect upon the attachments.

Lingual bracing arms are most effective methods of providing additional guide planes. They help the patient find the correct path of insertion, protect the lateral surfaces of the attachment when mistakes occur, and aid the patient to insert and remove the prosthesis. The vertical wall should be of the greatest possible extent and aligned with the attachment (Fig. 249). Where lingual space is restricted, the step can be made near the occlusal surface and a skirt of gold carried down the lingual surface of the tooth (Fig. 250). Where space permits, two steps can be made in the lingual surface to strengthen the arm. If possible, the lingual arm should be carried around the tooth above the next proximal space (Fig. 251). Making a groove for the free end of the bar will strengthen this component and aid retention. It will also resist any tendency to distort the attachment in a mesiodistal direction.

Wear of an attachment in the mouth is usually caused by inadequate heat treatment and by its resistance to horizontal and ro-

tational displacing forces. While these forces may cause the attachments to wear, the effect they may have on the supporting structures of the teeth and denture-bearing areas are more serious. This is one reason why careful planning is so important, for only in this way can the prosthesis be designed and constructed so that it carries out its functions while being subjected to the minimum of displacing forces. Loads falling on the prosthesis can be reduced by attention to jaw relationship records and by keeping the occlusal table as narrow as possible, for this decreases the force required to penetrate a bolus of food. It also reduces the torques resulting from masticatory and non-masticatory contacts (Fig. 252). A short occlusal table reduces the leverages of vertical and horizontal loads applied to the attachments of distal extension prostheses (Fig. 253).

Nearly all vertical and horizontal loads applied to the base will be transmitted to the abutment tooth through the neck of the male attachment. The severest loads are likely to be applied when the patient inserts and removes the prosthesis, especially before he has learnt to find the path of insertion. While an attachment of adequate neck width must be chosen, Figure 254 shows that a wide neck considerably decreases the amount of contact area available for retention. In making the compromise, the functions served by the attachment must be borne in mind. For example, an attachment retaining a distal extension prosthesis is likely to be subjected to far greater loads than one joining two sections of a fixed prosthesis.

Aligning the female sections of the attachments within their respective crowns finally determines the path of insertion of the

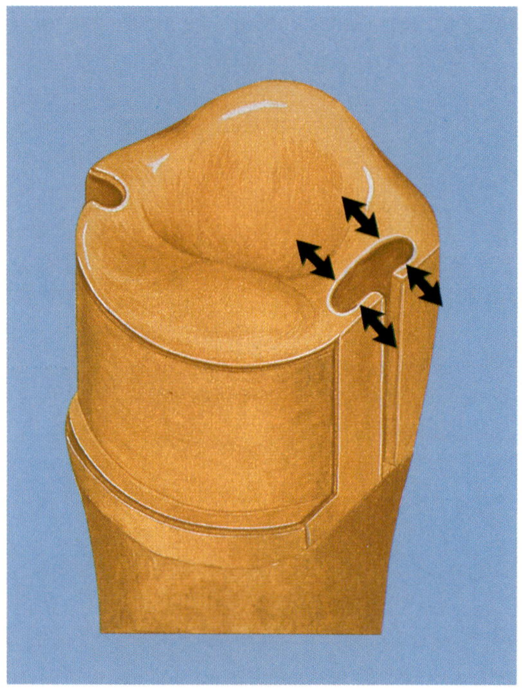

Fig. 248 The occlusal section of the slot is most prone to distortion.

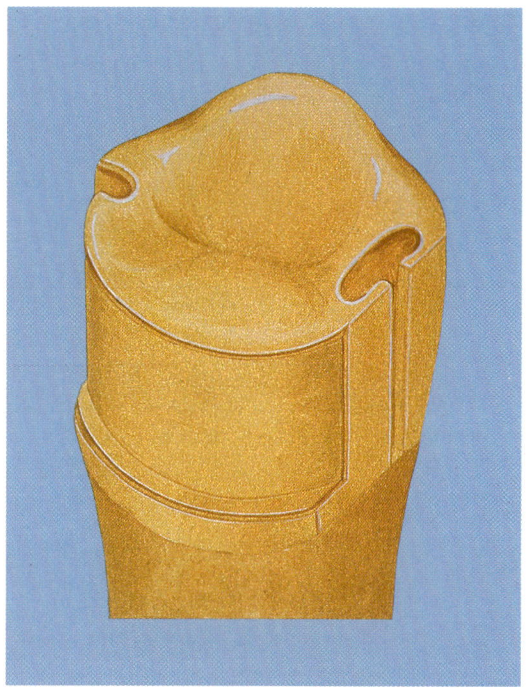

Fig. 249 The lingual bracing arm should be of the greatest possible vertical extent with an additional groove to aid retention. The groove contributes to a more rigid arm.

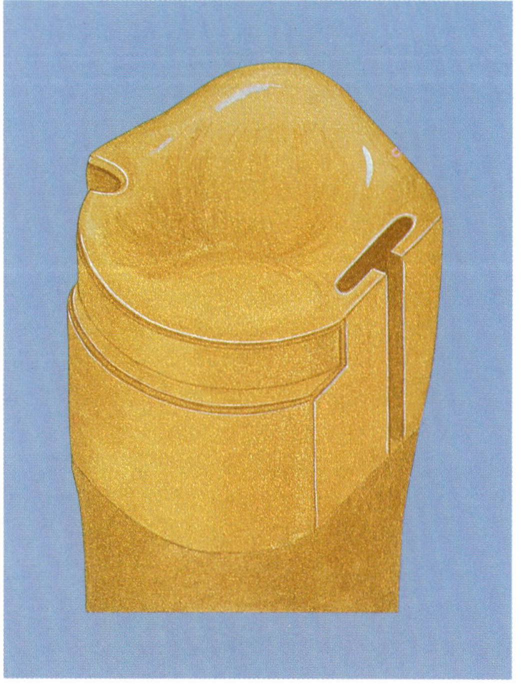

Fig. 250 Step placed near occlusal surface reduces buccolingual space requirements.

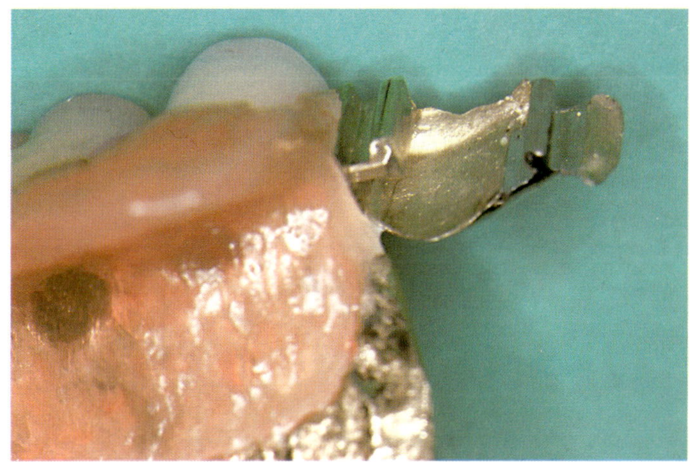

Fig. 251 Extended lingual bracing arm.

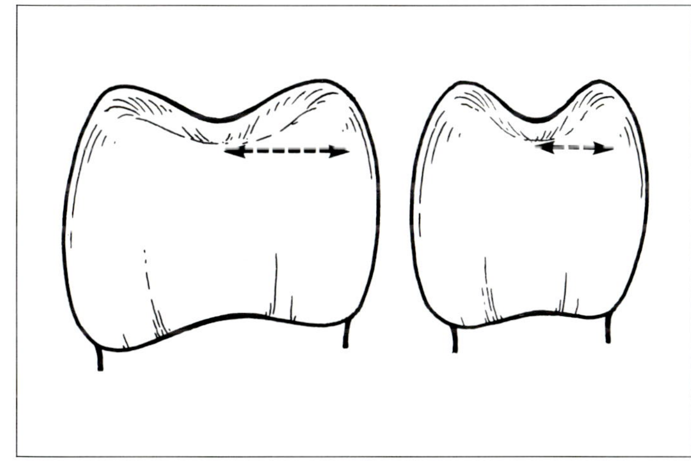

Fig. 252 The force required to penetrate a bolus of food is reduced if the occlusal table is kept narrow. The torques resulting from masticatory and nonmasticatory contacts are also lessened.

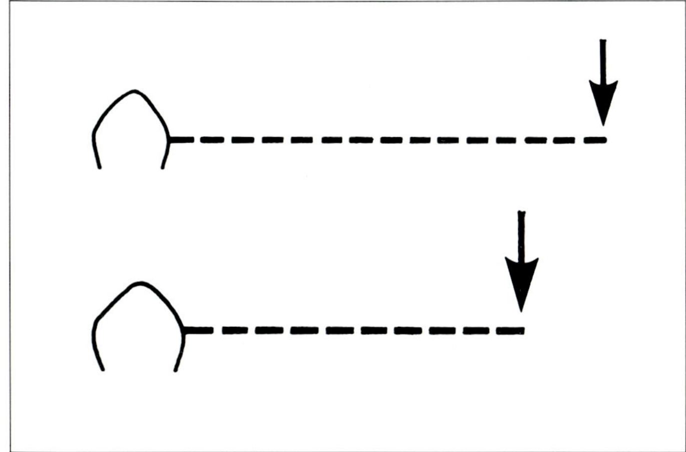

Fig. 253 Where possible, a distal extension prosthesis should have a short artificial occlusal table, for it reduces the leverages exerted by vertical and horizontal loads.

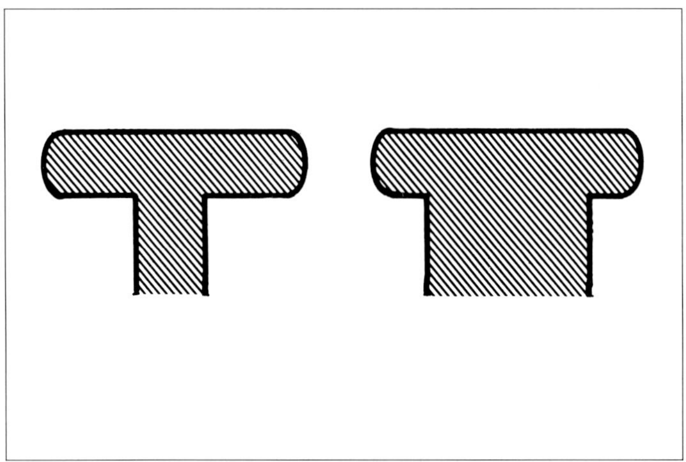

Fig. 254 A wide neck decreases the contact area available for the attachment.

denture. It is a critical stage carried out in the laboratory on the mounting base of an absolutely rigid surveyor. The path of insertion is chosen at the treatment planning stage and should be clearly marked on both the side and back of the diagnostic cast to show the degree of antero-posterior and lateral tilt required. In selecting the path of insertion, the contours of the edentulous areas must be considered (Fig. 255). If this is not carried out, the denture base extension will be jeopardised. Small alterations to this path may be necessary to make up for minor discrepancies between the alignment of the preparations and their planned alignment.

Most manufacturers provide a small surveying rod, modified to fit the female attachment at one end and the surveyor arm at the other, so that with the aid of this mounting jig, the attachment can be carried into place (Fig. 256).

If each attachment is carefully positioned in its waxed-up crown in this manner, all the attachments will be mutually parallel pro-

vided that no movement of the mounting table has occurred. Of course, the cast must be solidly clamped to the surveyor table, while the table itself must lock rigidly in place.

This is the stage at which the step should be cut in the lingual surface of the waxed-up crown to accommodate the bracing arm.

The female part of the attachment can be soldered to the cast crown, or the crown can be cast around the attachment. The first method is more straightforward, but cannot be used with platinised golds. The female part of the attachment is slid out of the waxed-up crown, leaving behind a rectangular space. The crown is then cast and the final localisation of the attachment is carried out on the surveyor when the attachment is carefully inserted into its rectangular box. The attachment is then held in place with Duralay* or inlay wax, so that

* Reliant Dental Mfg. Co. Worth, Illinois, USA.

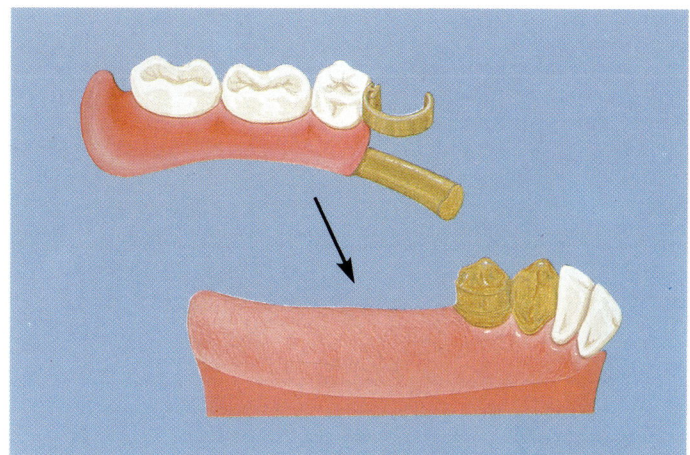

Fig. 255 The contours of the denture base area must be considered when deciding upon the path of insertion.

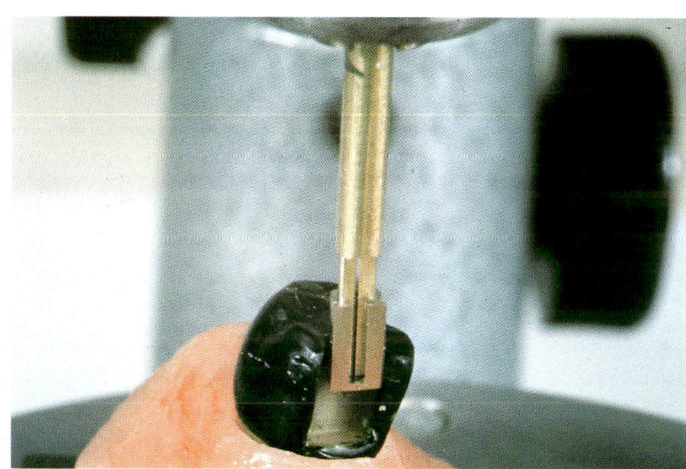

Fig. 256 The attachment is carried into place in the waxed-up crown by means of a special surveying rod fitting the attachment at one end and the surveyor arm at the other.

it can be invested and soldered. This technique gives the technician greater control of the final localisation and removes any possibility of inaccuracies due to the attachment moving during the casting process. Accidental flow of gold into the attachment is also prevented. In fact, this technique has to be used for most of the normal yellow gold alloys.

Attachments made of highly-platinised alloys, such as those used with bonded porcelain/gold, usually require a different technique. In this case the crown is cast around the attachment, taking care to ensure that the internal surface of the attachment is filled with investment or a suitably shaped carbon rod. This removes the need to use a special solder with its potential difficulties in bonding.

Carbon rods are provided by some manu-

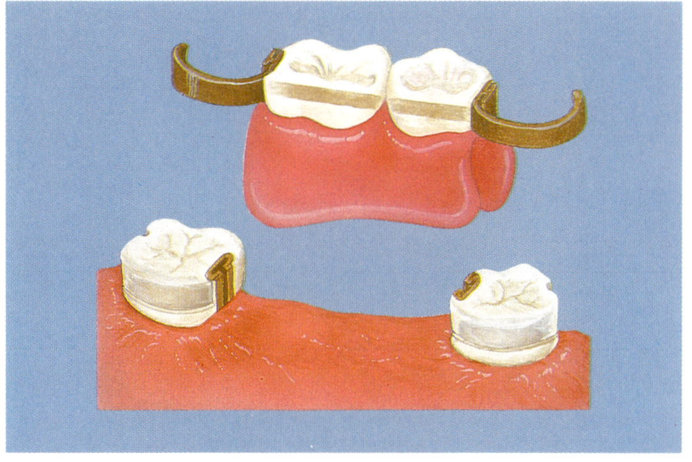

Fig. 257 The male attachments either end of a unilateral prosthesis may be soldered to a metal structure running the length of the restoration.

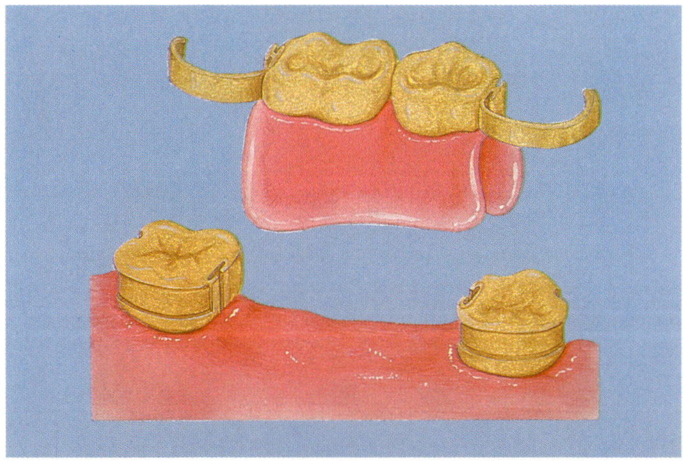

Fig. 258 The attachments can be soldered to gold occlusal surfaces.

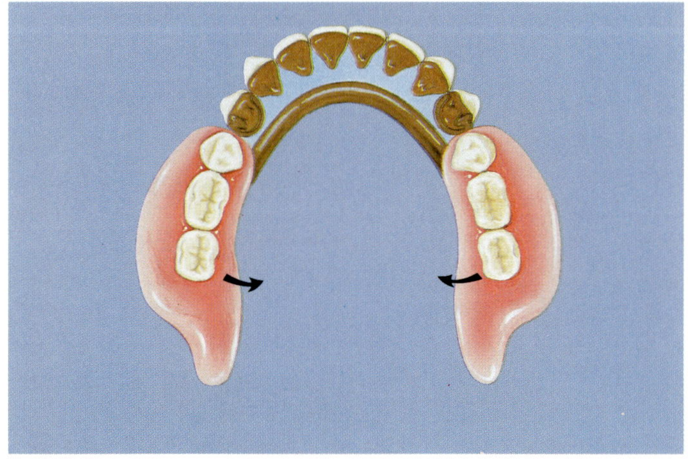

Fig. 259 A bilateral prosthesis is able to resist horizontal loads between the teeth and mucosa of both sides, while rotational loads applied to one side are resisted by the retainers of the opposite side acting with considerable mechanical advantage.

facturers to hold the attachment in the investment and prevent the flow of gold within the attachment.

When constructing a unilateral prosthesis, the male attachments on either end of the base may be joined by a gold bar running its entire length (Fig. 257).

A more satisfactory and neater method is to join the attachments to the metal of a gold occlusal surface (Fig. 258). By connecting the male attachments the following advantages are gained:

1. The retention of the attachments to the acrylic resin is improved. There is then little danger of the patient tearing the denture base away from the male attachments.
2. Processing changes of the acrylic resin will have minimal effect on the location of the attachments.
3. Accidental breakages of the acrylic resin of the base are unlikely to affect the all-important location of the attachments.

Where bilateral prostheses are concerned, the major connector provides valuable cross-arch bracing. As a result of this bracing action, horizontal loads are resisted by an increased surface area, and rotational loads applied to one side of the jaw are resisted by the retainers of the opposite side, acting with a considerable mechanical advantage (Fig. 259).

The major connector can only serve these functions if it is sufficiently rigid, while the attachments should be joined to the major connector. Small joining bars within the denture base may be necessary for this purpose. The connector must be able to resist forces applied when the patient inserts and removes the prosthesis.

Incorrect heat treatment of attachments is a common cause of failure. The required procedures differ according to the gold alloys employed, but manufacturers invariably give precise recommendations. Salt baths or other instruments for careful control of these procedures should have a place in any laboratory concerned with attachment work. There can be little excuse for lack of attention to these details which, if ignored, can result in speedy failure of complex and costly restorations. The heat treatment techniques therefore merit a great deal of care.

References and further reading

Abrams L. and Feber M. (1962).
Periodontal considerations for removable prostheses. Alpha Omega Fraternity (Sept).

Baker J. L. and Goodkind R. J. (1981).
Theory and Practice of Removable Partial Dentures. C. V. Mosby, St. Louis, Mo.

Bartlett A. A. (1966).
Duplication of precision attachment partial dentures. J. Prosthet. Dent., 16, 6: 1111.

Becker C. M., Campbell H. C. and Williams D. L. (1978).
The Thompson dowel-rest system modified for chrome-cobalt removable partial denture frameworks J. Prosthet. Dent., 39, 4: 384.

Blatterfein L. (1969).
The use of the semi-precision rest in removable partial dentures. J. Prosthet. Dent., 22, 3: 307.

Brecker S. C. (1966).
Clinical Procedures in Occlusal Rehabilitation. Saunders, Philadelphia and London.

Brodbelt R. H. W. (1972).
A simple parallelling template for precision attachments. J. Prosthet. Dent., 27, 3: 285.

Brown D. (1973).
Factors affecting the dimensional stability of elastic impression materials. J. Dent., 1: 265.

Caldarone C. V. (1957).
Attachments for partial dentures without clasps. J. Prosthet. Dent., 7, 2: 206.

Carr C. M. (1898).
Anchored adjustable dentures. Dent. Cosmos., 40: 2119.

Chayes H. (1910).
Empiricism of bridgework. Dent. Items Interest, 32: 745.

Chayes H. (1915).
Principles, functions and construction of saddles in bridgework. Dent. Items Interest, 37: 831.

Chayes H. (1917).
System of movable, removable bridgework in conformity with the principle that 'teeth move in function'. Dent. Rev., 31: 87.

Craig R. G. (1977).
Status report on polyether impression materials. JADA, 95: 126.

Eich F. A. (1962).
The role of partial dentures in the destruction of the natural dentition. Dent. Clin. N. Amer., 717.

Evans G. (1888).
A Practical Treatise on Artificial Crown and Bridge Work. The S. S. White Metal Mfg. Co., Philadelphia.

Evans G. E. (1905).
A Practical Treatise on Artificial Crown, Bridge and Porcelain Work. pp. 304–314. S. S. White Dental Mfg. Co., Philadelphia.

Gilmore S. F. (1913).
A method of retention. Council of Allied Dental Soc., 8: 118.

Goldman H. M. and Burket L. W. (1959).
Treatment Planning in the Practice of Dentistry. C. V. Mosby, St. Louis, Mo.

Goslee H. J. (1912).
Removable bridgework. Dent. Items Interest, 34: 731.

Grosser D. (1953).
The dynamics of internal precision attachments. J. Prosthet. Dent., 3, 3: 393.

Harris F. N. (1955).
The precision dowel rest attachment J. Prosthet. Dent., 5, 1: 43.

Hollenback E. A. and Oaks S. (1950).
Role of precision attachments in partial denture prosthesis. J. Amer. Dent. Ass., 41: 173.

Knowles L. E. (1963).
A dowel attachment removable partial denture. J. Prosthet. Dent., 13, 4: 679.

Koper A. (1973).
An intracoronal semi-precision retainer for removable partial dentures: the Thompson dowel. J. Prosthet. Dent., 30, 5: 759.

McCollum B. B. and Stuart C. E. (1955).
A Research Report: Basic Course in Postgraduate Gnathology, pp 45–46. Scientific Press, South Pasadena.

McCracken W. L. (1964).
Partial Denture Construction. 2nd Edn. p. 167. C. V. Mosby,. St. Louis, Mo.

McLeod N. S. (1977).
A theoretical analysis of the mechanics of the Thompson dowel semi-precision intracoronal retainer. J. Prosthet. Dent., 27, 1: 19.

Miller C. J. (1963).
Intracoronal attachments for removable partial dentures. Dent. Clin. N. Amer., 779.

Morison M. L. (1962).
Internal precision attachment retainers for partial dentures. J. Amer. Dent. Assoc., 64: 209.

Neurohr F. G. (1939).
Partial Dentures. Lea and Febiger, Philadelphia.

Parr M. (1888).
Removable Bridges. In A Practical Treatise on Artificial Crown and Bridge Work (Evans, G., ed.) The S. S. White Metal Mfg. Co., Philadelphia.

Peeso F. A. (1894).
Metal cap for the anchorage of a bridge. Busy Dentist, 1: 36.

Peeso F. A. (1916).
Crown and Bridgework for Students and Practitioners. Lea and Febiger, Philadelphia.

Preiskel H. W. (1966).
The use of internal attachments. Brit. Dent. J., 121: 564.

Preiskel H. W. (1979).
Precision Attachments. 3rd Edn. Henry Kimpton, London.

Schuyler C. G. (1953).
An analysis of the use and relative value of precision attachment and the clasp in partial denture planning. J. Prosthet. Dent., 3, 5: 711.

Sherer J. W. (1949).
Sherer spring lock attachment. Dent. Digest, 55: 163.

Singer F. and Schon F. (1966).
Partial Dentures. Henry Kimpton, London.

Steiger A. and Boitel R. (1959).
Precision Work for Partial Dentures. Stebo, Zurich.

Terrel W. H. (1951).
Specialised frictional attachments and their role in partial denture construction. J. Prosthet. Dent., 3: 339.

Thompson M. J. (1949).
Reversible hydrocolloid impression material: its treatment and use In operative prosthetic dentistry. J. Amer. Dent. Assoc., 39: 708.

Thompson M. J. (1957).
Solution for specific problems in replacing missing teeth with partial denture. Ill. Dent. J., 26: 251.

Chapter 7

Extracoronal Attachments

Units with part or all of their mechanism outside the contour of a tooth are known as extracoronal attachments. These increasingly popular and versatile devices have their main application with distal extension prostheses, although they may be used to retain restorations for bounded spaces. Plaque control problems, space considerations and mechanical effectiveness are major influences upon design. For descriptive purposes, three groups of extracoronal attachments can be described: projection, connecting and combined units.

Projection units

This is by far the largest and most popular group of extracoronal attachments. Since they project from the abutment crowns, no box preparation is required but the projections themselves complicate plaque control. Projection units can, in turn, be divided into two subgroups:

1. Rigid projection units.
2. Projection units allowing play between the two sections.

Connecting units

These units provide a joint between two sections of a removable prothesis; they do not anchor a prosthesis to a tooth. The joint commonly allows movement between the two sections of the denture. The axial rotation and rotation joints designed by Steiger and Boitel are good examples.

Combined units

Combined units consist of two attachments; a hinge-type of connecting element outside the tooth joined directly to an intracoronal attachment. The male sections of combined attachments may be interchangeable with those of an equivalent intracoronal attachment. No projection remains when the denture is removed, but box preparations are required. By their very nature these units tend to be complex, cumbersome and of limited application.

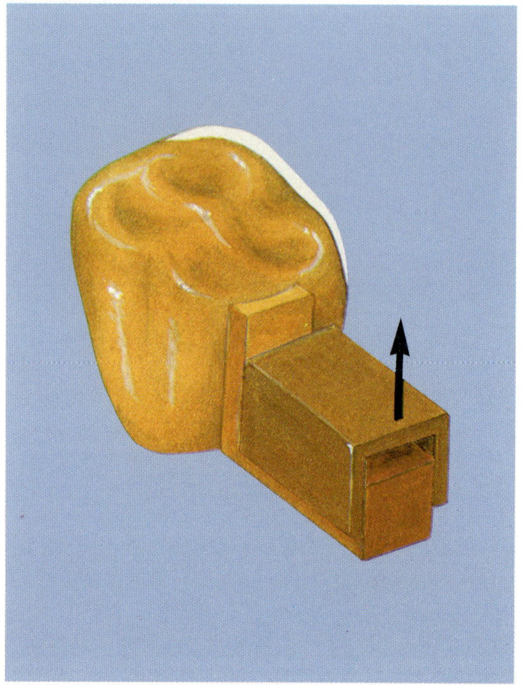

Fig. 260 Hypothetical rectangular unit. The height of the projection governs the length of the path of insertion, and influences the retention available.

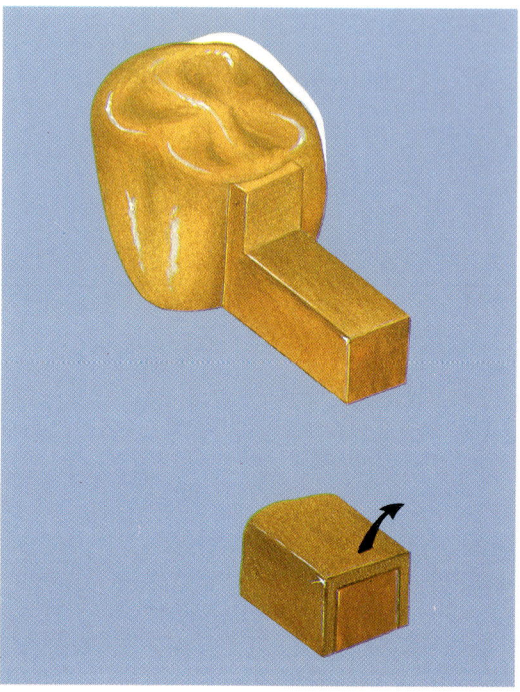

Fig. 261 The height also governs the ability to resist rotational loads around the sagittal axis. Furthermore, the lateral facing surfaces counteract side-to-side movement of the denture base.

Projection units

The design of most units is a compromise between conflicting requirements. The problems are best understood by considering a hypothetical parallel-sided block soldered to the distal aspect of an abutment crown for the retention of a distal extension prosthesis. A closely fitting female unit engages this rectangular projection.

The height of the projection governs the length of the path of insertion, the retention available and its ability to resist rotational loads around a sagittal axis. Apart from retention, the height of the unit is an important feature of wear resistance (Fig. 260).
The lateral surface area counteracts side-to-side and 'fish-tail' movements of the denture base. This surface area is a function of height and length. The width of the attachment affects its strength and also

Fig. 262 (a) A component of the attachment assembly should prevent the removable prosthesis sliding away from the abutment tooth. (b) Ideally, hinge movement around the abutment should be restricted or even eliminated.

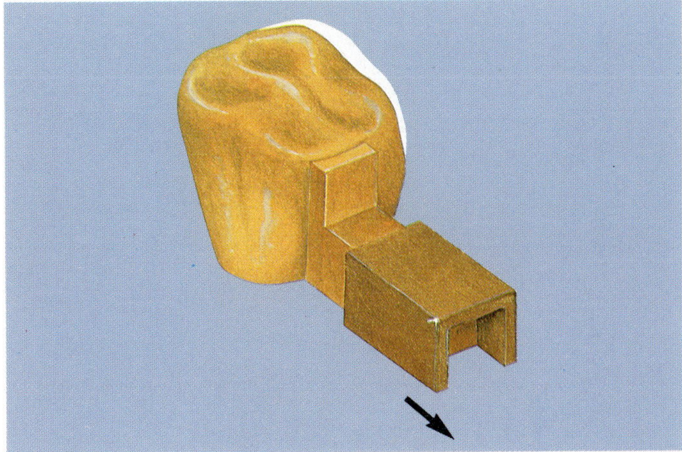

Figure 262 a

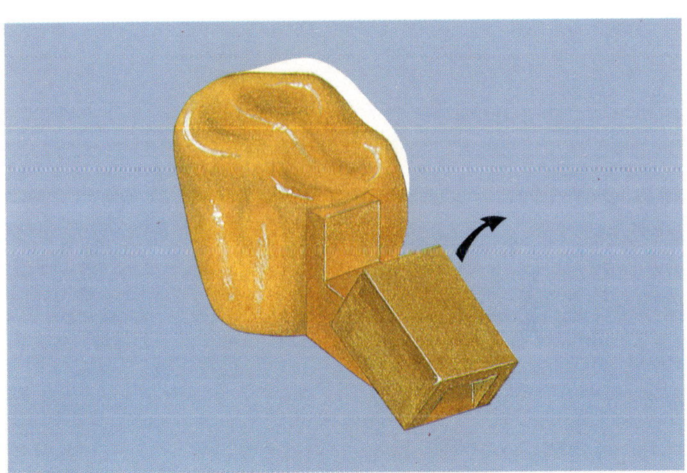

Figure 262 b

provides bulk for the incorporation of retaining devices (Fig. 261). The shape of unit will need to be modified to prevent sliding or undesirable tilting movements (Fig. 262 a, b).

While bulky extracoronal units may look impressive on specially constructed demonstration models, the restrictions of the mouth must be considered.

Vertical space is a precious commodity and the cry is often heard for shorter and still shorter attachments. Careful design may overcome some of the drawbacks of short attachments. Incorporation of bracing arms may compensate for the reduced lateral surface area, while meticulous construction of the attached denture base will reduce the forces applied. Metal occlusal and lingual surfaces around the attachment will further reduce the overall space requirements.

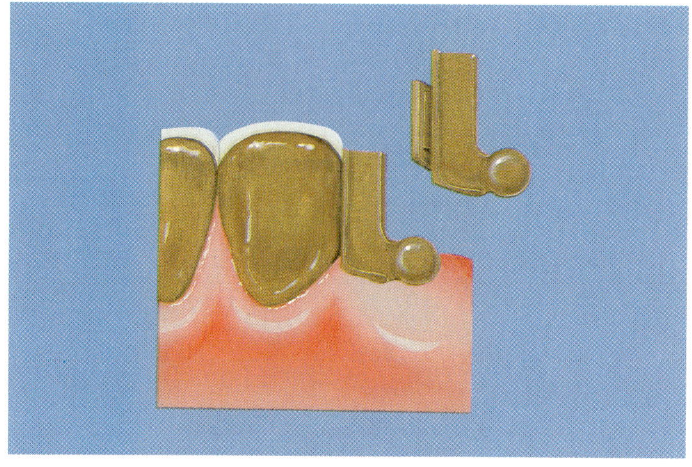

Fig. 263 Although extracoronal attachments may not require large box, or shoulder preparations, some space within the crown contour is required for the retaining plate.

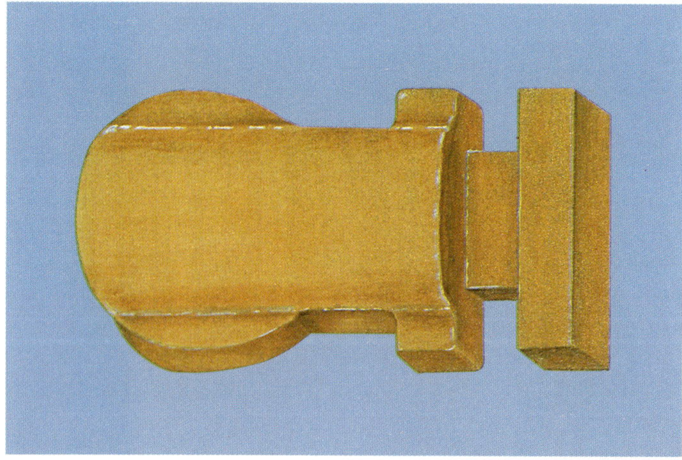

Fig. 264 Rounding the base of the attachment will be helpful to plaque control.

The mechanical advantages of a long attachment and corresponding large lateral surface areas have been mentioned, but when applied to the mouth the drawbacks may be intolerable. First of all the problems of plaque control increase with the length of unit. Secondly, a greater length requires more space within the prosthesis for the attachment. If the attachment is not aligned with the long axis of the edentulous ridge, as is frequently the case, the longer attachment may produce an unacceptable lingual bulge in the prosthesis.

The additional lateral surface contact area provided by a bracing arm is a useful way of overcoming the effects of reducing the length of the attachment. The problems of pulpal space are not completely eliminated by using extracoronal attachments. Units that are produced for 'cast on' techniques will incorporate a retentive element to be surrounded by the metal of the

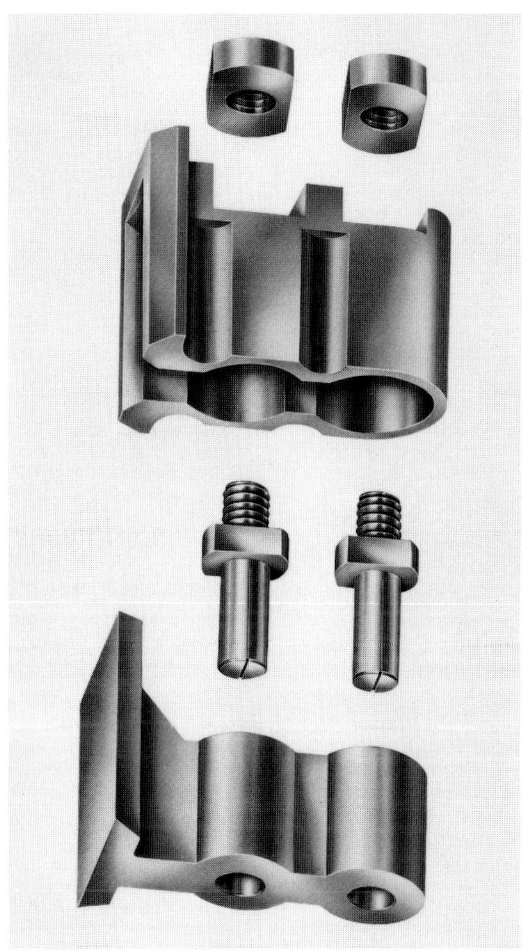

Fig. 265   The Stabilex attachment, to show removable male pins.

crown. Space needs to be provided for these elements within the crown contour to prevent overcontouring of the restoration. A bevelled shoulder or chamfer edge finish will normally suffice (Fig. 263).
The width of the attachment is limited by two considerations, the buccolingual space available and difficulties of plaque control. Rounding the base of the attachment may be helpful in this respect (Fig. 264). If some of the difficulties of designing

projection units are understood, the way is clear to appreciate the correct application of projection units.
Rigid extracoronal attachments tend to be somewhat more bulky than those allowing a degree of play. If the lateral surfaces of these units are sufficiently large and parallel-sided, they may be used in conjunction with intracoronal attachments, useful for certain types of unilateral distal extension prostheses. Other applications

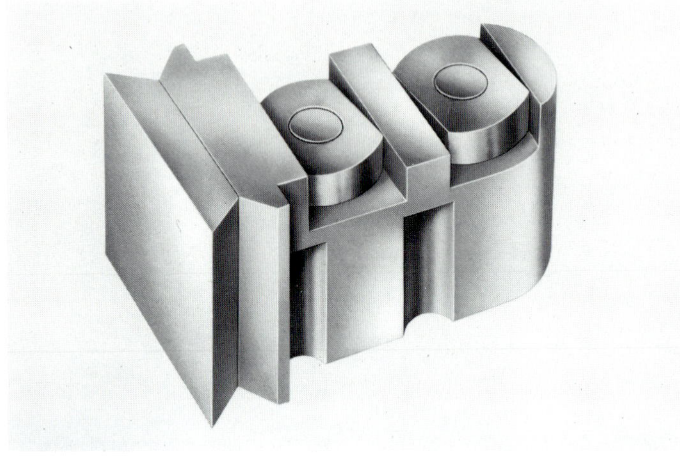

Fig. 266   The attachment assembled.

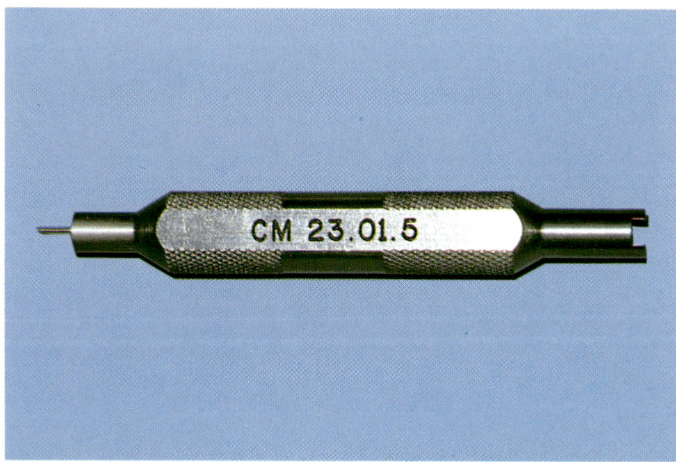

Fig. 267   Screwdriver   for changing the pins.

include the restoration of bounded spaces and of bilateral distal extension gaps.
If one takes, for example, the Stabilex unit, the mechanical efficiency of the attachment is self-evident (Figs. 265 to 267). It provides a rigid connection between male and female sections, with additional retention provided by pins. The retention of the pins is adjustable, but the pin may be unscrewed and replaced if necessary. A special screwdriver is made for the purpose. While this robust attachment provides extremely effective retention, it is bulky. Plaque control is difficult, as the attachment requires more than 4 mm of vertical space. Perhaps the greatest drawback is its length that complicates the construction of the prosthesis, together with subsequent plaque control and restricts application to situations in which there is

Fig. 268 (a) The Conex attachment. A series of refinements has reduced its bulk, facilitated plaque control, and improved retention. (b) The Conex attachment with modified retaining pin. This modified pin improves retention still further. (c) The attachment assembled. The female section is designed for incorporation within the acrylic resin of the denture base.

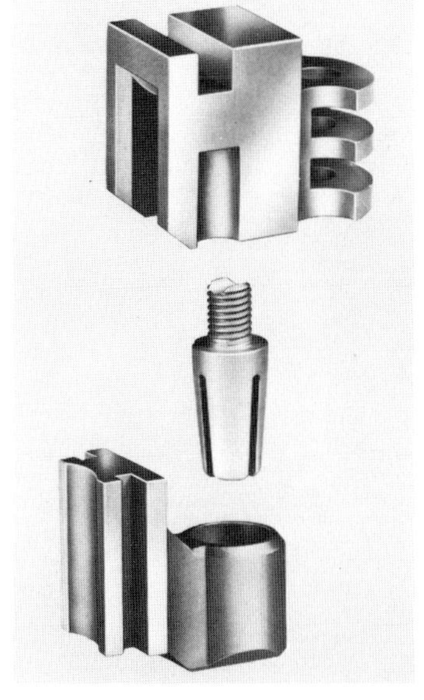
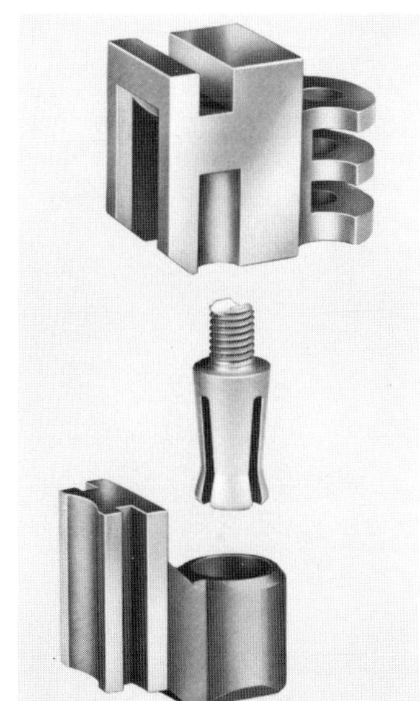

Figure 268 a   Figure 268 b

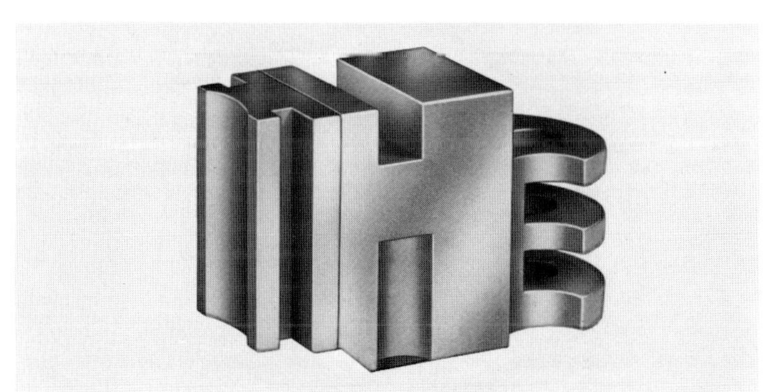

Figure 268 c

generous space available.

The Conex attachment (Fig. 268 a, b, c) shares a common ancestry with the Stabilex, but is far smaller mesiodistally. A series of refinements has reduced the bulk of the unit, facilitated plaque control and improved retention. Its applications and popularity have thereby grown. The parallel sides provide a precise path of insertion that resist rotational forces. The central retaining pin may be unscrewed and replaced. Two types of pin may be employed (Fig. 269 a), providing frictional retention or a mechanical lock. Where buccolingual space permits, a lingual bracing arm is recommended (Fig. 269 b). The retention can be so effective that a special separation device is produced to help part the two sections (Fig. 270). The retention of the central pin may be adjusted by insert-

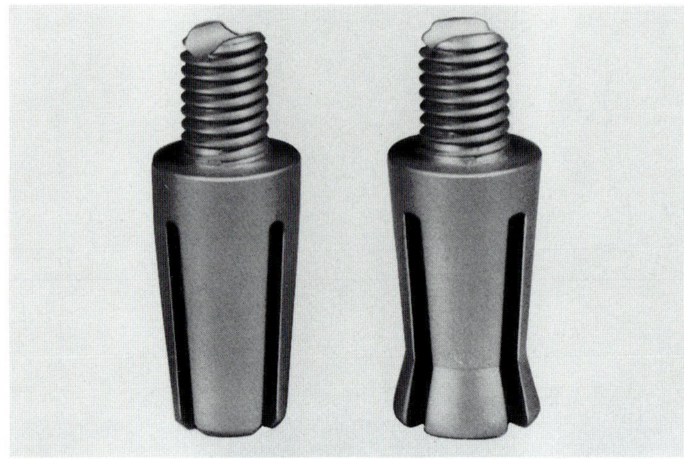

Fig. 269 (a) Two models of retaining pin are available producing frictional retention (left) or an additional mechanical lock (right). (b) Lateral rotational forces are resisted by metal to metal contact. A bracing arm is, nevertheless, advisable.

Figure 269 a

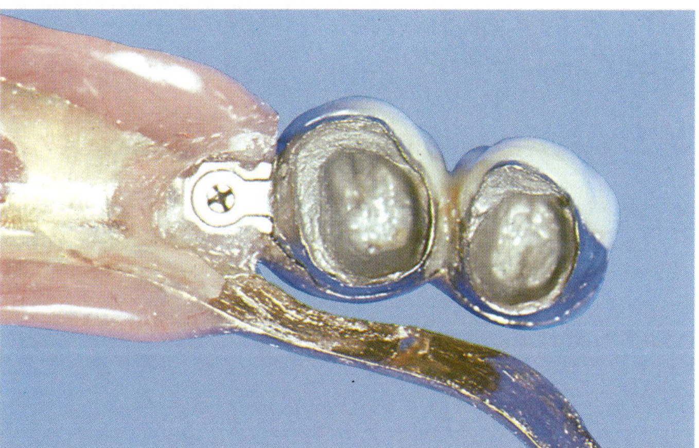

Figure 269 b

ing a special instrument, the opposite end of which may be used to unscrew the pin (Figs. 271 to 273). The manufacturers do not recommend soldering to the removable section of the attachment. Instead, special additional tagging is produced for soldering purposes. The additional tagging is screwed to the back of the attachment (Fig. 274).

A modified Conex attachment is now produced that enables the operator to screw the removable section of the prosthesis in place (Fig. 275). This may have application for certain tooth-supported prostheses, provided that adequate plaque control is possible. The retention of the special pin is adjusted with the longer screw. This longer screw is also used to hold the pin in place. In exceptional circumstances, the attachment can be converted to a removable unit by cutting off the screw extension (Fig. 276).

Fig. 270 Separation device to allow the dental surgeon and technician to part the two sections of the attachment in the laboratory.

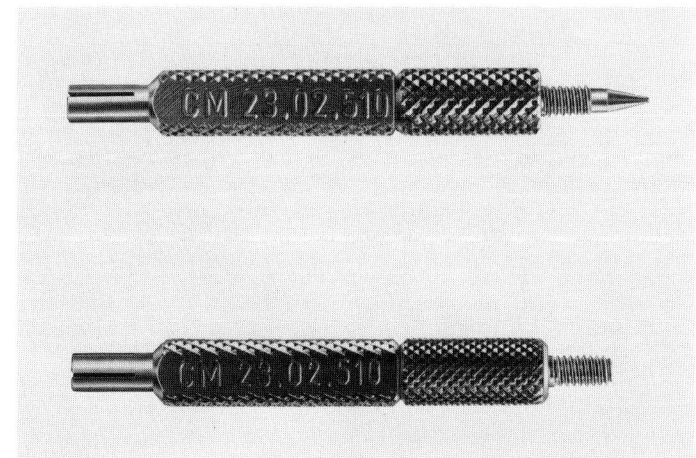

Fig. 271 Conex adjusting tool. The pointed end spreads the retaining pins and increases retention. The opposite end unscrews the pin. When not in use, the pointed end should be protected within the tool using the screw threads available.

Most Conex applications will be for the retention of removable prostheses, especially distal extension dentures. Where unilateral distal extension spaces are to be restored, the parallel sides of the Conex allow it to be used in conjunction with intracoronal attachments on the contralateral side (Fig. 277).

The manufacturers feel that bracing arms are unnecessary due to the generous lateral surface area of the attachment. They may well be correct, but where buccolingual space permits, the arm helps with seating and removing the restoration (Figs. 278 and 279).

When employed correctly, Conex attachments provide excellent results, and plaque control presents few problems (Fig. 280). Other uses of these attachments include the retention of small restorations for bounded spaces (Fig. 281). Conex attachments may be used in conjunction with

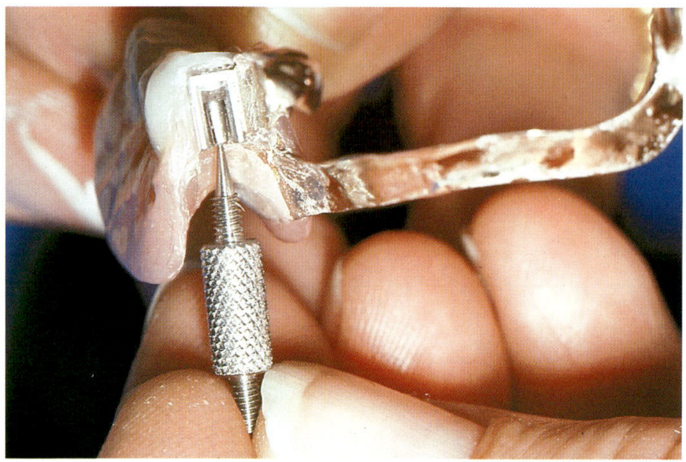

Fig. 272   Increasing the retention of a Conex attachment.

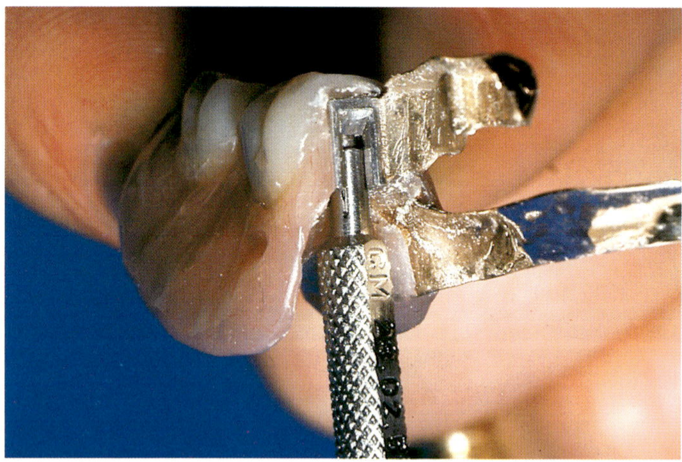

Fig. 273   Unscrewing the retaining pin of a Conex attachment.

intracoronal attachments and parallel-sided telescopic crowns.

The Scott attachment is a laboratory-produced extracoronal system that may be rigid, or allow movement, depending on the inclusion of an axial-rotational joint. There are few restrictions to its use, provided that abutments of adequate strength are present and sufficient vertical and bucco-lingual space exists for the attachment. The design allows the projecting unit (the connector) to be placed away from the gingival margin with considerable advantages to oral hygiene practice (Fig. 282). This section of the prosthesis may be purchased as a plastic blank that may be cut to size on the master cast (Fig. 283). Retention is provided by the frictional grip of the removable telescopic crown on the tapered connector. This arrangement compensates for wear, as the outer section simply slides further down over its counter-

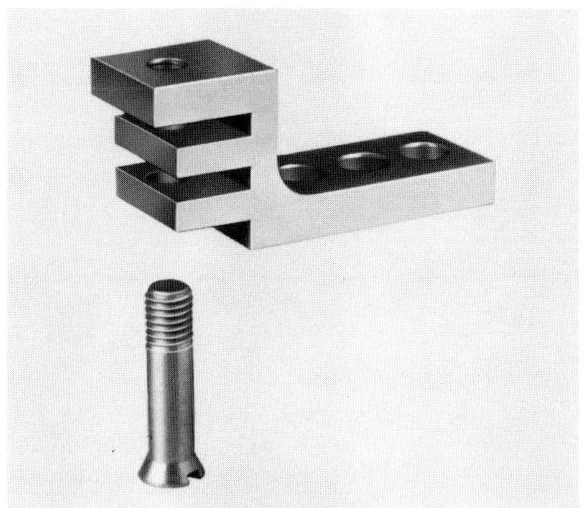

Figure 274

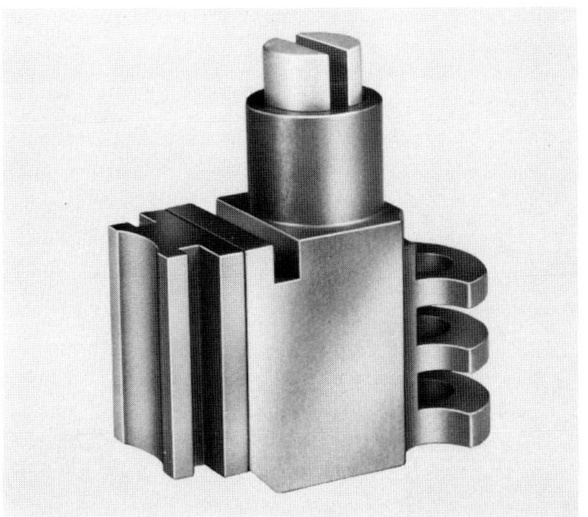

Figure 275

Fig. 274   Additional tagging may be bolted to the Conex female unit. This tagging may be soldered to the major connector.

Fig. 275   Modified Conex allowing the construction of a screw-retained fixed prosthesis.

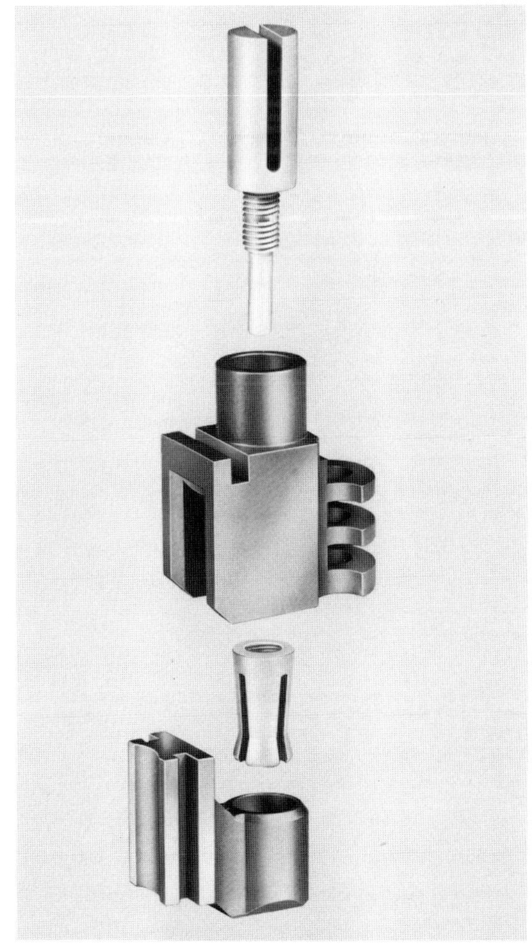

Fig. 276   Component parts of the modified Conex attachment.

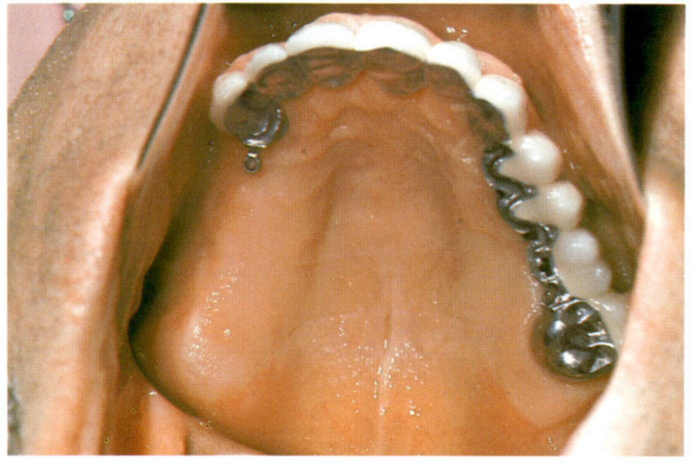

Fig. 277 The parallel sides of the Conex attachment permit it to be used in conjunction with intracoronal attachments.

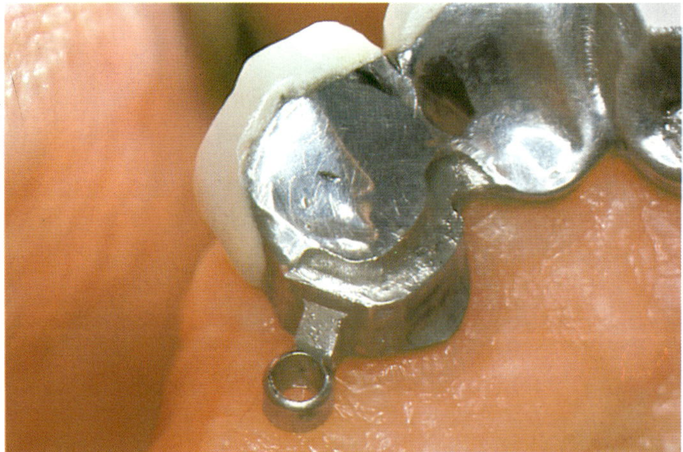

Fig. 278 Abutment crowns with recess for bracing arm.

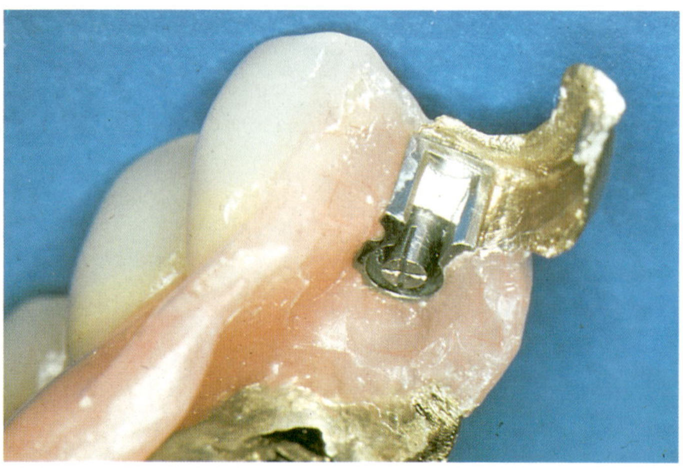

Fig. 279 Bracing arm on denture.

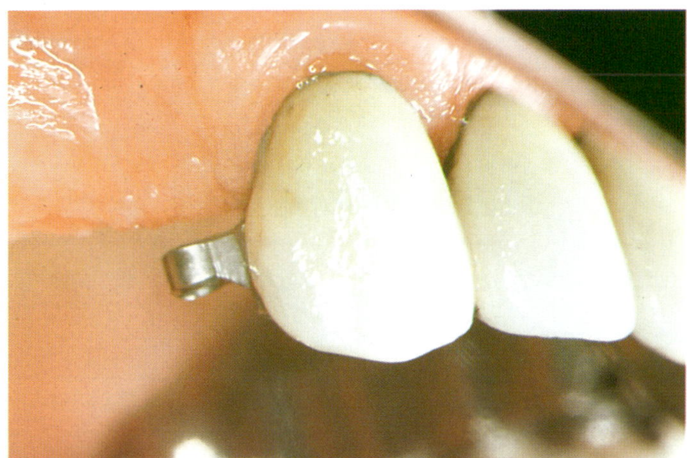

Fig. 280 Eighteen month post-insertion result. Given sufficient vertical space, adequate plaque control is straightforward.

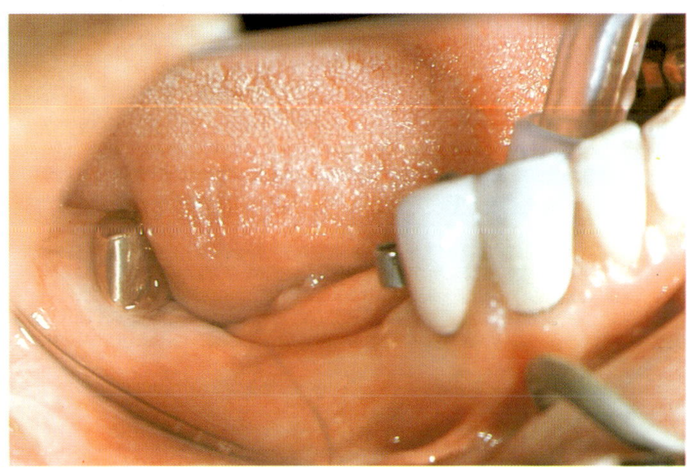

Fig. 281 Conex units may be used to retain unilateral restorations for bounded spaces. They may be employed in conjunction with intracoronal attachments or parallel-sided telescopic crowns.

part. Supplemental retention is provided by parallel-sided iridio-platinum pins supplied with the attachment and these are incorporated when the pattern of the removable section (telescopic crown) is constructed in wax. *Scott* (1968) felt the attachment with play had applications where distal extension prostheses are concerned. Apart from the retention of distal extension prostheses, this versatile unit may be used to retain removable anterior prostheses (Figs. 284 to 288). Its design allows close adaptation to the underlying mucosa.

Extracoronal projection units with play between the components have become extremely popular. While it is only possible to describe a small number, the principles involved apply to the entire group.

Any movement occurring between two sections of the attachment may well decrease loads applied to the abutment

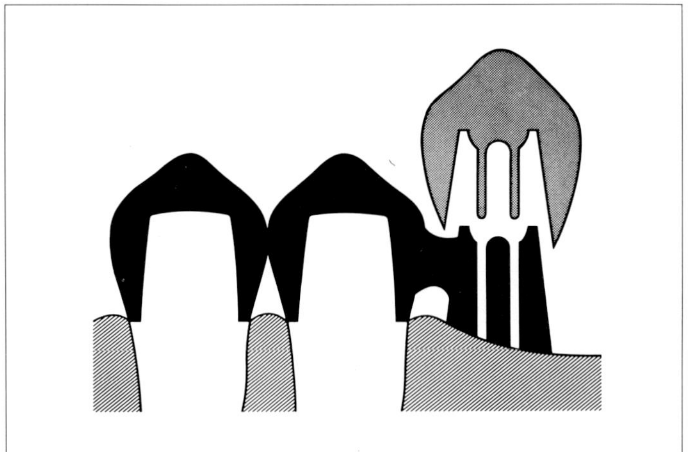

Fig. 282 The Scott attachment. The projecting unit may be placed away from the gingival margins with considerable advantages to plaque control.

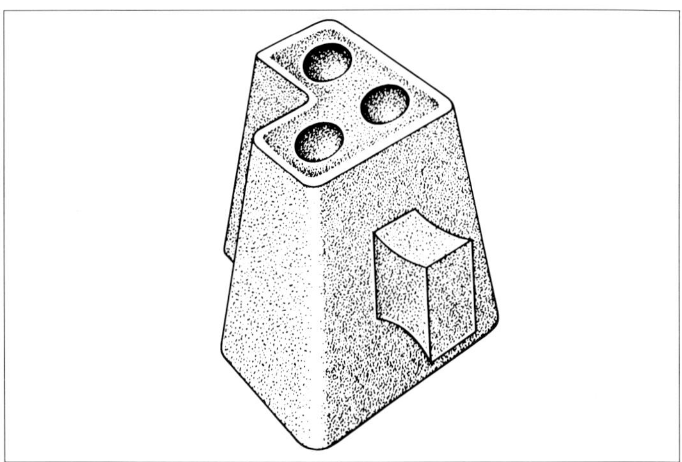

Fig. 283 Diagram of the projecting unit of the Scott attachment. This unit may be obtained as a plastic blank and cut to size on the master cast.

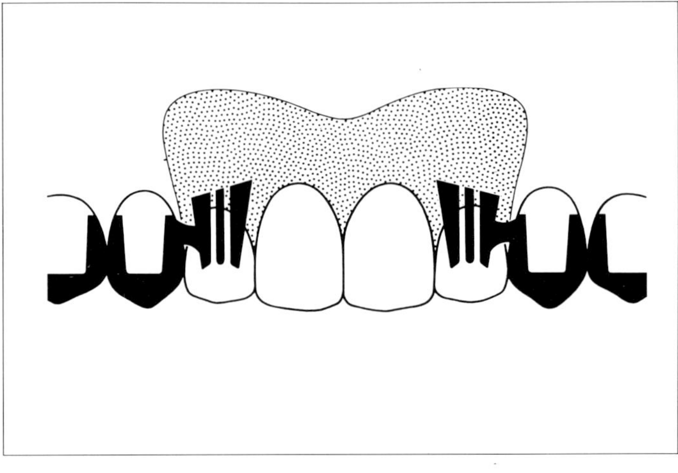

Fig. 284 The Scott attachment used to retain a removeable anterior restoration. Its design allows close adaptation to the underlying mucosa.

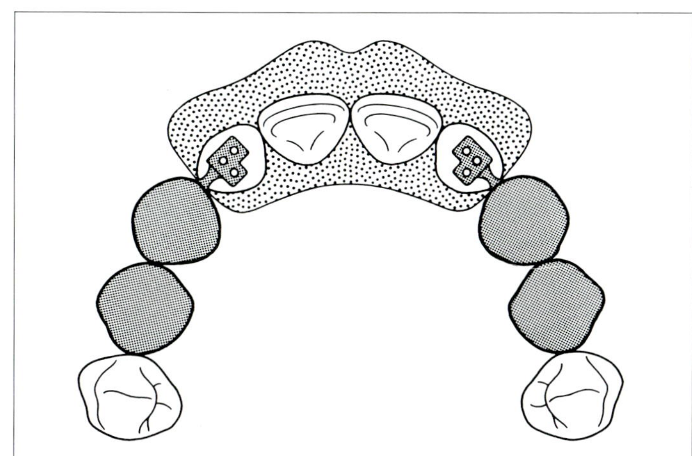

Fig. 285   Diagram of the prosthesis in place.

Fig. 286 (a) (b)   Occlusal view of Scott attachment in the mouth.

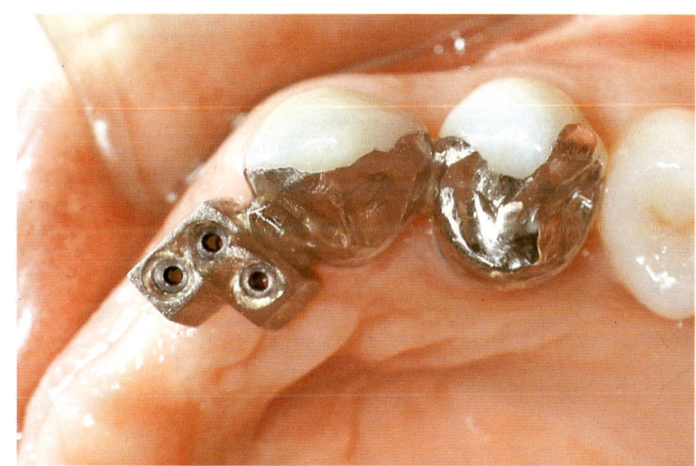

Figure 286 a

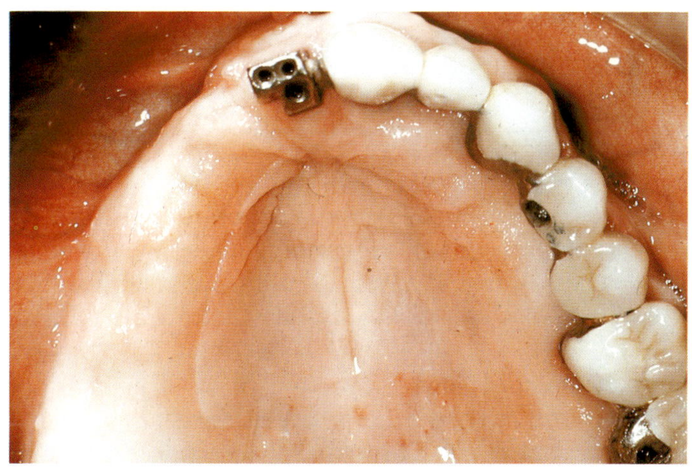

Figure 286 b

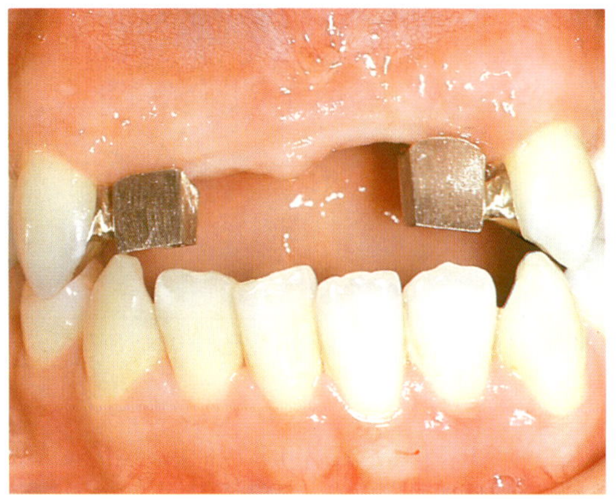

Fig. 287 (a)   Labial view of Scott attachment.

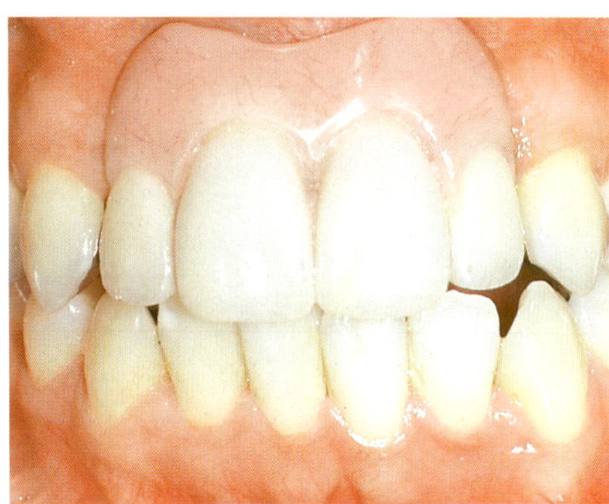

Figure 287 (b) The restoration assembled.

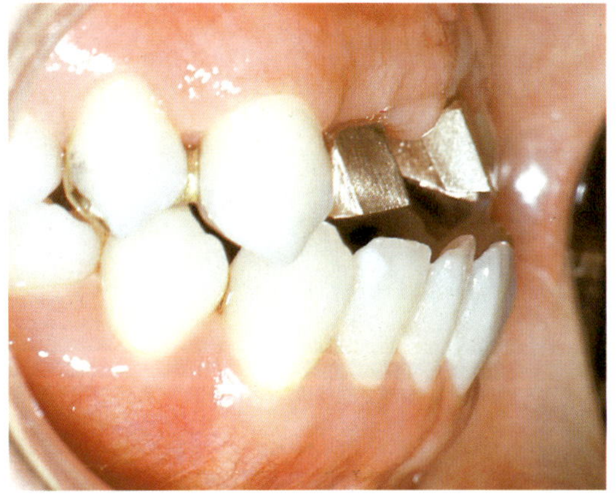

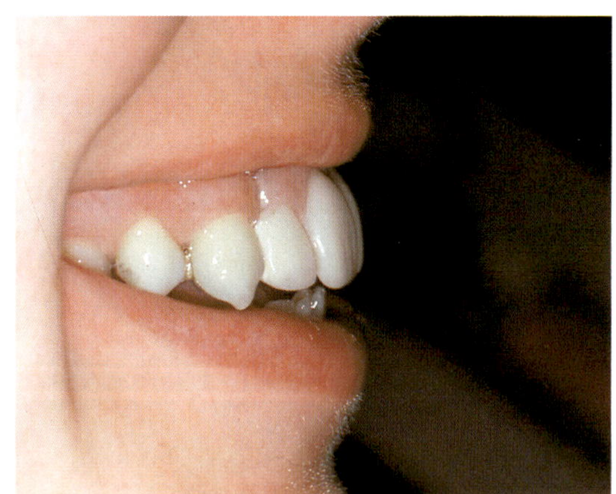

Fig. 288 (a) (b)   Lateral view of restoration.

crowns. Instead of being applied to the periodontal tissues, additional load will be placed on the edentulous ridge, a structure prone to resorption. Furthermore, many units, such as hinges, allow a degree of movement without significant limitation so that a vicious circle may be initiated. Increased denture base movement contributes to further resorption and yet more base movement. This problem becomes worse when the movements allowed are in more than one plane. Why are these types of attachment so popular? The answer lies in the compact size and versatility of many of them. However, possible drawbacks must be appreciated.

Consider a hypothetical attachment allowing vertical play. The denture base is entirely-mucosal supported until load is transmitted through the attachment. Now

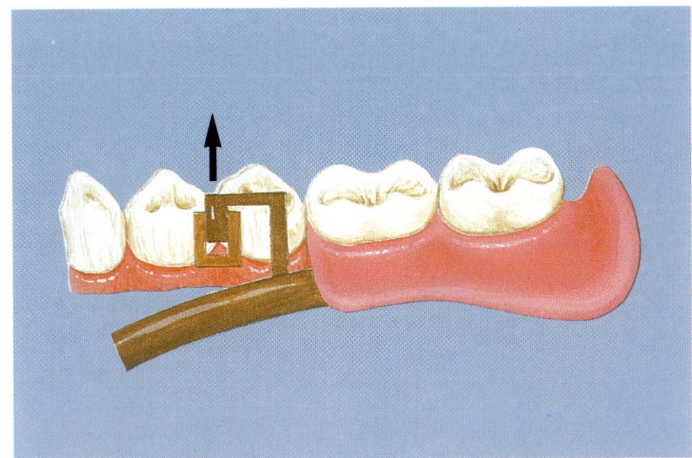

Fig. 289 A replacement spring slightly too long would have a tendency to lift the base away from the mucosa.

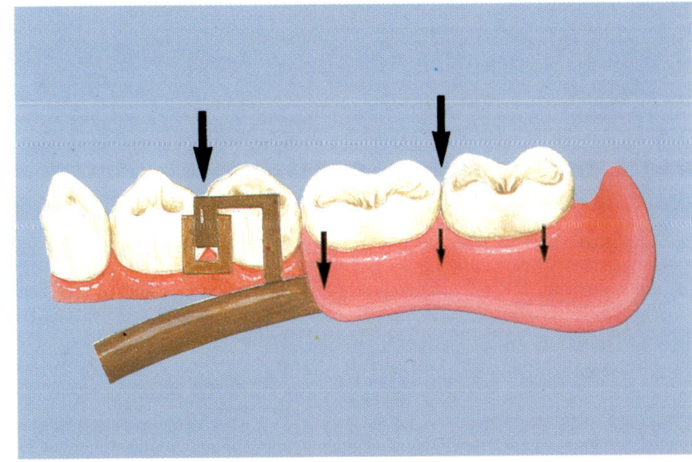

Fig. 290 If a spring loses its resiliency and becomes deformed, damaging loads can be applied to the gingivae and to the mucosa distal to the abutments.

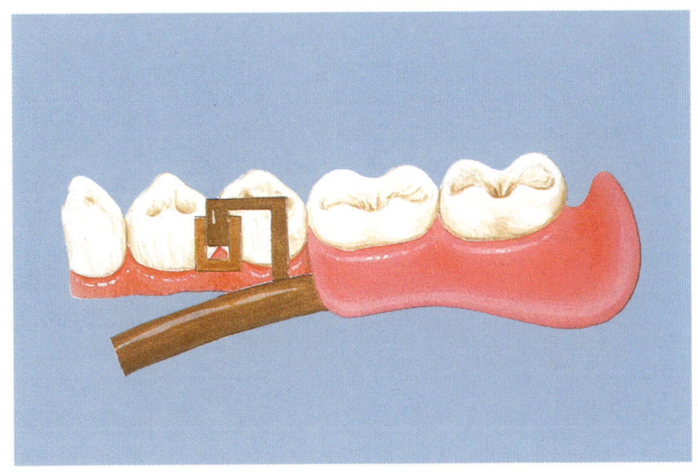

Fig. 291 The hazards of springs must be appreciated. They will need to be changed at regular intervals with a maximum period of 6 months.

suppose this hypothetical sliding attachment is spring controlled. A replacement spring slightly too long would result in the entire denture base being lifted out of contact with the mucosa (Fig. 289). On the other hand, a spring that had become permanently deformed would transmit little load to the abutment teeth. The partial denture, now without its occlusal support, would then be likely to damage the mesial section of the edentulous ridge. Unfortunately, the minute size of attachment springs and the forces applied often result in speedy permanent deformation (Fig. 290). Since this type of mishap can occur with all types of spring-controlled attachments, it is essential that springs be changed regularly, usually at 6-monthly intervals. Attachment manufacturers carefully control the spring lengths; nevertheless it is most important to ensure that the ends of the springs have not been damaged, and that the springs are pushed completely home.

Now examine hinge movement. While the distal abutment gingivae may be spared occlusal load, plaque control will be complicated by the projection. In theory, load distribution will be uneven, with more load applied to the distal section of the edentulous ridge than mesially. For a well-made denture, with negligible base movement, this point may be of academic interest. However, many hinges wear with time and then allow a degree of lateral play and rock that is far from satisfactory.

The alignment of hinges has been the subject of controversy for sometime. The views of the two rival camps deserve further thought and may be expressed as follows:

1. The hinges should be aligned with the sagittal plane to prevent jamming of the hinges during rotation.
2. The hinges should be aligned with the midline of the ridges so that no buccal or lingual movement of the base accompanies rotation.

There is little doubt that hinges aligned with the sagittal plane will not jam and will provide unrestricted movement. But what price is paid for sagittally aligned hinges, and is this sacrifice worthwhile? First of all, a lingual bulge is produced in the denture; the longer the hinge the bigger the bulge (Fig. 292). Secondly, the bases either side may not be of equal length. In that case, a cantilevered pontic would be necessary to align the attachments. To join an extracoronal attachment to a cantilevered pontic is to produce a cantilevered extension of nearly two units, to which a distal extension prosthesis is attached. This arrangement is not only unnecessary, but contributes to a most unfavourable prognosis of the distal abutment.

The argument for sagitally aligned hinges is based on the presumption of an entirely rigid major connector. However, *Heckneby's* (1969) work has shown that neither the denture base resin nor a lower major connector can be considered rigid under load, particularly as the total base movement should not exceed 0.3 mm (Fig. 293). Occasionally, tales are told of patients who chew simultaneously on both sides. Such freaks, if they exist, have yet to be found. While many of the pleas for sagitally aligned hinges do not stand careful scrutiny, this does not mean that hinge-type attachments can be twisted at any angle to each other (Fig. 294). Provided the denture has been well-made, divergencies of up to 20° should produce little problem.

Fig. 292 (a) (b) Hinges aligned with the sagittal plane provide unrestricted movement. However, a lingual bulge may be produced in the denture and the justification for such an arrangement is questionable.

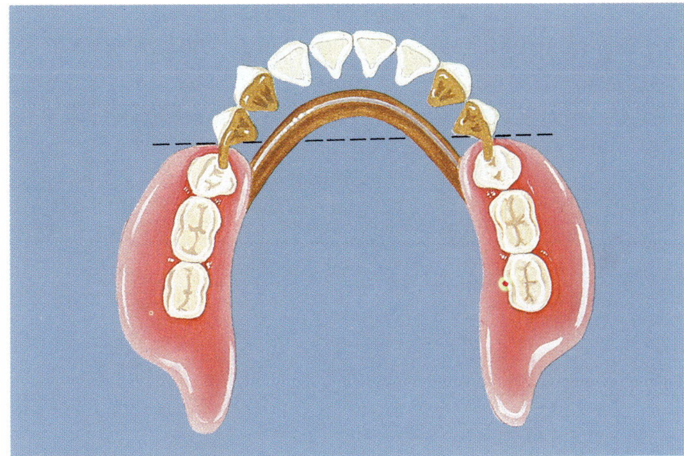

Figure 292 a

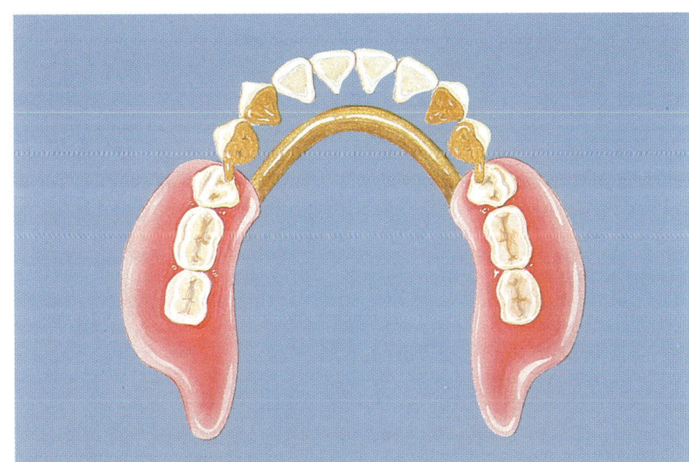

Figure 292 b

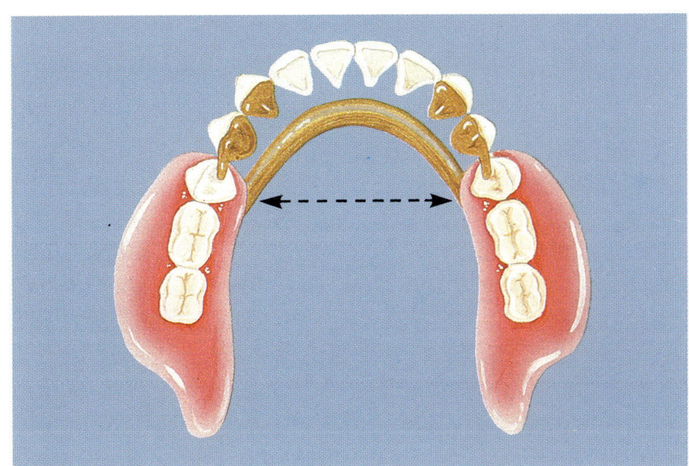

Fig. 293 Only a minute flexion of the major connector of the denture base is necessary to permit distal base movement of 0.3 mm.

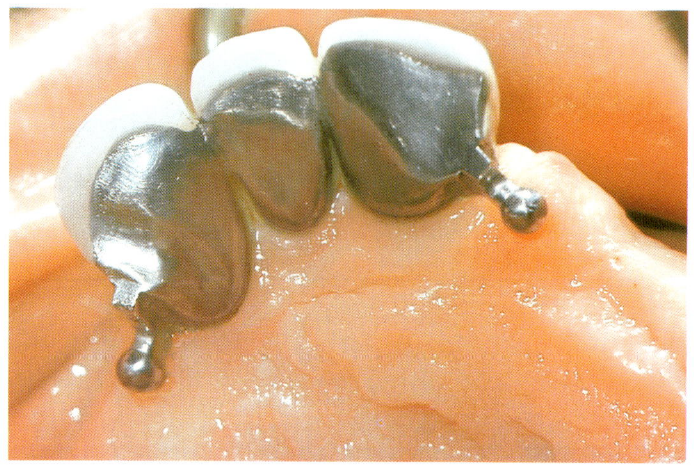

Fig. 294 Twisting hinges at more than 60° to each other changes load distribution to their surfaces and can result in damage to the attachment and a poorly retained prosthesis.

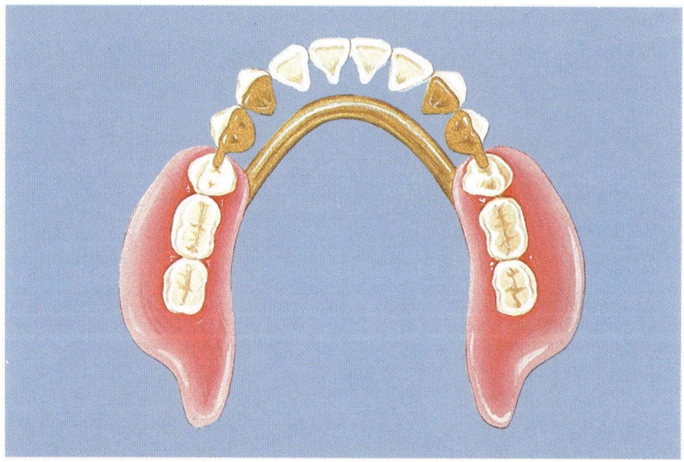

Fig. 295 Aligning hinges with edentulous ridges reduces buccolingual space requirements, but often complicates plaque control.

Once this figure is exceeded, vertical loads and tilting forces may be applied to parts of the attachment unable to resist these forces. A loose denture and damaged attachment might ensue.

Aligning the attachment with the edentulous ridge reduces the buccolingual space required (Fig. 295). In the days of large denture base movements, this arrangement ensured there was no lingual component to the rotation of the denture. The only practical problem today is that the entire base of the attachment may be in contact with the mucosa, and this may complicate plaque control.

Twisting the attachments to an alignment slightly lingual to the ridges is a sensible compromise (Fig. 296). It introduces few mechanical problems and simplifies plaque control as the distal section of the attachment will overlie the distal slope of the mucosa.

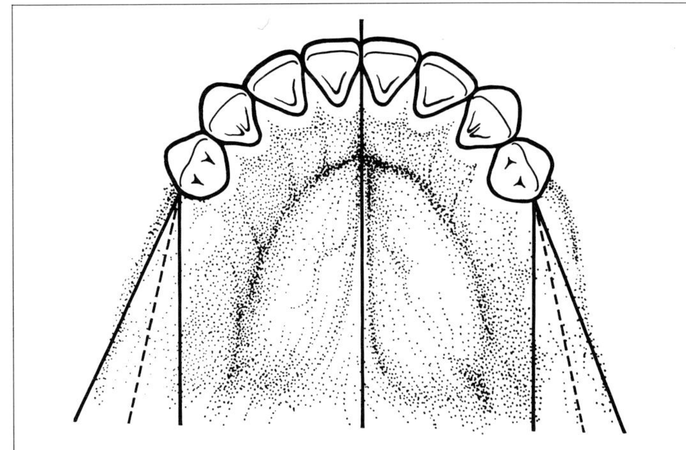

Fig. 296 Bisecting the angle between the edentulous ridge and the sagittal plane is usually a sensible compromise. Plaque control is simplified without the problem of lingual space involvement.

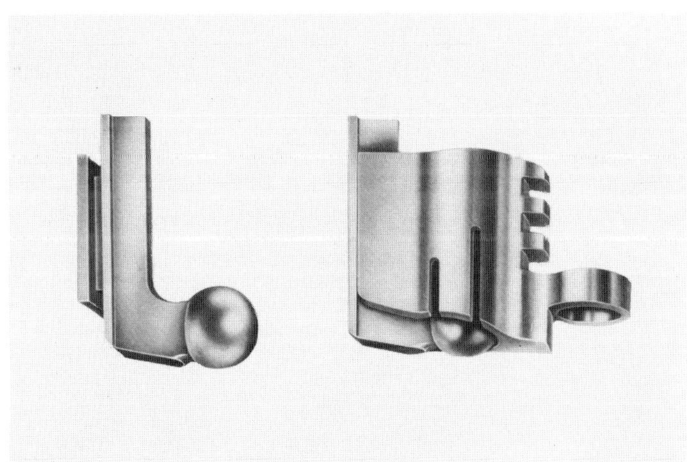

Fig. 297 The Dalbo extracoronal attachment.

The Dalbo extracoronal attachments are excellent examples of units allowing play between the two sections. Manufacture has been refined over quarter of a century, during which time the attachments have shown themselves to be versatile and robust. The male unit is soldered to the surface of the abutment crowns, forming a projection to which the female element, buried within the denture, can be joined. The male portion of the Dalbo design projects as an L-shaped bar with a ball joint on the lower extremity. The female section fits over the bar and engages the sides of the ball connection of the male (Figs. 297 and 298). This lock between the socket and the ball provides the direct retention of the unit, which is adjustable by gently bending the finger springs around the open end of the socket. Dalbo units are available in two sizes, with a matrix height of 5 mm or 6 mm. Each of

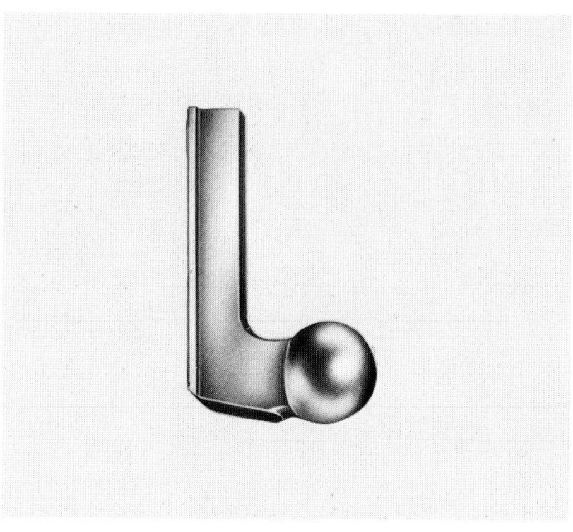

Figure 298 a

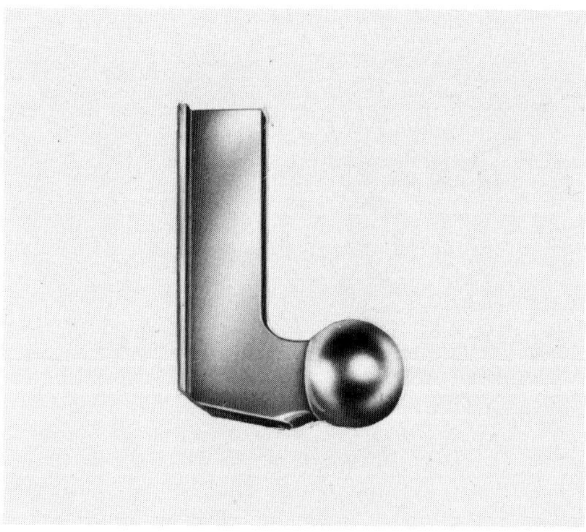

Figure 298 b

Fig. 298   The Dalbo male attachment. (a) The 'bilateral' model. (b) The 'unilateral' model.

these attachment heights is available in two configurations with the base of the L-shaped male unit longer in one than the other. The increased lateral surface area of the longer unit provides additional resistance to rotational and lateral displacing forces, at the expense of additional bulk. These two configurations are sometimes known as 'bilateral' and 'unilateral'. However, it would be an unwise operator who attached a unilateral distal extension prosthesis without a major connector to even the largest of these units—or to any other for that matter.

Dalbo units provide excellent resistance to both distal and lateral displacing forces. Furthermore, they incorporate a most effective tilt-preventing device that maintains the denture base in contact with the mucosa (Fig. 299). This is one of their important advantages over a clasp retainer that requires auxiliary indirect retention.

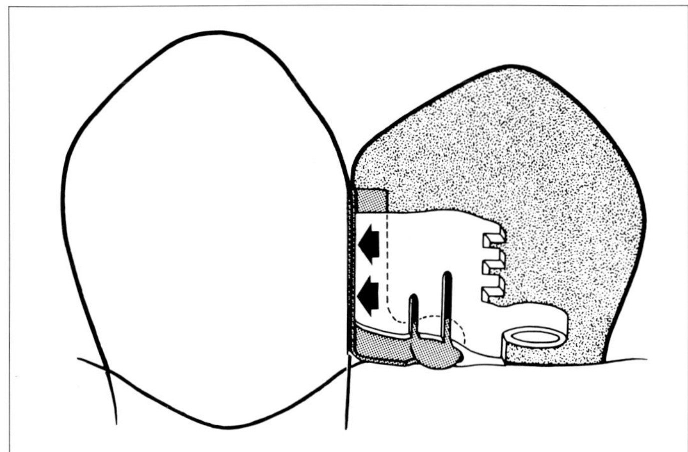

Fig. 299   Contact between the vertical surfaces prevents the distal denture base rotating away from the mucosa.

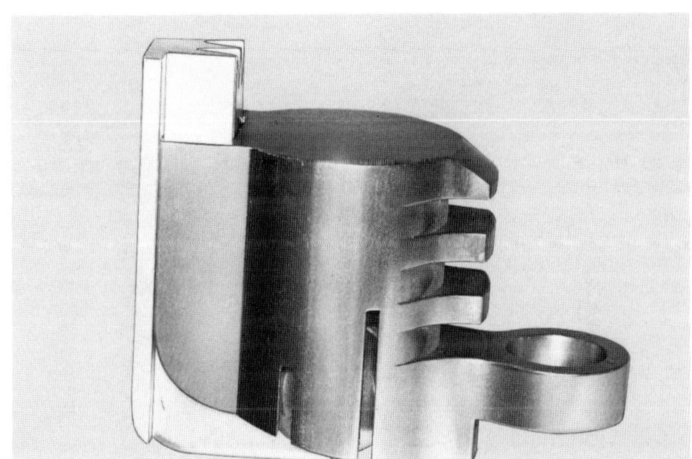

Fig. 300   Contact between lateral facing surfaces provides excellent resistance to lateral forces.

Tilt prevention is achieved by contact of the two flanges of the attachment, so that if a satisfactory impression technique has been used, the denture is both well-retained and stable. It is, of course, necessary to provide adequate and splinted abutments.

The design of the conventional Dalbo attachment allows some vertical play, for loads in this direction are transmitted through a coil spring to the ball connector of the male attachment. The Shoulder Dalbo is a modification of the spring-controlled Dalbo in which the vertical travel is restricted by metal to metal contacts (Figs. 301 to 304). The spring controls only hinge movement and the advantages of this arrangement are apparent in that loss or damage to the spring does not completely destroy occlusal support. The different sizes of Dalbo have dissimilar springs, and containers for spares should

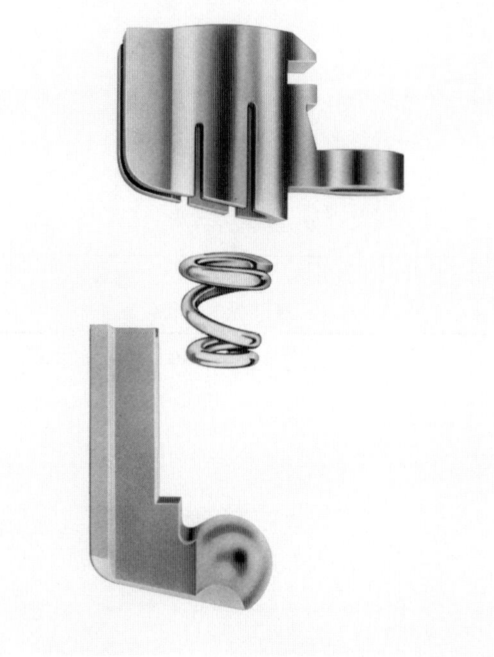

Fig. 301   An exploded view showing the components of the Shoulder Dalbo.

be clearly marked (Fig. 305 a). An important check is to ensure that a polished facet on top of the ball is visible to show that loads are being applied to it; otherwise the prosthesis is mucosal-borne. Springs introduce maintenance problems and complicate jaw relation recording and rebasing procedures. A solid spacer may be used to replace the spring (Fig. 305 b).

Another addition to the range is the miniaturised female section without the spring chamber (Fig. 306 a, b). The complications of the spring are removed, and the vertical space required for the attachment virtually halved. Small wonder this unit is becoming one of the most popular denture retainers. The male attachments employed are identical with the conventional variety, so that

it is possible to replace conventional Dalbo units with the miniaturised variety (Fig. 307).

The drawbacks, however, must be understood. The reduced height of the female unit decreases the lateral surface area of contact and the attachment is weaker than its conventional counterpart and less able to resist lateral loads. It is for this reason that the manufacturers recommend the longer 'unilateral' variety of miniaturised Dalbo attachment, as the increased length helps counteract the effect of the decreased height. When using the 'bilateral' miniaturised Dalbo, it is apparent that exceptional care must be taken to ensure the minimum of lateral forces are applied. This is an extremely useful attachment with

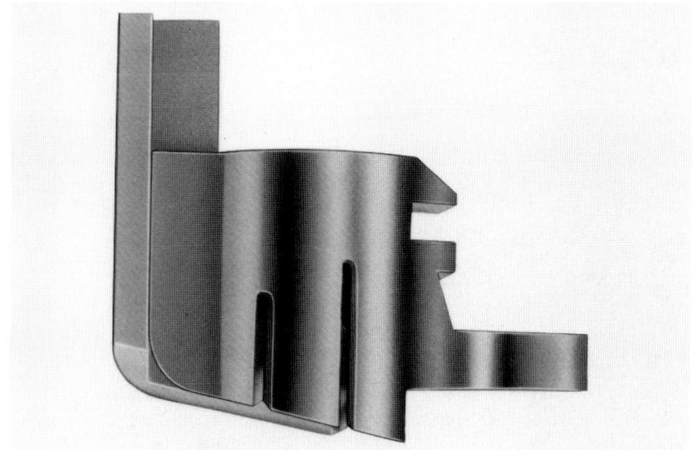

Fig. 302   The Shoulder Dalbo attachment assembly. The contours of the male and female components have been refined.

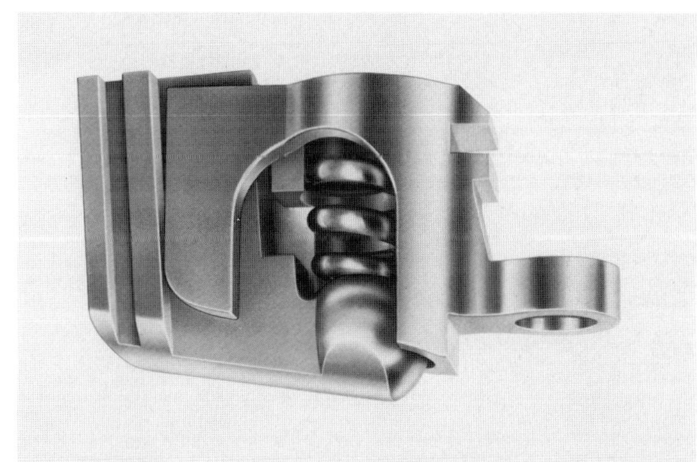

Fig. 303   Cut-away view of the Shoulder Dalbo without occlusal load.

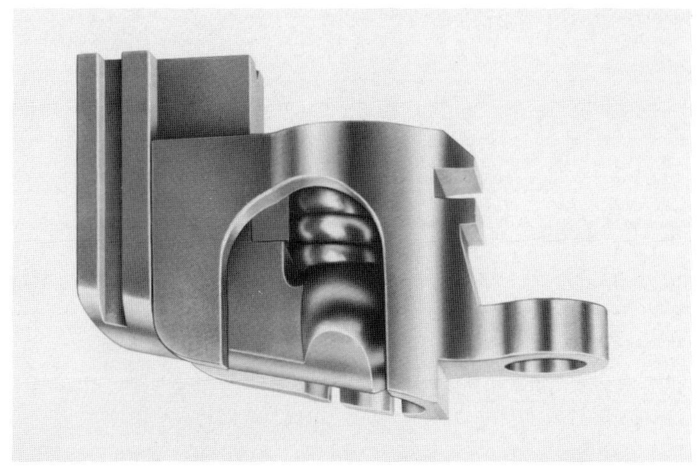

Fig. 304   Under occlusal load vertical travel is limited by contact of the shoulder.

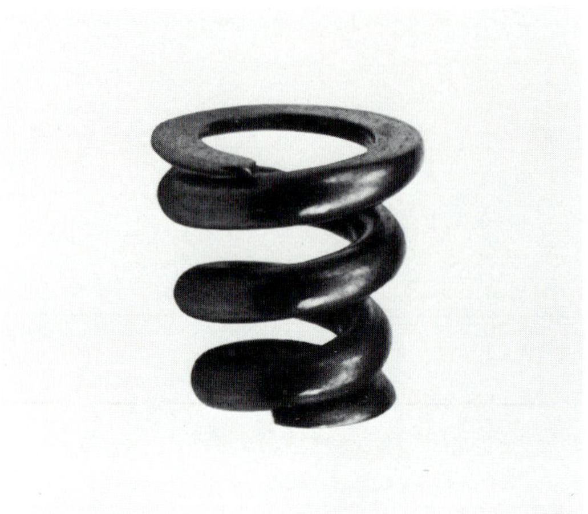

Figure 305 a

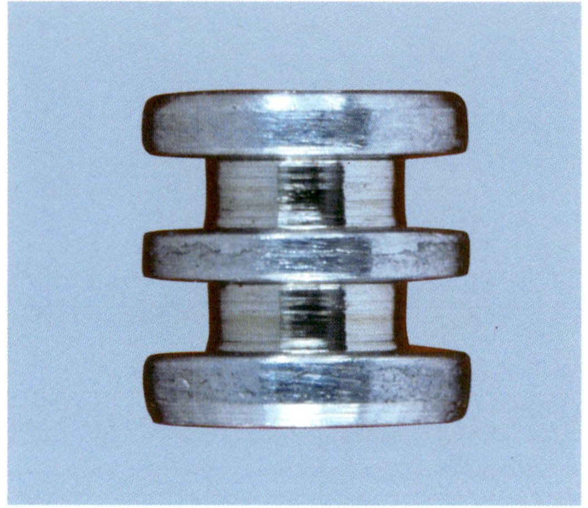

Figure 305 b

Fig. 305 (a)   Magnified view of a Dalbo spring. (b) A solid metal spacer may be used to replace the spring.

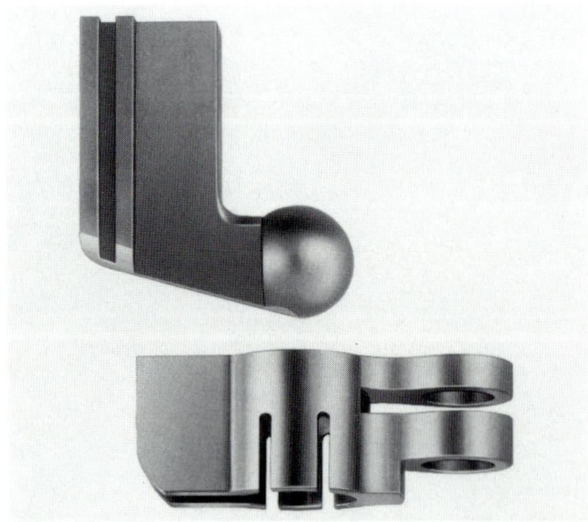

Figure 306 a

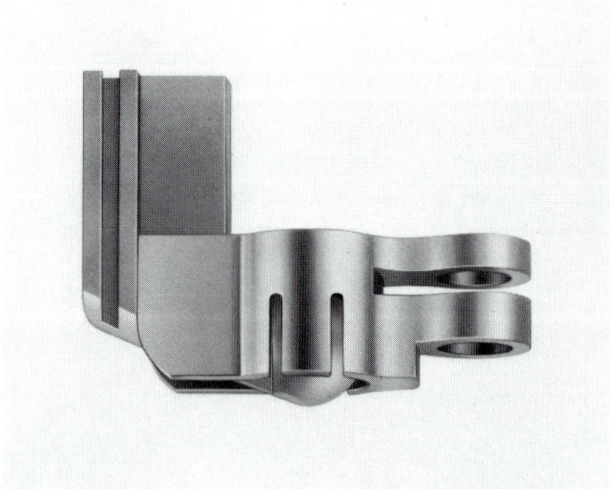

Figure 306 b

Fig. 306 (a)   The miniature Dalbo extracoronal attachment. Spring complications are removed and vertical space requirements virtually halved. (b) The assembled unit. Note the gain in vertical space achieved by the modified female.

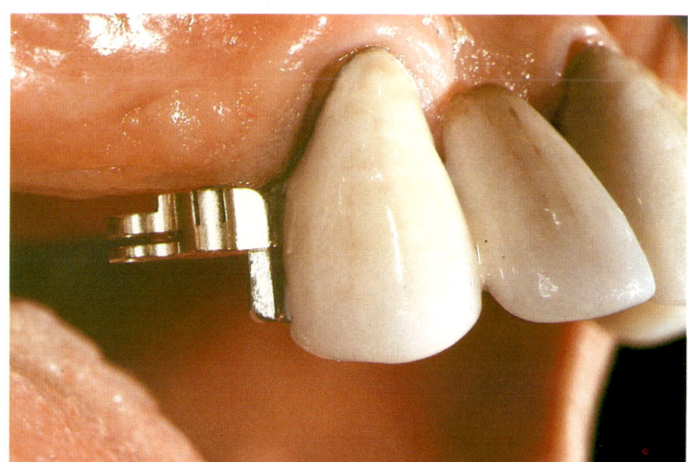

Fig. 307 Miniature Dalbo replacing conventional unit. The reduced vertical space requirement is apparent.

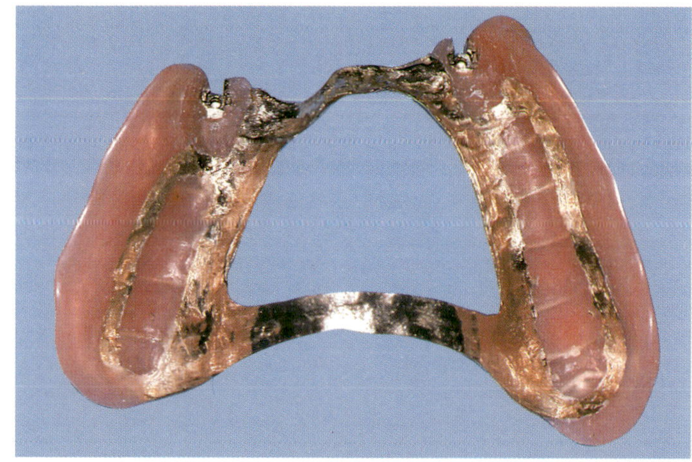

Fig. 308 An old example of an upper partial denture retained by two Dalbo extracoronal attachments. Had palatal support been required, a plate connector would have been necessary.

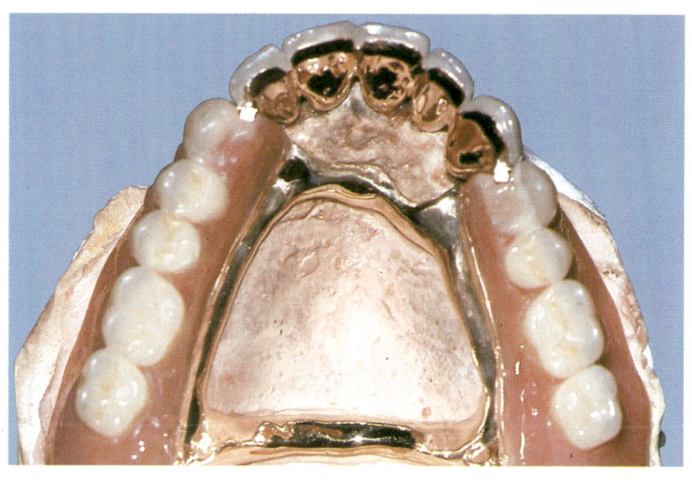

Fig. 309 A clasp-retained denture made for this situation might have been unsightly and poorly retained.

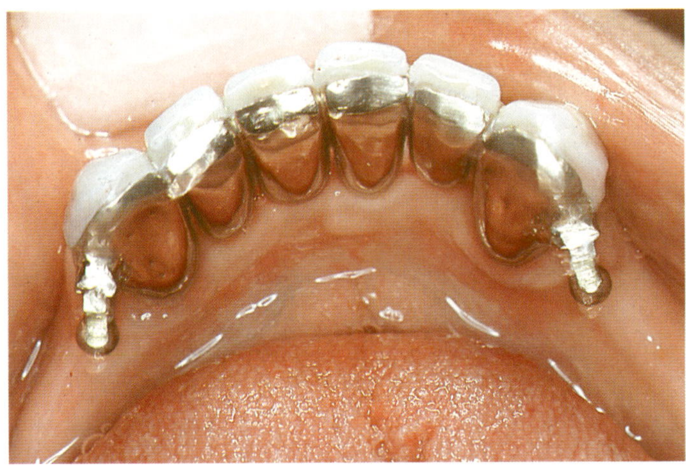

Fig. 310 Extracoronal attachments are particularly useful where lower canines are the abutments. The shape of these teeth generally precludes the use of introcoronal attachments.

which to replace a conventional unit that is causing problems through lack of vertical space.

Dalbo extracoronal attachments require no buccal retainers or lingual bracing arms. The appearance of the completed restoration should be excellent, while the retention and tilt-preventing properties are extremely effective. Since the attachments do not interfere with the apparent contour of the abutment crown, they are particularly useful where buccolingual space is restricted (Figs. 308 and 309). Common examples are lower canine teeth that are frequently too thin to accommodate an intracoronal attachment (Figs. 310 and 311). Patients learn to handle Dalbo attachments remarkably quickly and require less skill in handling them than intracoronal attachments.

Like other extracoronal attachments, vertical loads are transmitted away from the long axes of the abutment teeth and require the use of splinted abutments and a well-constructed denture. This problem should not be accentuated by placing the attachment on the distal aspect of a cantilevered pontic.

A notable feature of this attachment is that laterally applied and tilting forces are resisted by metal-to-metal contact; not by acrylic resin to metal contact. This feature must contribute to the strength for which the attachment is well-known.

The projection across the gingivae is a complication shared with other extracoronal units. With the base of the attachment in contact with the mucosa, one must avoid small and irregular spaces that are difficult to clean (Fig. 312). A slight lingual twist to the attachment increases the slope at which the mucosa falls away, and simplifies plaque control (Fig. 313).

While alignment with the sagittal plane is not recommended, it is essential that the attachments align with each other in the vertical plane. This is achieved with a rigid surveyor, using a paralleling mandrel supplied by the manufacturer. The path is normally selected to give an approach from

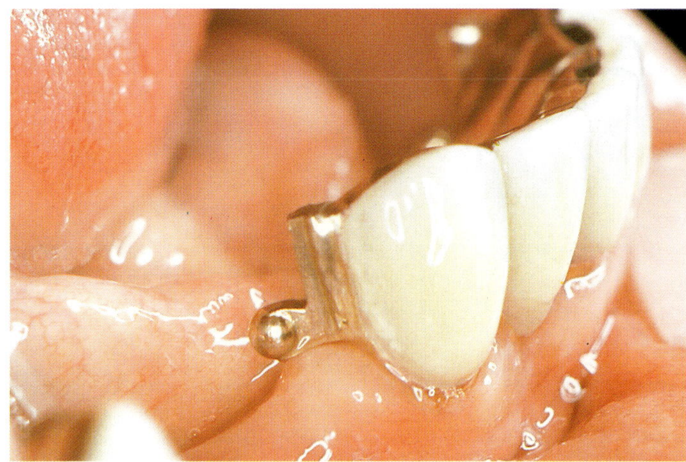

Fig. 311 Abutments 8 years later.

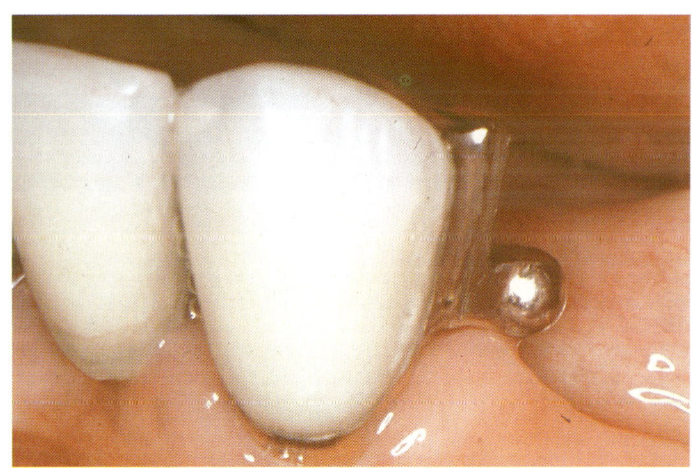

Fig. 312 With more than a decade of use this attachment continues to provide satisfactory service.

the distal aspect of the abutments to facilitate positioning of the attachment.

Extracoronal attachments are extremely sensitive to poor plaque control (Fig. 314), yet there is one point that is so often overlooked—denture hygiene. If the acrylic resin of the denture is cut away from the attachment to leave a 'relief chamber', the space will fill with debris and plaque that will be difficult to remove.

Space requirements often dictate that the base of the attachment be placed in contact with the mucosa. The curved base, however, helps to simplify plaque control and covers a relatively small area—far less than an inadequately recessed intracoronal attachment. Sound periodontal tissues before prosthodontic therapy and adequate maintenance subsequently are essential for success. Patterns of wear on the occlusal surface are desirable features, provided they are not excessive. They

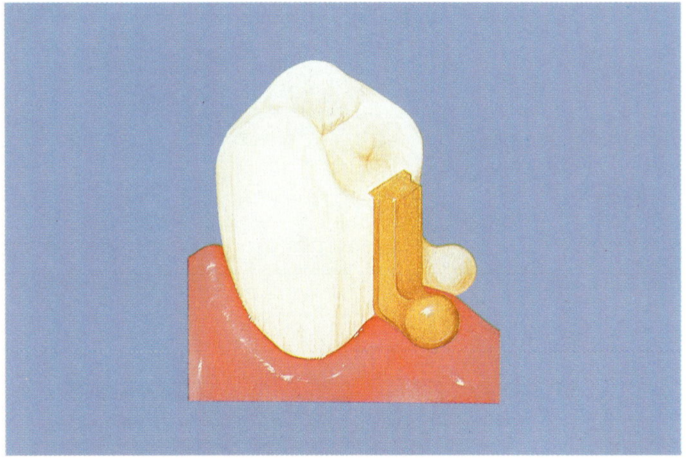

Fig. 313 Aligning the attachment lingual to the midline of the ridge increases the slope at which the mucosa falls away from the base of the unit and simplifies plaque control.

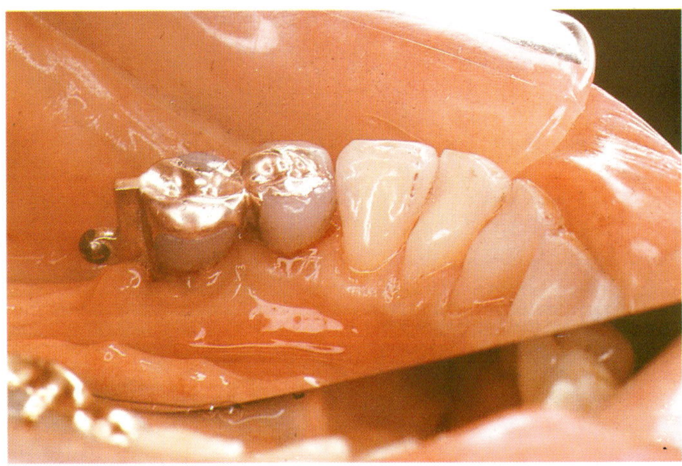

Fig. 314 Inadequate plaque control combined with continual denture movement frequently lead to this type of denture damage.

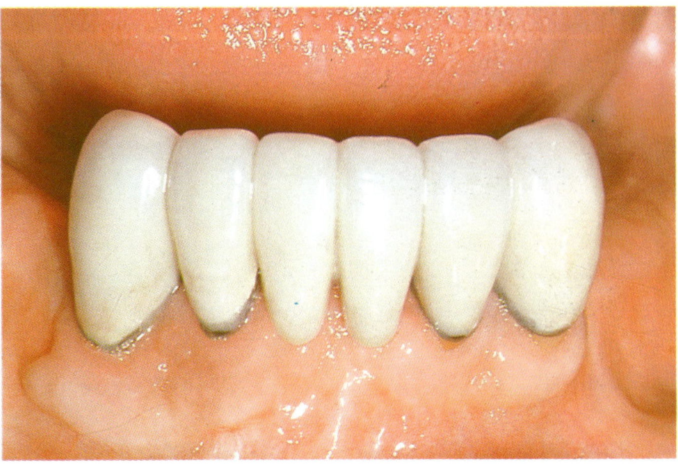

Fig. 315 Dalbo retained denture illustrating free mucosal graft 3 years post-operatively.

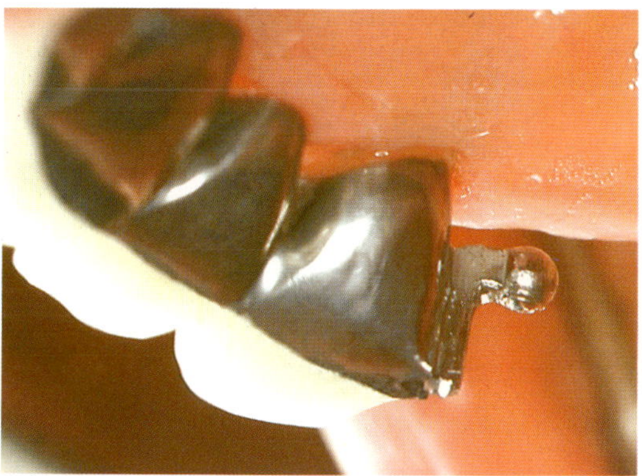

Figure 316 a

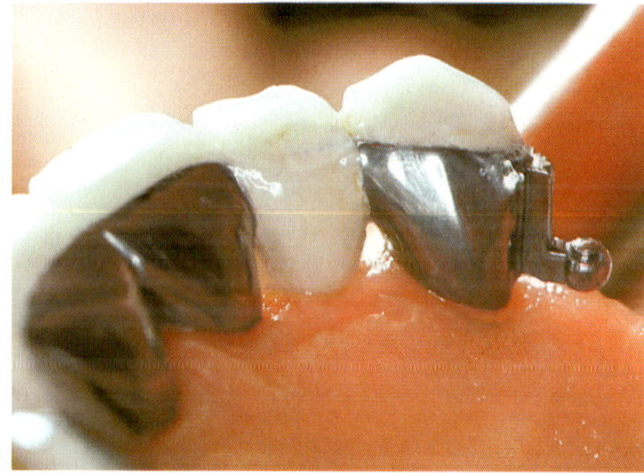

Figure 316 b

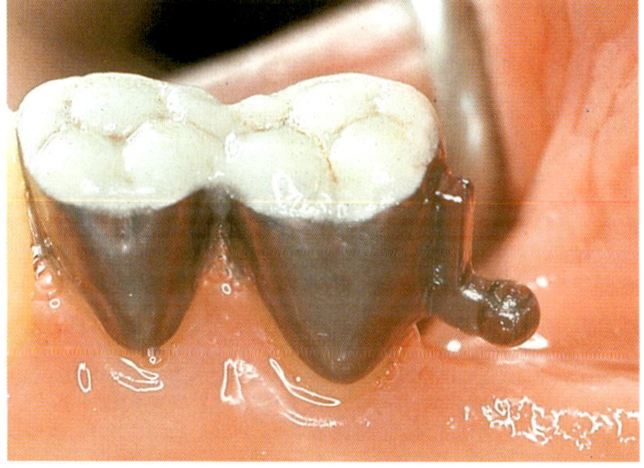

Figure 316 c

Figure 316 d

Fig. 316 (a-d)   Seven year results. Note the slight wear of the attachment sides and the wear of the occlusal surface by the spring. Wear patterns on the occlusal surface are desirable, if small, demonstrating transmission of vertical occlusal forces.

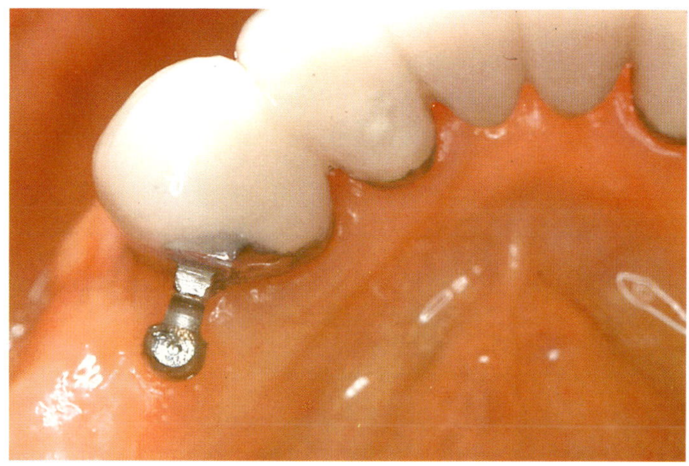

Fig. 317   Transmission of vertical occlusal forces through the miniature attachment produces slight flattening of the occlusal surface.

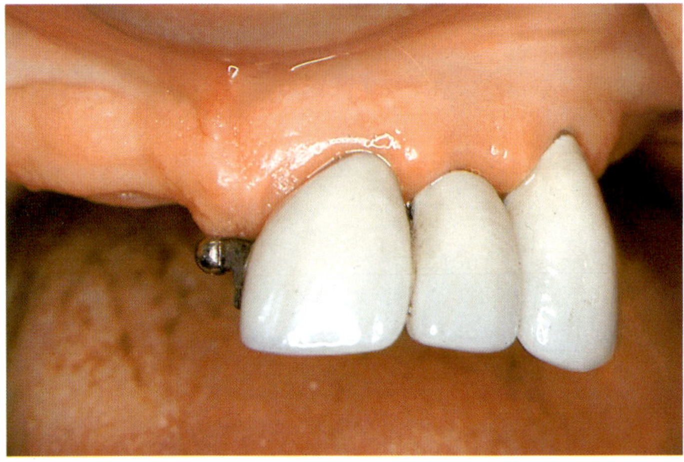

Fig. 318 Gross misalignment of Dalbo attachment that completely alters the designed load distribution to the unit.

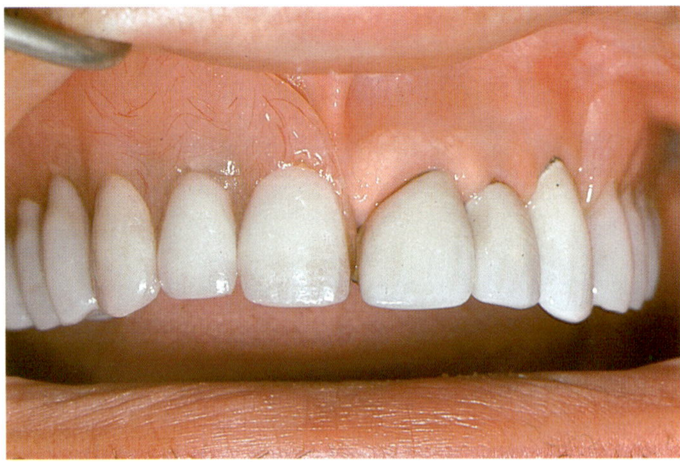

Fig. 319 A surprisingly well-retained restoration.

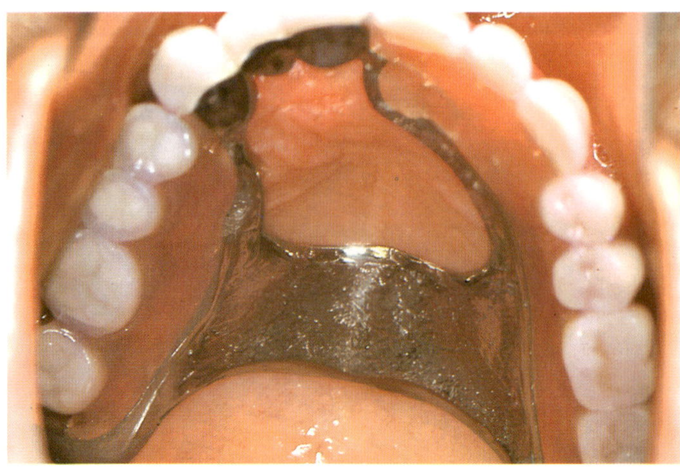

Fig. 320 Note the palatal bulge caused by the incisor attachment.

demonstrate that the denture is partly tooth supported (Figs. 315 to 317).

The Dalbo units are straightforward to use, but the nature of their construction also make them prone to misuse. While the axes of the hinges do not require alignment, divergencies of 60° are sometimes attempted. In these circumstances, the entire load distribution to the unit is altered and there is little to prevent tilting of the denture following distortion of the female section of the attachment (Figs. 318 to 321). The miniature females are more prone to this type of mishap.

Like other extracoronal units, the shape of the Dalbo units make them useful for combined restorations where, for example, there is an anterior space between two small groups of teeth. Even a well-made partial denture will have a tendency to rock around the abutments in this situation, but a poorly constructed denture is capable of causing appreciable damage (Figs. 322 and 323). A better approach is to restore the anterior space with a fixed prosthesis, thereby splinting the remaining teeth (Fig. 324). Extracoronal attachments can be employed to retain the bilateral distal extension denture (Figs. 325 to 327). A similar restoration can also be constructed when only two lower canines remain, provided their bone support is adequate. This type of restoration is frequently opposed to a complete upper denture. It is essential that this complete denture be stable when the entire restoration has been completed; it would hardly be satisfactory to provide a complex lower prosthesis that made the upper denture unwearable. Stability in this case can be achieved only with correctly positioned teeth arranged to provide a balanced ar-

ticulation. It cannot be achieved if the metal framework of the fixed prosthesis is completed before the jaw relation records are made, for this framework actually determines the position of the lower anterior teeth.

The jaw relationship records and trial insertions should be carried out as if the lower restoration were to be simply a partial denture, and the correct position of the teeth recorded in this way. Their position can be recorded on the master cast by means of a plaster mask, and the metal structure then completed. When the assembled restoration is first inserted a check record is essential.

Dalbo attachments may be used to restore bounded spaces, virtually as substitutes for intracoronal attachments. When applied in this way they lose their hinge action potential, and their vertical movement is best prevented. The advantage of not requiring an abutment box preparation makes them useful for anterior prostheses in younger patients, and occasionally posterior ones as well, provided there is sufficient vertical space for the attachment. The advantages and disadvantages of fixed and removable prostheses are discussed in Chapter 1 and 4, and apply to these extracoronal units. Extracoronal attachments, like the Dalbo, should not be used where the abutment teeth on either side of the saddle tilt towards each other. An impossible plaque control problem results leading to gingival and periodontal damage (Figs. 328 and 329).

When used correctly, extracoronal attachments provide a neat, well-retained restoration, with many of the advantages of a partial denture. Mucosal coverage is possible, the restoration may be removed

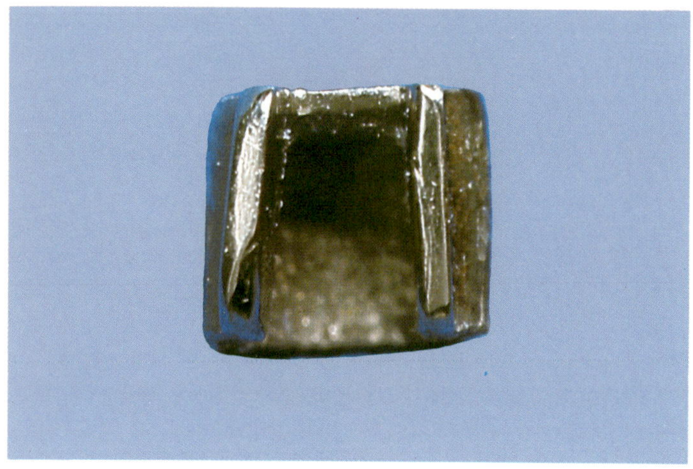

Fig. 321 Damage to the walls of the female attachment section caused by misuse. These walls were originally parallel.

for cleaning, and it may be rebased should further alveolar resorption occur (Fig. 330).

Some attachments require individual technical procedures, but the majority follow remarkably similar patterns. The abutments are surveyed to check for misalignment (Fig. 331), corrections carried out and the impression made in the material of choice. The crowns are then waxed-up (Fig. 332), and the attachments carried into place with the aid of a special mandrel (Fig. 333). Where bonded porcelain to gold techniques are employed, the attachments are left in the waxed-up crowns which are then cast (Figs. 334 and 335). With conventional yellow gold alloys the attachments are removed from the waxed-up crowns and subsequently soldered in place after casting.

Following construction of the major connector, an important clinical task is to ensure that the location of the two sections of the attachments is identical in the mouth and on the master cast.

Retention

Thanks to its effective ball and socket connection the Dalbo attachment is remarkably wear-resistant. With the aid of a carving instrument the edges of the lamellae can be bent inwards by a minute amount. This procedure should be carried out in careful stages, one attachment at a time, and the prosthesis reinserted after each adjustment. Excess acrylic resin may jam the lamellae of the attachment. No attempt should be made to remove it with a rotating instrument. Instead, an old discarded probe should be taken, heated over a flame, and the excess resin burnt away with its tip as the instrument is run along the outside edge of the attachment. Rotating instruments tend to skid off the gold, damage the attachment and remove too much resin.

Occlusal support

This vital aspect is one of the weaker points of the conventional spring-con-

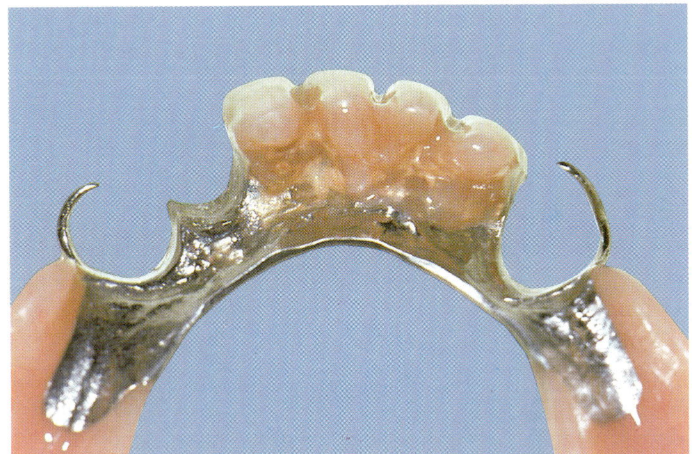

Fig. 322 A poorly designed partial denture.

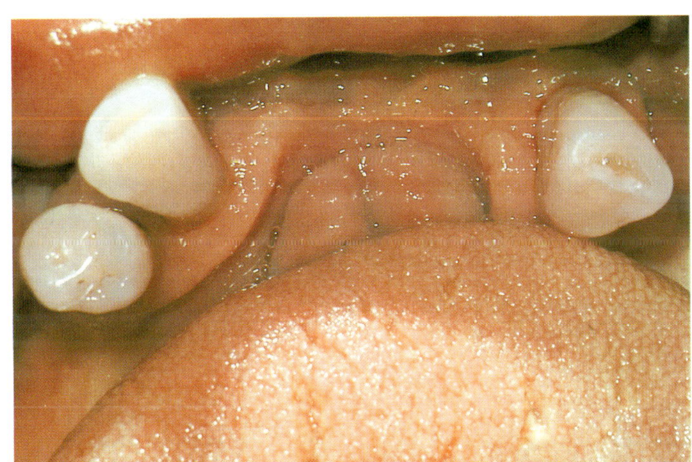

Fig. 323 The resulting damage in the mouth.

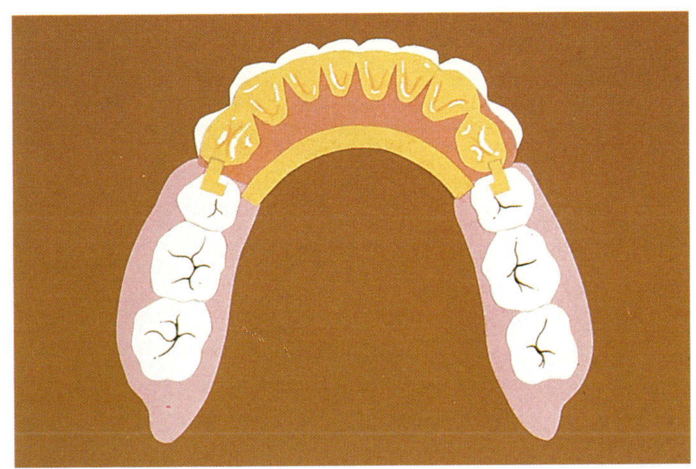

Fig. 324 Ideally the anterior spaces should be restored with a fixed prosthesis and the distal spaces with a bilateral distal extension denture.

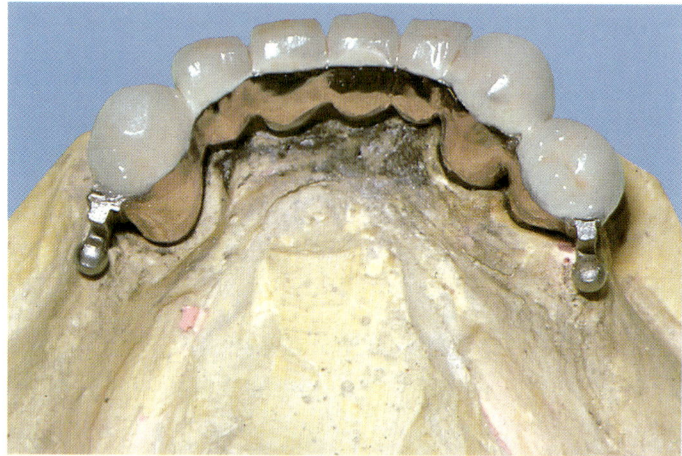

Fig. 325 The anterior space can be restored by a fixed prosthesis.

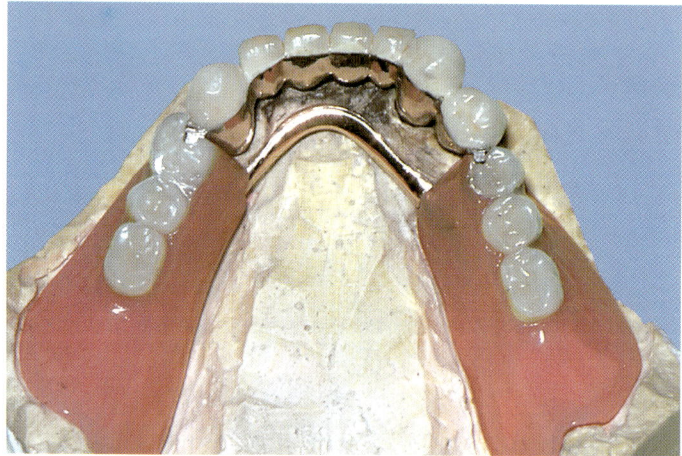

Fig. 326 The restoration on the master cast.

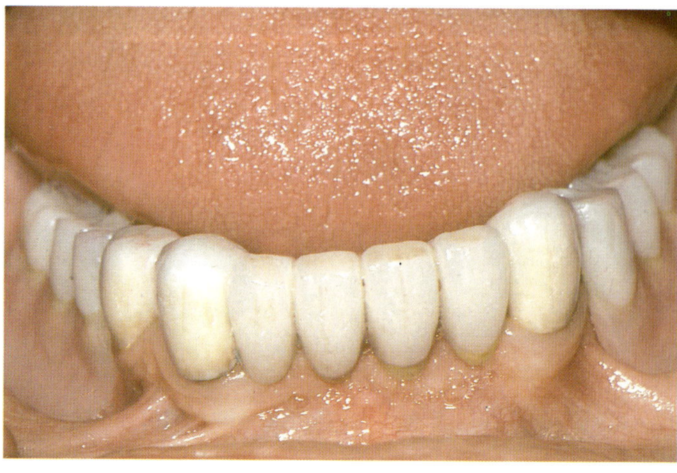

Fig. 327 The restoration in the mouth.

Fig. 328 Where the abutments either side of a space tilt towards each other, the attachments have to project a considerable distance from the crowns of the abutments. These are most unsuitable situations for extracoronal retainers.

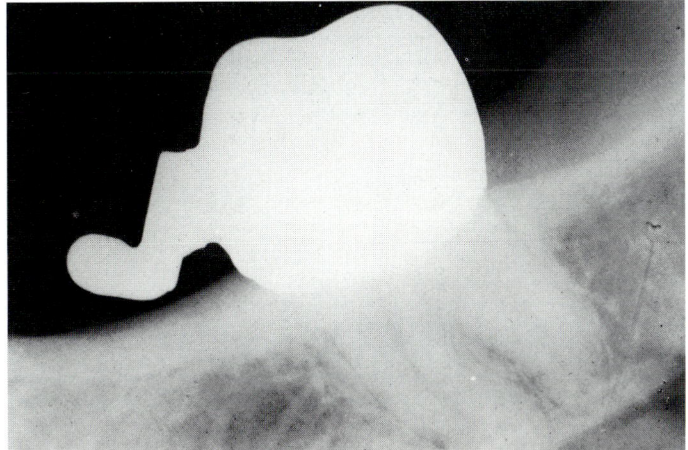

Fig. 329 Lingual view of abutment crown.

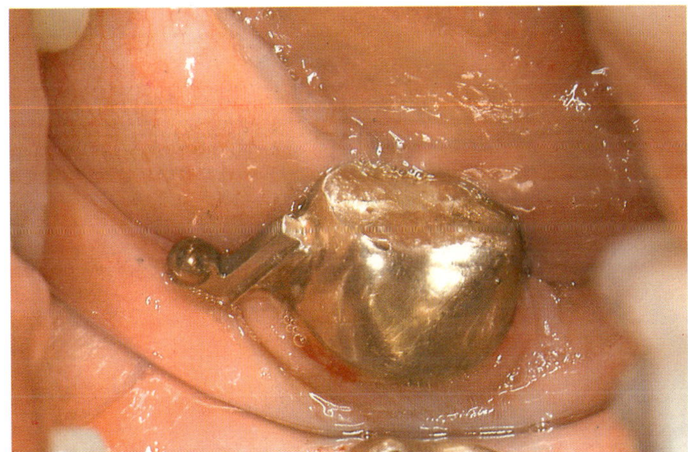

Fig. 330 An example of a removable anterior prosthesis retained by two extracoronal attachments.

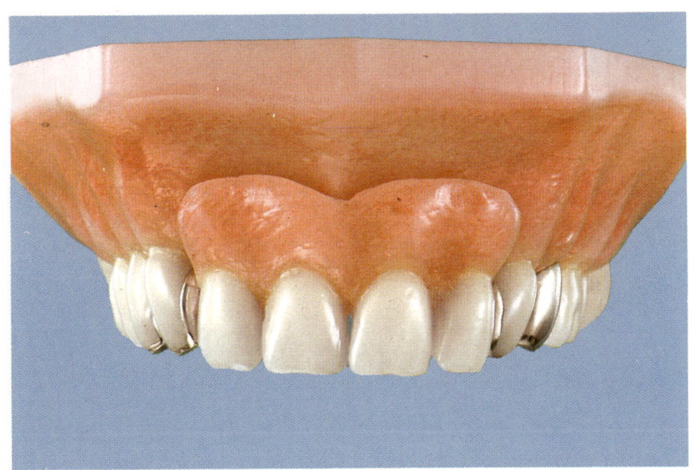

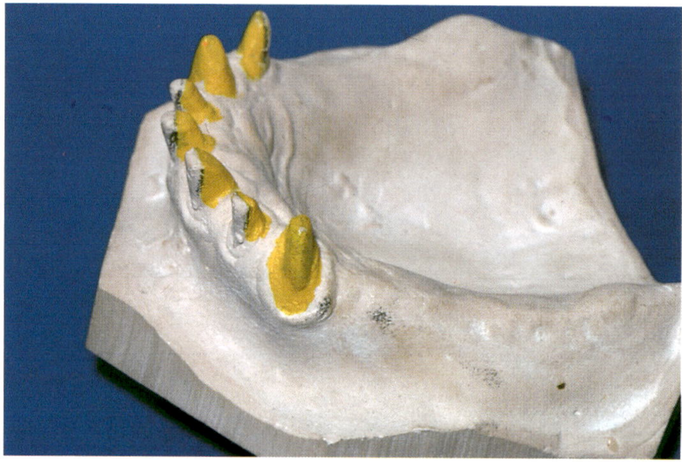

Fig. 331 Checking the alignment of the preparations.

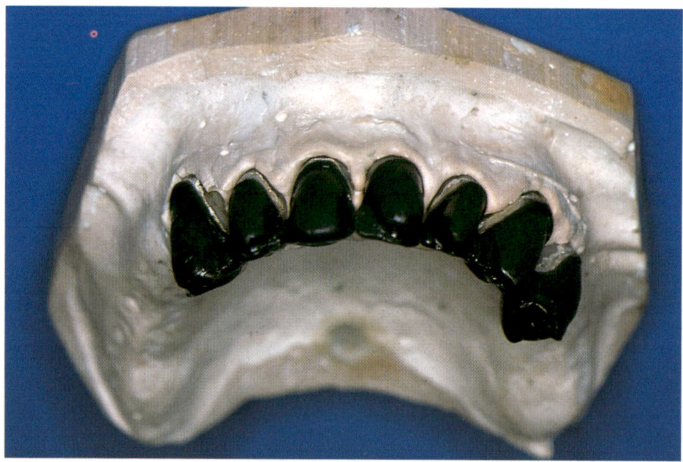

Fig. 332 The crowns waxed-up.

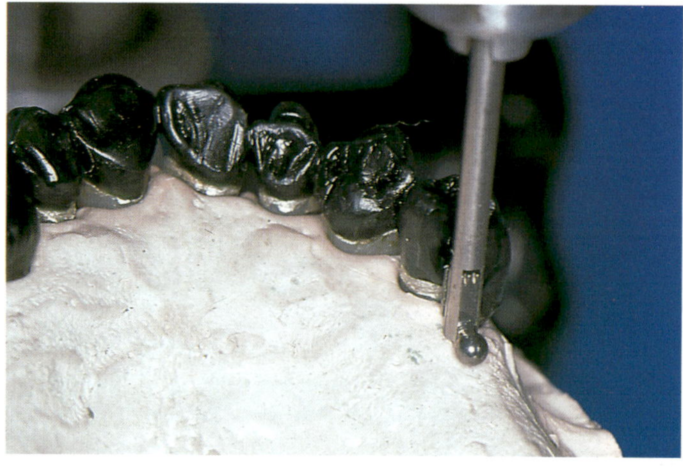

Fig. 333 Alignment of the attachments with a paralleling mandrel.

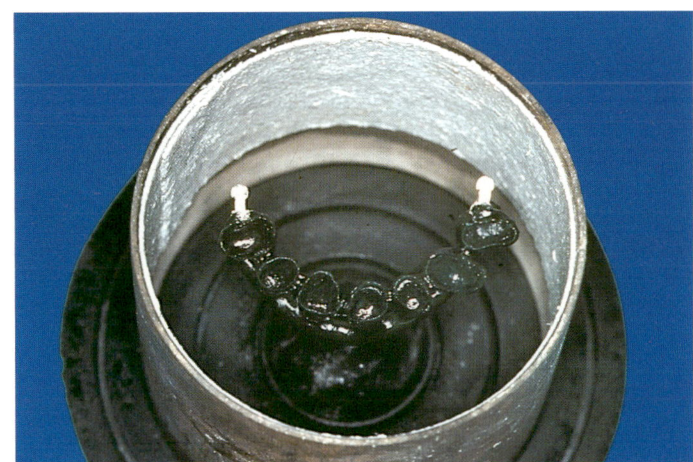

Fig. 334 The waxed-up crowns prior to investment (bonded gold to porcelain).

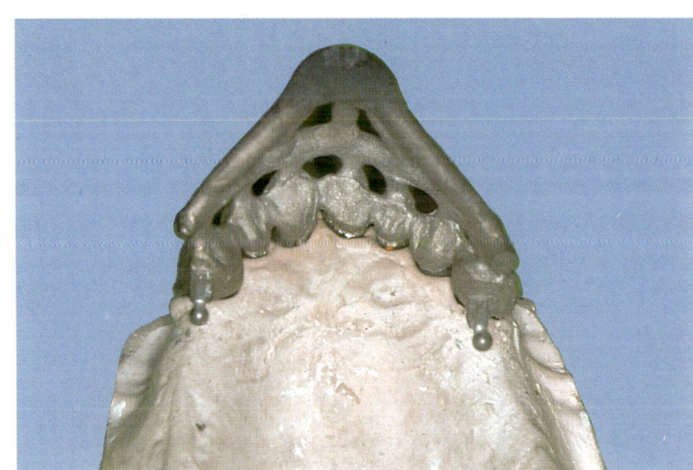

Fig. 335 The sprues in place following casting with platinised gold. For yellow gold techniques the attachments are removed before the crowns are cast and subsequently soldered.

trolled attachment. Permanent deformation of the spring is insidious, is seldom noticed by patients, and results in the denture becoming entirely mucosal-borne. Problems with springs is the one criticism levelled at the unit by *Rantanen* (1972) in his survey of attachment-retained partial dentures. Springs may not just deform, they may break or fall out. The period between spring changes varies with the loads applied, but 6 months should be re-garded as the maximum (Fig. 336). Spring damage or loss can be detected by careful examination of the articulation, as it results in the mesial denture tooth coming out of occlusion (Fig. 337). Some wear of the ball is both normal and desirable, showing that it is carrying load. Failure to check this important point can lead to the prosthesis losing tooth support, resulting in damage to the edentulous ridge (Fig. 338).

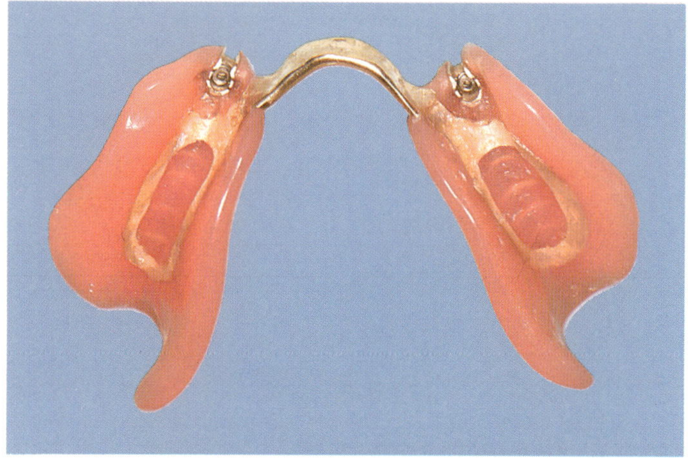

Fig. 336 Springs should be changed at no longer than 6 monthly intervals.

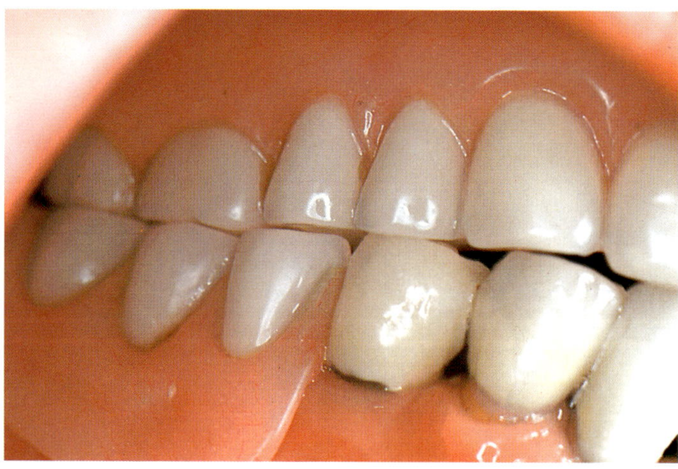

Fig. 337 Deformation of spring has lead to the mesial artifical tooth becoming out of occlusion.

The old spring is simply removed with a well-used probe, and the chamber examined to ensure that no broken pieces or debris remain. The new spring can then be carried into place on the shank of an old bur from which the head has been removed. The wider end of the spring is inserted first. Spring containers must be carefully marked to ensure the two sizes are not confused.

In view of the complexities of springs, operators may prefer to substitute the metal spacer where loads dictate the use of conventional Dalbo attachments. The miniature attachments do not suffer from this problem, but it is unwise to use them for long bases opposed by natural teeth. Even miniature Dalbo attachments should be inspected to ensure that a shiny spot is present that shows occlusal loads are being transmitted through the attachment.

Fig. 338 (a) (b) Two examples illustrating the results of lack of maintenance.

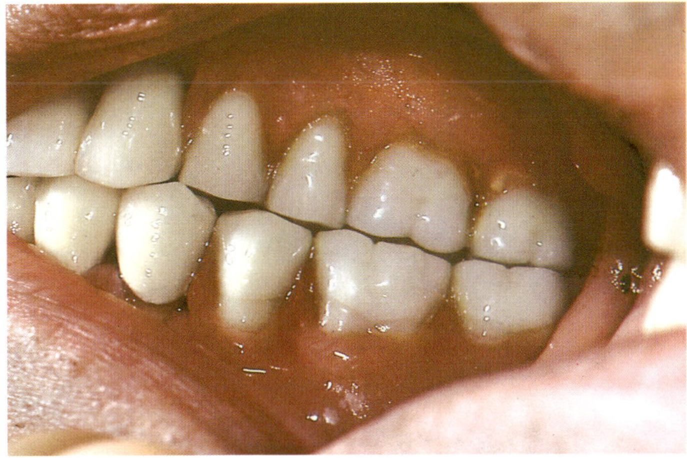

Figure 338 a

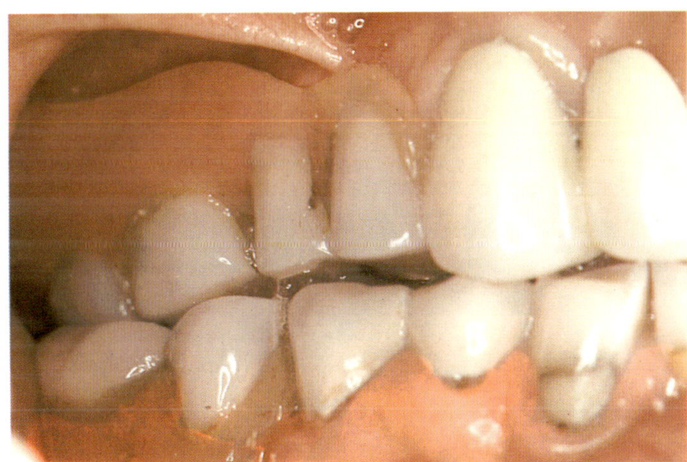

Figure 338 b

Rebasing

Partial dentures retained by intracoronal or rigid extracoronal attachments can be rebased like clasp-retained prostheses. The precise path of insertion of the units, together with lack of movement potential, ensures that the denture framework is in its correct relationship to the abutment crowns when it is completely seated. The Dalbo, and other similar extracoronal at-tachments, do not have this advantage. While vertical play can be prevented by using the metal spacer, the distal hinge movement is virtually uncontrolled. Ingenious modifications of the Dalbo, such as the Pin-Dalbo (Fig. 339) and Dalbo M (*Mensor* 1968), have been developed to prevent such evil fortune. Since it is only natural to apply load to the artificial teeth when making the impression, some hinge movement will inevitably occur. With the

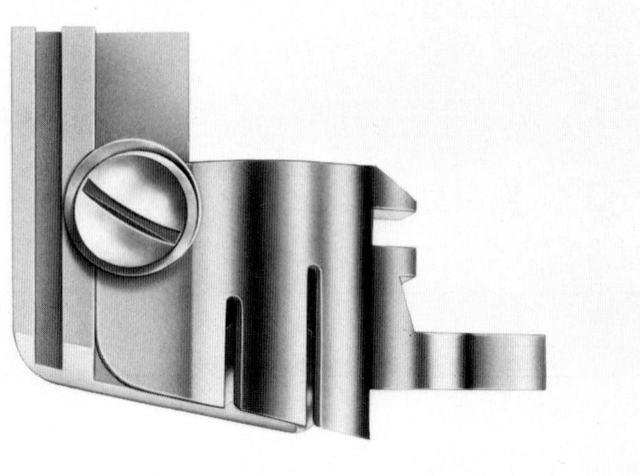

Fig. 339 The Pin-Dalbo. A modified Dalbo attachment allowing the two sections to be locked together during impression or rebasing techniques.

Dalbo attachments the two flanges will now be separated. If the resin is then processed with the flanges in this relationship, the denture will be free to rotate away from the mucosa until the flanges touch (Fig. 340). Apart from derangement of the occlusion, this allows the back of an upper denture to drop, or a lower denture to lift. Rebasing is not a 5 minute operation. It is an exacting and demanding technique requiring considerable time and clinical expertise.

The resin should be cut away from the occlusal and lingual aspect of the female attachment. Occasionally, the buccal facing may need to be sacrificed. It will now be possible to see the precise relationship of the two sections of the attachment when the denture is seated. Furthermore, seating load can be applied directly to the attachment and never to a point distal to it. The rebase impression can now be made, ensuring that the relationship between the attachment sections remains undisturbed.

This relationship is even more critical with the miniature units, in view of the small contact area and the relatively large leverages around them (Fig. 341). Once the material has set, excess is removed from the region of the attachment and the abutment crowns, together with the attachment relationship, is then examined with care. As an additional safeguard, the denture base can be checked for movement. The denture is then removed in an overall alginate impression that records details of the entire arch. Before the impression is cast, dowels are placed in each attachment and become incorporated in the cast. These locating dowels prevent movement of the attachment during processing (Fig. 342 a, b)

Most manufacturers produce such dowels for their attachments. Without them the alignment will be disturbed during processing.

Once the laboratory phase is completed the denture should be minutely examined

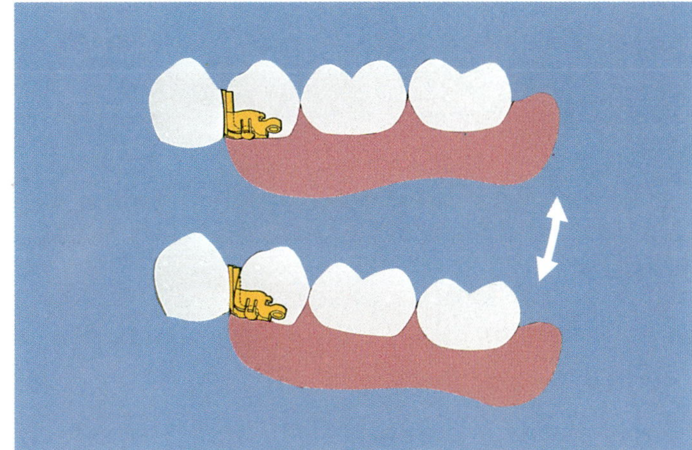

Fig. 340   Hinge movement occurring during rebasing or relocating procedures will allow the base to lift away from the mucosa subsequently until the two sections of the flange engage.

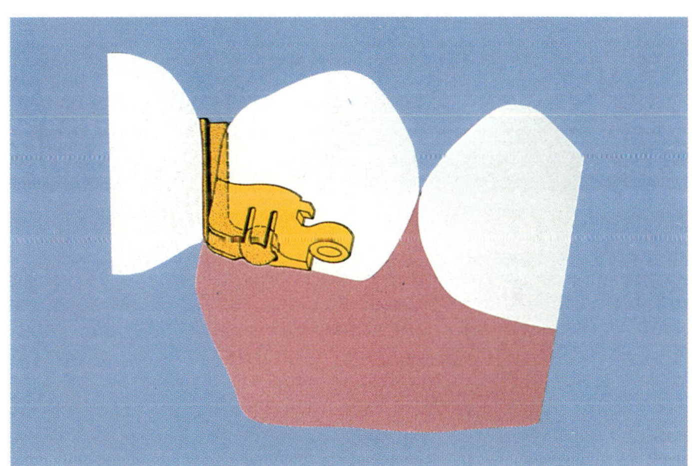

Fig. 341   The miniature attachments require considerable care as it is difficult to detect small rotations.

for irregularities on the impression surface, paying particular attention to the attachment area.

Replacing the denture in the mouth requires three important checks:

1. *Does the denture base seat correctly?*
   Ensure that no acrylic resin flash jams against the distal crown or attachment. No perceptible movement should occur when load is applied to the artificial teeth. The adaptation of the base can be checked with disclosing material.

2. *Do the attachments engage?*
   The slight click of the sockets engaging the ball should be felt. In the case of other similar attachments one should be able to feel the two sections lock together. In the absence of a satisfactory connection, examine the attachments for debris or acrylic resin that may prevent them seating. Make a small adjust-

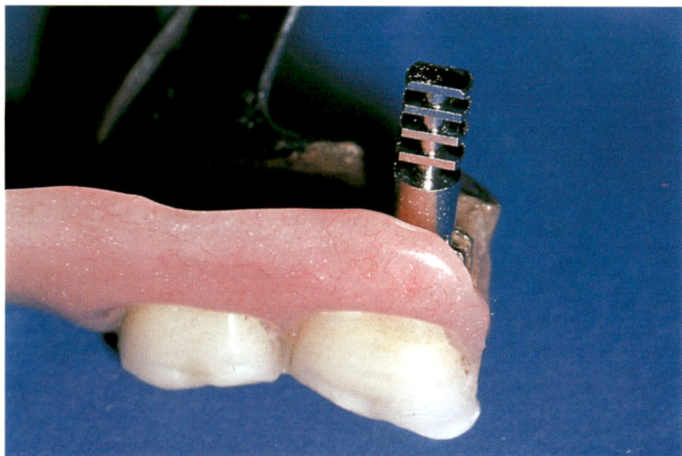

Fig. 342 (a) Locating dowel placed in attachment. These devices maintain the location of the attachments during processing. (b) Locating dowels incorporated in the master cast.

Figure 342 a

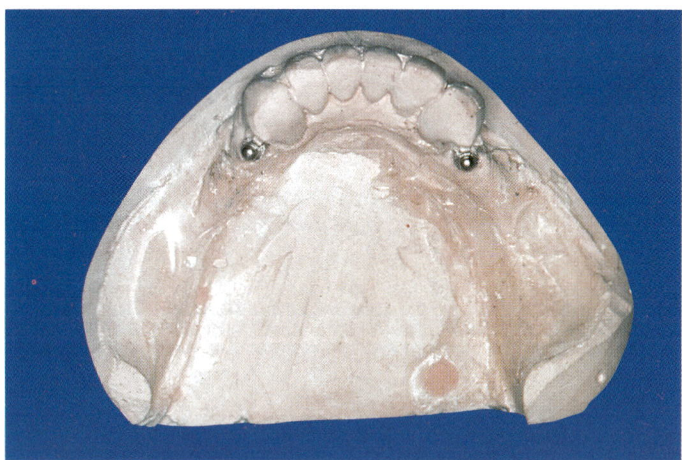

Figure 342 b

ment to the retention in case this has been altered during processing. If the attachments still do not engage, it is due to one or both of them having moved in the denture base during processing, usually as a result of failure to employ a rebasing jig or locating dowel. A relocating procedure will be required and this is described below.

3. *Check the occlusion and articulation.* This is best achieved using a check record and remount procedure. In the case of a lower restoration, a centric relation record is made and the record stone or wax left on the occlusal surfaces of the denture in the mouth. The denture is removed in a full-arch alginate impression. When this impression is cast, it is mounted with the centric relation record against a cast of the opposing jaw that has been positioned with a facebow. Eccentric records can then

be made and the occlusion and articulation perfected. Only minor corrections should be necessary unless an error in attachment locating has occurred.

Relocating procedure

The aim of this difficult procedure is to correct the alignment of an attachment when all other aspects of the construction are correct. The process has to be carried out in the mouth.

First of all the offending attachment is cut out of the denture, taking care to damage neither the buccal facing nor the attachment. A lingual window is cut out of the acrylic resin to allow subsequent inspection of the relationship of the flanges (Fig. 343), and to ensure that the denture will not foul the attachment when subsequently reinserted. The denture is then inserted in the mouth, minus the attachment, to ensure it seats correctly and that the occlusion and articulation are correct.

Space under the projection of the male unit is blocked with soft wax or, better still, plaster (Fig. 344). Any self-polymerising resin that flows into this space will lock the denture firmly in place, making subsequent removal time-consuming, destructive and painful for all concerned. Only those who have suffered this misfortune can know the problems a small amount of acrylic resin in the wrong place can cause.

The gingivae and surrounding mucosa are protected with vaseline and the attachment positioned on its counterpart. Check to ensure sufficient resin was removed to allow the denture to seat into its correct position without applying load to, or tilting, the attachment. The most common problem is slight load to the retention ring of the attachment causing tilting. Further resin will need to be removed in this instance and it is at times like this we appreciate the bulk occupied by different attachments. The location of miniature Dalbos and other small devices is particularly critical. Suppose the top of the flange failed to touch by 0.2 mm. The number of degrees the base was free to rotate would be about double compared with a similar error on the conventional Dalbo unit.

With the denture firmly seated and the attachment correctly located, lock the two together with the aid of a small amount of self-polymerising resin inserted through the lingual window (Fig. 345). When the resin has completely covered the denture, ensure that adequate retention has been obtained and that the location is correct. The remaining defect in the denture resin can then be repaired in stages, thereby minimising the effects of acrylic resin contraction.

Finally, remove excess resin from the free edges of the socket using a heated blunt probe.

The proper use of rebasing dowels will virtually eliminate the need to relocate attachments after rebasing. Accidents apart, the relocating procedure will be required when attachments need to be replaced and is frequently employed when a second denture is to be made after the abutment crowns have been cemented.

The PR extracoronal attachment must be one of the most robust constructed (Fig. 346 to 348). It features very large lateral surfaces. Retention is provided by a spring-loaded plunger, mounted lingually, engaging a dimple in the male section. A retraction slot is prepared to guide the plunger into place. The two small projec-

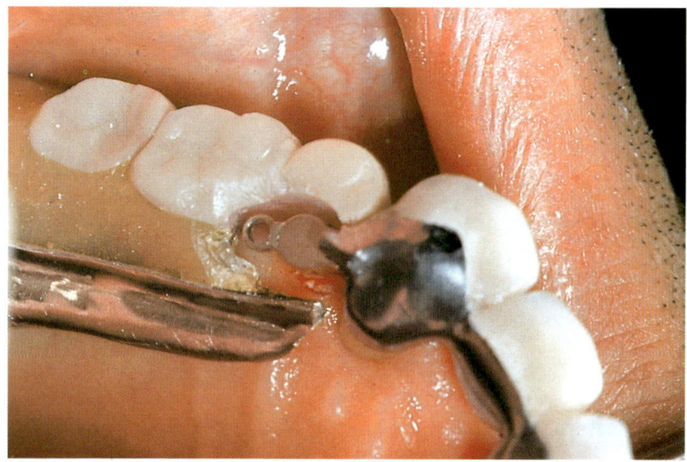

Fig. 343 Female section cut away from denture with a lingual window prepared to allow inspection of the two sections of the attachment.

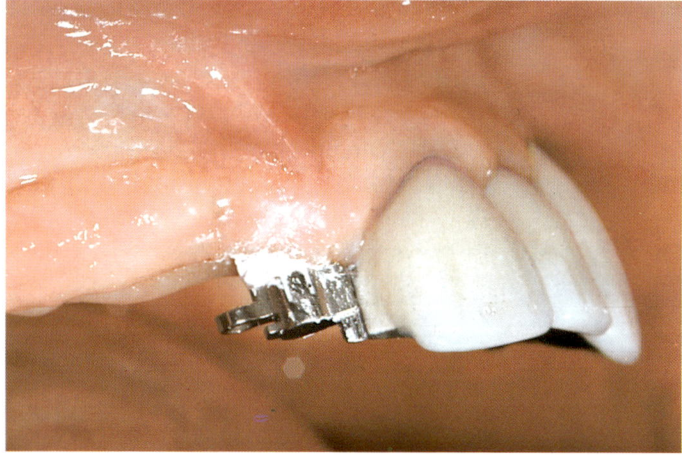

Fig. 344 Space under the attachment is blocked out with wax, or preferably plaster.

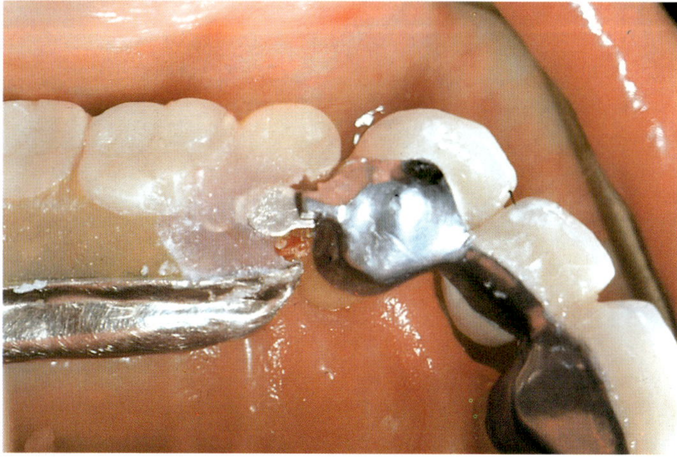

Fig. 345 Relocating the attachment to the denture with self-polymerising acrylic resin.

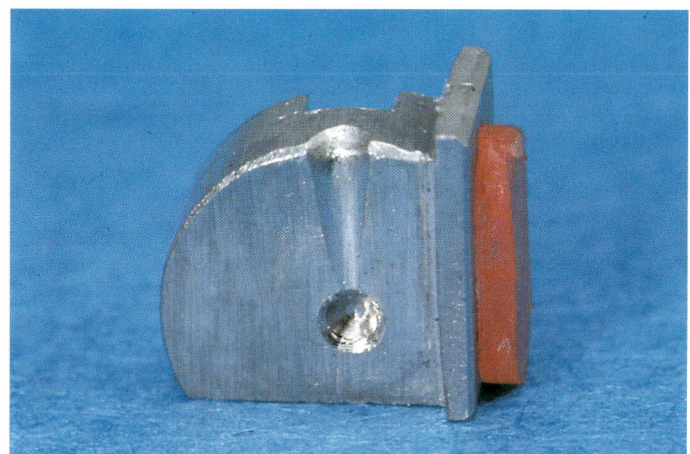

Fig. 346 Lingual view of PR male section showing dimple for retaining plunger and retraction slot. Note the large lateral facing surface.

Fig. 347 (a) PR attachment: anterior view of female section. (b) PR attachment embedded in a denture. The retaining plunger is on the left and the two locating projections on the right.

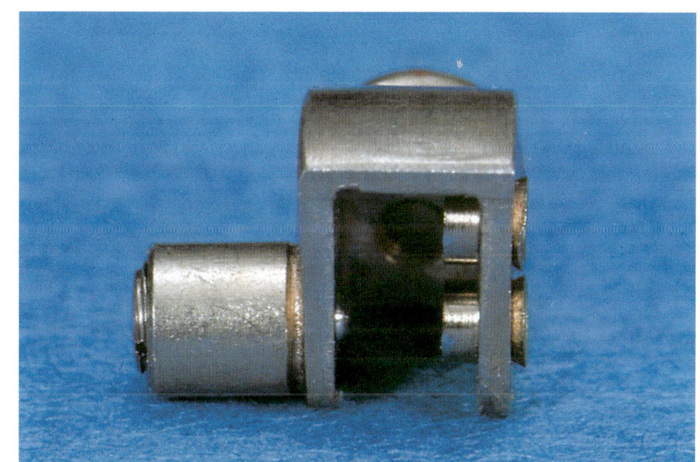

Figure 347 a

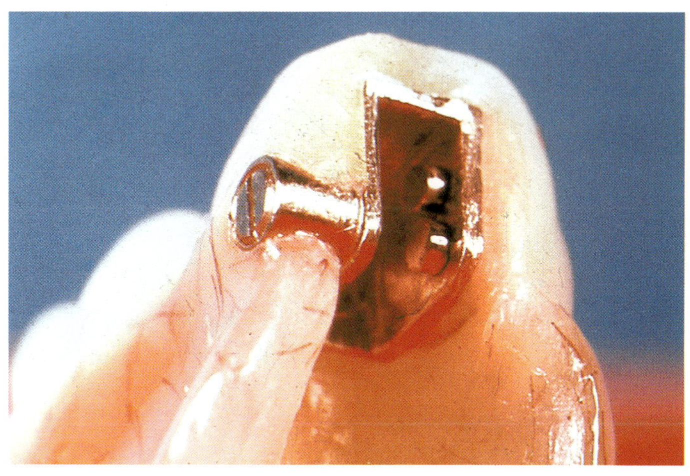

Figure 347 b

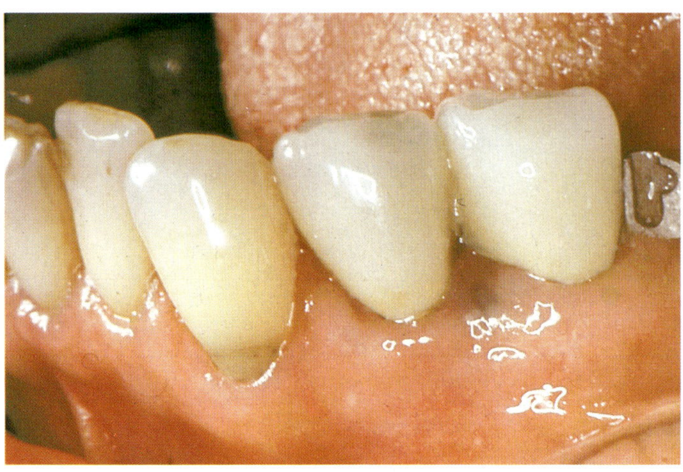

Fig. 348 Buccal view of the receptacles for locating projections of the PR attachment.

tions on the buccal side of the female unit govern the movement potential. The lower projection limits the vertical travel and the upper one restricts hinge movement. From the mechanical point of view the attachment has obvious advantages, particularly as a range of useful ancillary devices is available.

Plaque control and size restrictions are the limiting factors. The smaller of the two attachments is 4.5 mm tall, 5 mm long, and 5.4 mm wide. The larger unit measures 5.5 mm × 6 mm × 5.9 mm. Where space permits, these units have obvious merit. Left and right-sided units are made, and elements compatible with yellow gold or bonded procelain to gold are available.

The Ceka Attachment System

The Ceka attachment system has gained steadily in popularity and has been subjected to a process of continual modification and improvement. It is among the most versatile of all attachments and is based on the Ceka attachment unit that consists of a male pin engaging the centre of a circular retaining element. When used as an extracoronal retainer, the male retaining pin is attached to the denture and engages the centre of the retaining element that is joined to the abutment tooth. The retaining pin is conical in shape, while the female section is tapered from top to bottom (Figs. 349 and 350). Although a large range of these units is available, the dimensions of the female retaining element are standard.

As with other attachments, space considerations are essential. At least 5 mm of vertical space is required (Fig. 351) for the full size units, while there must be sufficient buccolingual space to allow the 4 mm diameter of the ring to be surrounded by an adequate thickness of denture base material. These dimensions can be reduced slightly by employing cast metal occlusal and lingual surfaces. Inadequate assessment of space requirement is a prime cause of denture fracture around the attachments. In practice, breakages are usually, and unfairly, blamed on the attachments.

Unlike some units, the Ceka attachment is primarily a direct retainer. Its circular shape will not prevent rotation around a vertical axis. For this reason an occlusal rest seat should be incorporated in the abutment crown contour. This occlusal rest seat will provide a positive stop in the transmission of occlusally directed forces and will also aid location of the denture in subsequent rebasing procedures. The lingual contour of the abutment crown should make provision for a lingual bracing arm. This arm will prevent lateral movement of the denture base and will help with seating the prosthesis in the mouth (Fig. 352 a, b). Guide planes in conjunction with the lateral bracing arms serve to provide the denture with a precise path of insertion and withdrawal, and help to prevent unwanted hinge movement. Guide planes are incorporated in some of the Ceka attachments and patterns.

A description of the various types of Ceka unit currently available is set out below. The manufacturer's terminology has been employed as far as possible.

600 series

The 600 series are resilient and must be used in conjunction with the correct retaining pin and spacers (Figs. 353 to 355). This series was derived from the original Ceka unit and it can be seen that the contours of the retaining pin allow vertical as well as rotational play. However, it should be understood that if these units are used in conjunction with a properly constructed bracing arm, together with an occlusal rest seat, the difference between

'rigid' and 'resilient' retaining pins become solely of academic interest.

700 series

The 700 series are comparatively rigid. The design of the male spring pin eliminates any vertical play. As with the 600 series, the male retaining pin may be unscrewed from its base thereby allowing replacement to be made without difficulty. A recent modification of the pin has been introduced that reduces its height by 0.3 mm while improving the stability of the connection formed within the attachment. The retention base for the pin is now only 2.1 mm high and the overall height of the 700 series unit has been reduced to 3.25 mm. Close scrutiny is required to recognise the new 700 series retaining pin. The taper on the pin commences immediately beneath the retaining base without the very small vertical collar found on the original 700 series. The new retention base does not permit interchange of the 600 and 700 retention pins, that was possible with the earlier models and allowed conversion from rigid to resilient units. The older 700 series retaining pins are still in production and are denoted by an 'X' on all labelling. It is apparent that great care must be taken to ensure that old and new pins are kept well separated.

300 series

The base of the male pin may be connected to the framework of the partial denture in one of three ways, and base type selected accordingly. The 'S' Type is designed for soldering to the framework of the partial denture. Soldering is the neatest and most effective method of connection

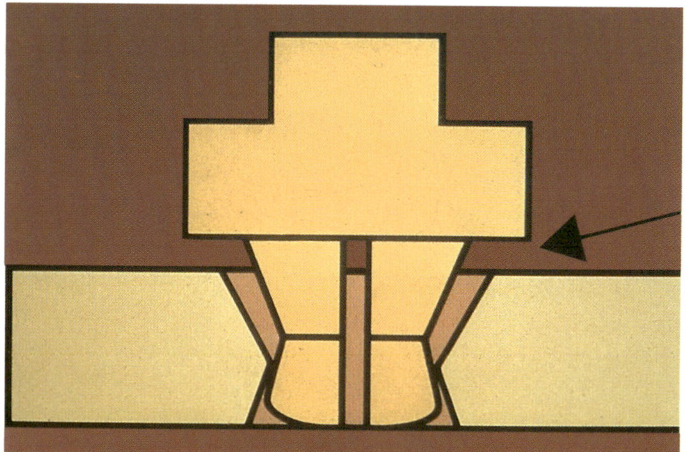

Fig. 349 Diagram of the Ceka attachment. (a) The resilient pin at rest. (b) The resilient pin under vertical load. (c) The resilient pin under rotational load.

Figure 349 a

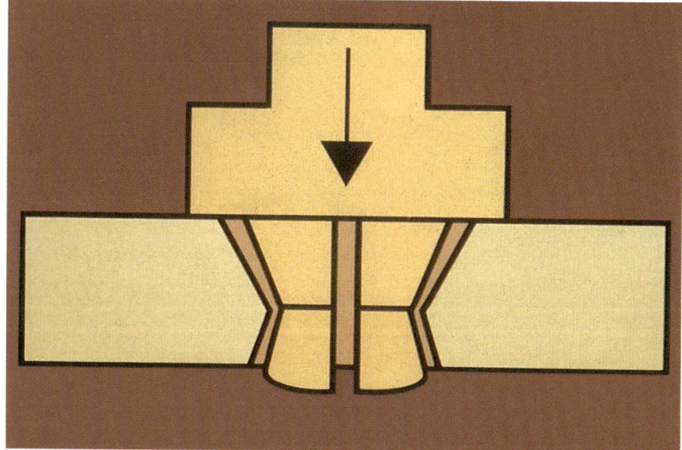

Figure 349 b

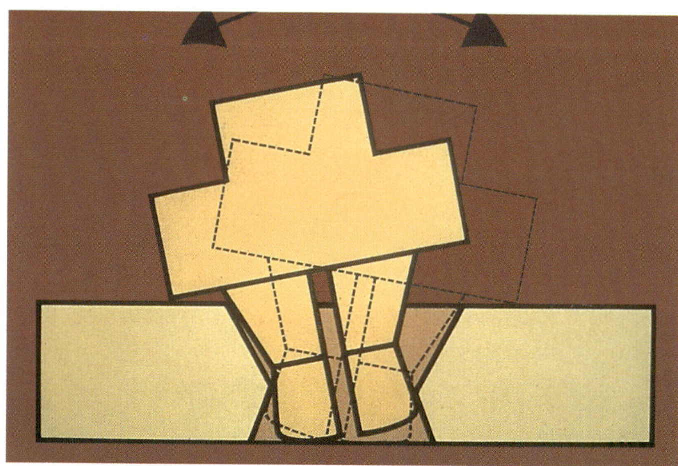

Figure 349 c

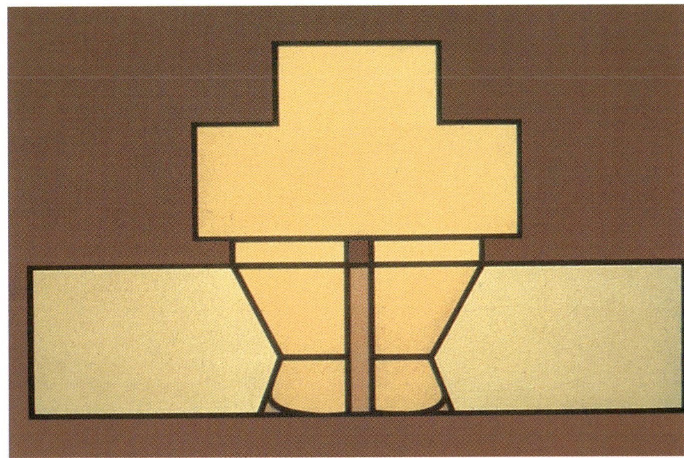

Fig. 350 The rigid pin assembly. The Ceka pin may be unscrewed for replacement.

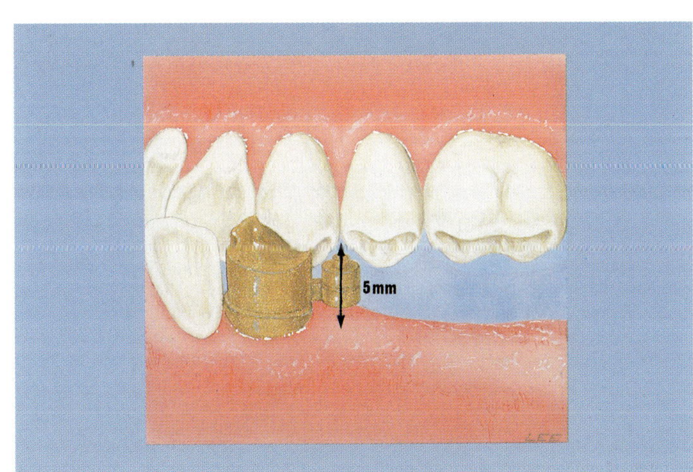

Fig. 351 At least 5 mm of vertical space is required for use of the full-sized Ceka unit.

once the technical problems of the soldering process have been mastered. The KS Type (Fig. 356) is designed to be buried in the acrylic resin of the denture base and includes retaining tags for the acrylic resin. The tags may be bent to reduce the space requirement. KS Type bases are available in a choice of yellow gold or stainless steel. The third method allows the attachment to be bolted to a minor connector of the partial denture (Fig. 357). The 300 series will be favoured by those who wish a direct metal-to-metal connection, but do not feel confident of the soldering techniques employed. While the union provided by the bolt connection is effective, it occupies additional space—a precious commodity in the region of the attachment.

Mini retaining unit

A new type of retaining pin has been introduced where vertical space is restricted. It is known as the mini retaining unit and to save space the retaining pin and base form one solid unit (Fig. 358). It should be pointed out that, unlike other male retaining

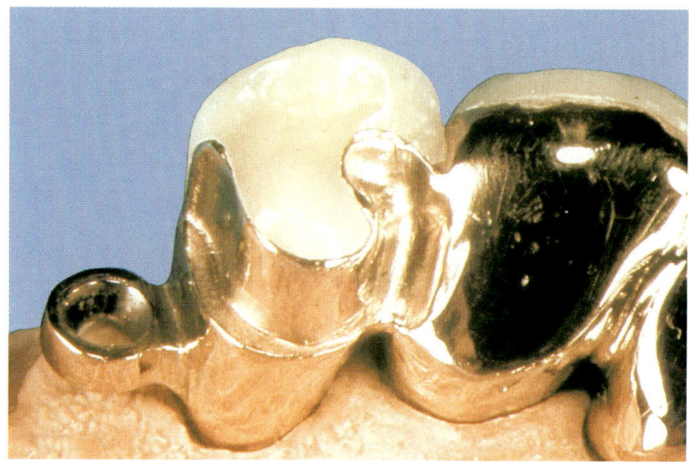

Fig. 352 (a) A modified design to show Ceka attachment with its associated guide plane, bracing arm and rest seat preparation. (b) The removable prosthesis in place.

Figure 352 a

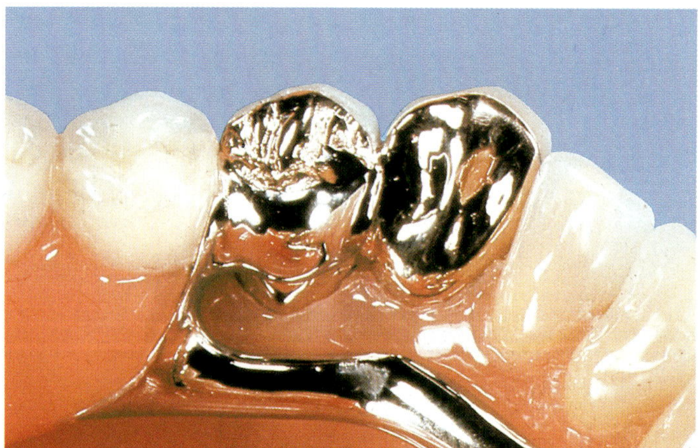

Figure 352 b

pins in the Ceka system, the miniature retaining pin cannot be separated from its base. The miniature configuration reduces the height of the retaining pin to 2.45 mm for the rigid and 2.75 mm for the resilient connection.

Female retaining rings

The female retaining rings of the Ceka units can be purchased as part of a precious metal bar that is sectioned close to the attachment by the technician. Palladium gold and yellow gold versions are available. The attachments manufactured in 'high heat' golds are available for use with porcelain bonded to gold techniques.

OL series

A recent addition to the range is a plastic pattern that can be invested and burnt out, allowing the attachment and crown to be cast on. The pattern includes a metal liner that becomes incorporated within the cast, thereby ensuring precision of fit with the male retention pin and adequate wear

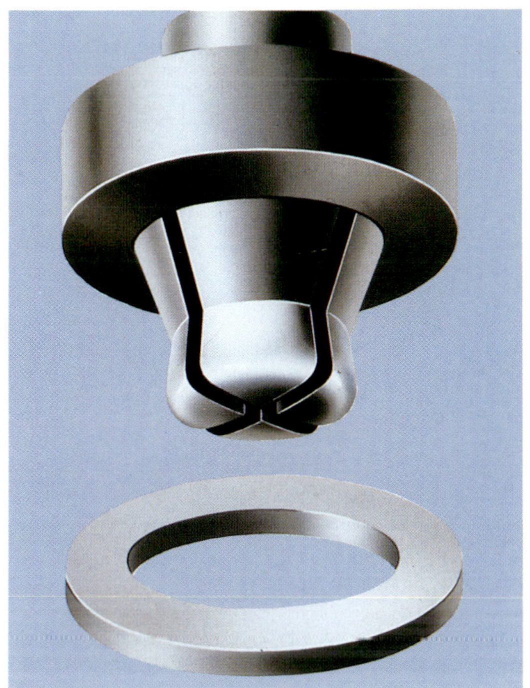

Fig. 353 The male section of the 'resilient' Ceka system showing the spacer that is incorporated during construction and rebasing procedures.

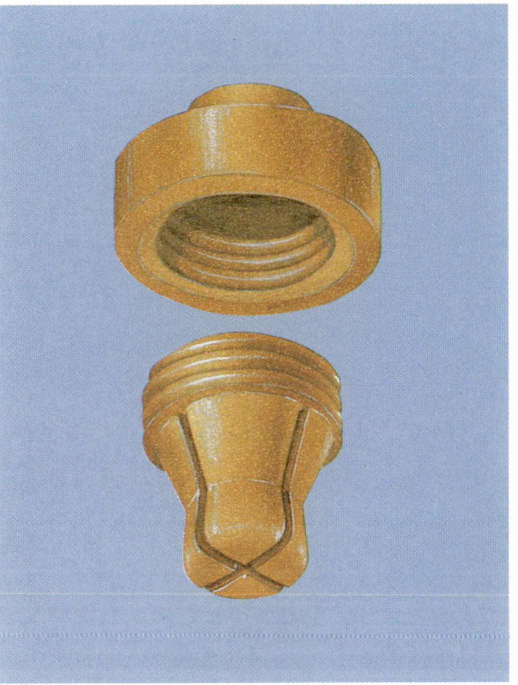

Fig. 354 The '600' series Ceka attachment for soldering to denture framework.

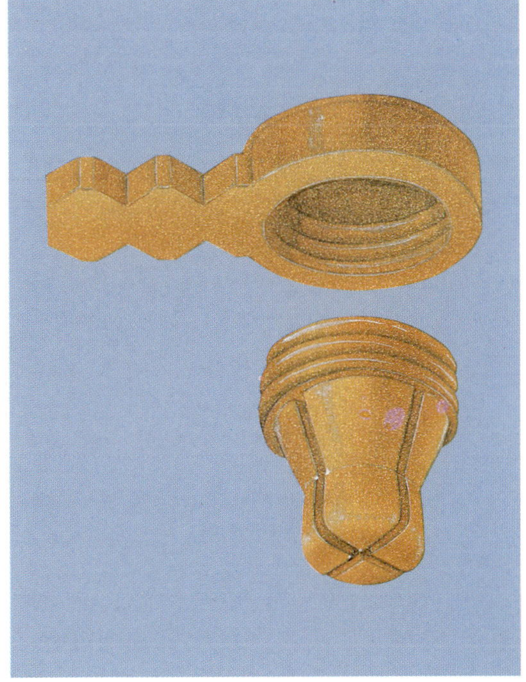

Fig. 355 The '600' series Ceka attachment for burying in acrylic resin.

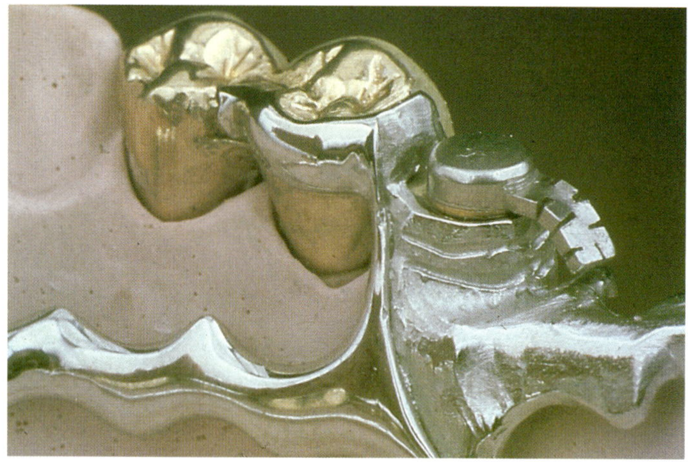

Fig. 356   Retention pins with bases for incorporation in acrylic resin of denture base (KS-type). Note that the tagging may be bent to accommodate it to the space available.

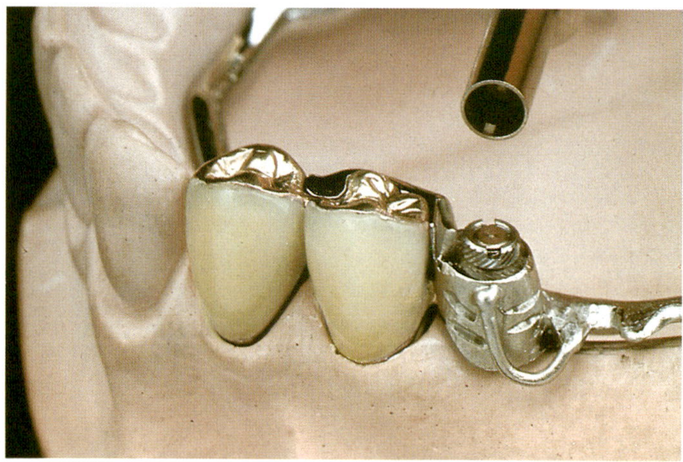

Fig. 357   Base of retention pin bolted to denture connector ('300' series). This tends to occupy a significant amount of vertical space.

resistance. This type is known as the OL series (Fig. 359). The plastic blanks in the OL series are colour-coded red and blue, although the dimensions of the patterns are identical. The red pattern incorporates a platinised alloy and is for use with precious metal alloys. The manufacturers produce one alloy, known as 'Irax', especially for this purpose. The blue pattern incorporates a liner for use with non-precious alloys and for this purpose the manufac-turers have produced one that is known as 'Noprax' that can be employed with porcelain bonding.

Ceka attachments with guide planes

A development of the Ceka attachment incorporates its own guide plane, sometimes known as a back plate. This unit is

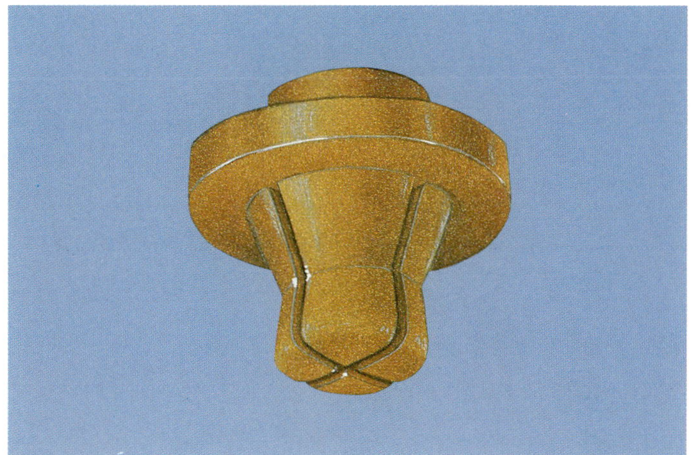

Fig. 358   The miniature retaining pin. The base and retaining pin form one solid unit, but the arrangement saves considerable vertical space.

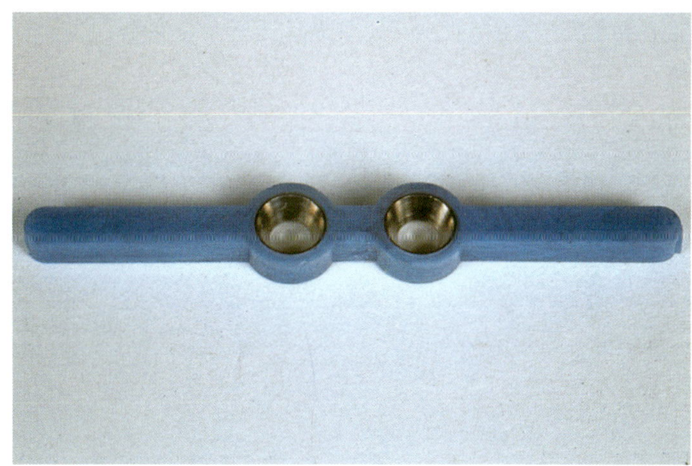

Fig. 359   The 'OL' series features a plastic pattern with a liner of metal. The blue pattern incorporates a liner for use with non-precious alloys.

available prefabricated in a high fusing alloy (Fig. 360) and a choice of male retaining pins allows either a resilient (696 series) or rigid (726 series) connection. Furthermore, 300 series, 400 series and Ceka mini male parts may be used in conjunction with it. This useful gadget is also available in plastic patterns, once again colour-coded for use with precious (red pattern) (Fig. 361) alloys or non-precious (blue pattern) alloys.

The Ceka attachments are versatile, robust and relatively simple to employ. Where buccal space is limited, the attachment can be positioned slightly lingual to its normal place and a lingual metal surface employed to reduce the bulk of the prosthesis. If buccolingual space is particularly restricted, it is not the best attachment for the situation.

When used to retain distal extension prostheses the applications are similar to other

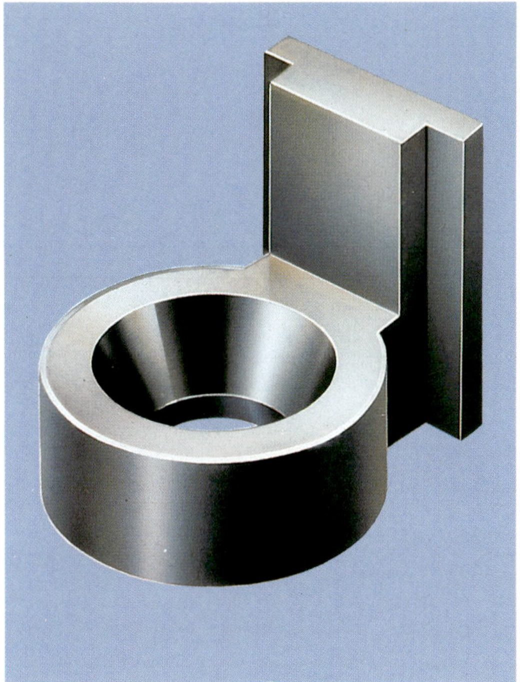

Fig. 360   The Ceka Lo-Cast attachment with back plate. This prefabricated Ceka unit incorporates its own guide plane for use with high fusing alloys.

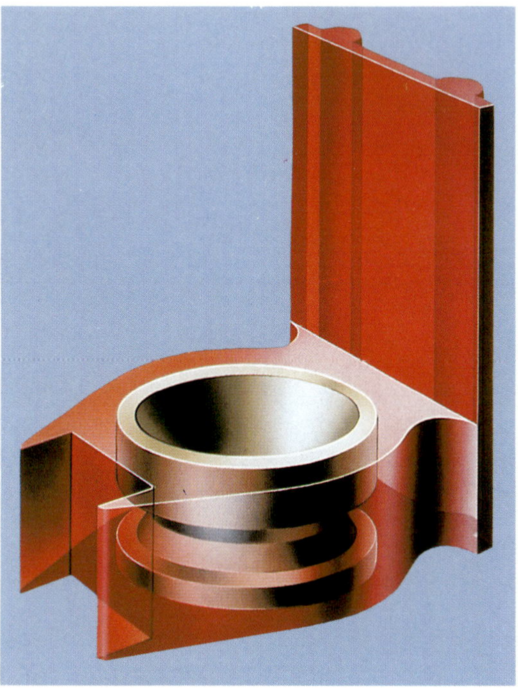

Fig. 361   Plastic pattern of Ceka attachment with its own guide plane. Red patterns are for use with precious metal alloys.

extracoronal units, apart from the need for bracing arms and some additional occlusal support (Fig. 362). The attachments need to be aligned in the vertical plane and this is achieved with a special mandrel (Fig. 363). The connecting strut between the attachment and abutment tooth must be kept as short as possible to reduce leverages applied to the abutments. As for vertical space, the female retaining ring should be placed as close as possible to the mucosa. The positioning of this ring should take into account ease of plaque control without which the prognosis of the restoration must be hopeless. Dental tape and proximal brushes are probably the most effective method for cleaning the attachment and its surroundings.

To obtain the best possible results from these attachments, the clinician must be familiar with some of the technical aspects of their use. The distal surface of the abutment crown should incorporate a guide plane against which the metal mesial section of the denture will fit. This adaptation will help prevent the distal section of

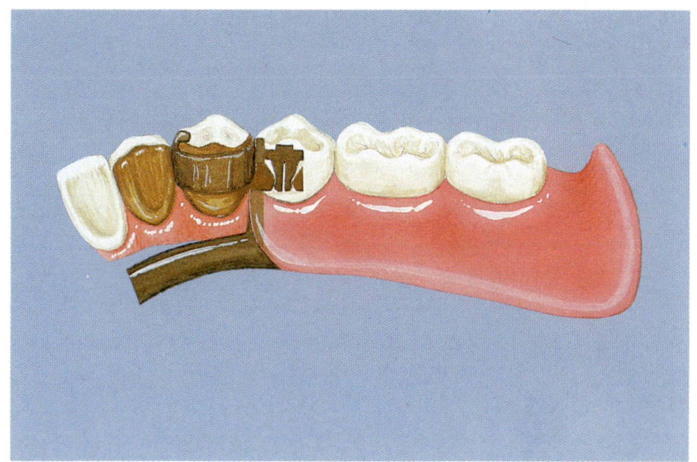

Fig. 362 The bracing arm, an essential feature of the design, provides stabilisation and additional occlusal support. It is particularly useful for rebasing and relocating procedures.

the denture base separating from the mucosa and the bracing arm will provide additional guide plane activity. In preparing the cast of the edentulous area, it is important that provision is made so that there is metal to mucosa contact immediately distal to the attachment. No wax spacer should be placed in this important region.

Once the crown assembly has been completed, an investment cast is produced that includes a dummy attachment in place (Fig. 364). This will allow the metal of the denture base to be adapted with accuracy around the attachment, the denture framework is then cast in the conventional manner (Figs. 365 and 366). Additional resistance to rotational forces is provided by carrying the metal framework around the ring. The metal surface simplifies cleansing. Thanks to an ingenious series of gadgets produced by the manufacturers, the technician is now able to wax up the framework around a special former and thereby produce a highly polished metal surface around the attachment (Fig. 367).

During acrylic processing and other laboratory procedures, the male retaining pin is replaced with a stainless steel dummy. In this way the mechanical properties of the retaining pin are not compromised by temperature changes or mechanical injury. One standard sized dummy, known as the HI, may be used for the 600 series; the new 700 series require an HIA dummy. The HIA dummy can be recognised by its black chrome finish. The mini retaining pin cannot, of course, be removed from its base. Once the dummy has been removed and the male spring pin inserted, a riveting procedure must be carried out to prevent accidental loosening in the mouth (Fig. 368). A special riveting tool is provided in the technician's and surgeon's kits.

The dentist is provided with a convenient accessory kit vital for routine adjustments and maintenance (Fig. 369). The technician is provided with one of the most compre-

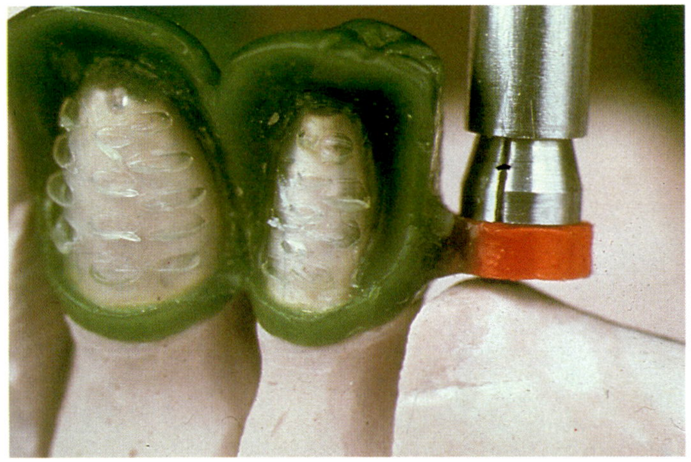

Fig. 363 Mandrel for alignment of attachment. Twisting the knurled knob releases the tension and allows it to be withdrawn without disturbing the ring in the waxed abutment.

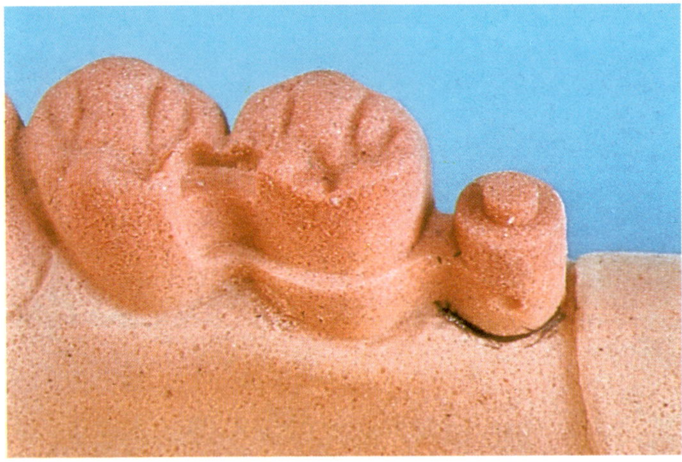

Fig. 364 Investment cast showing rest seat.

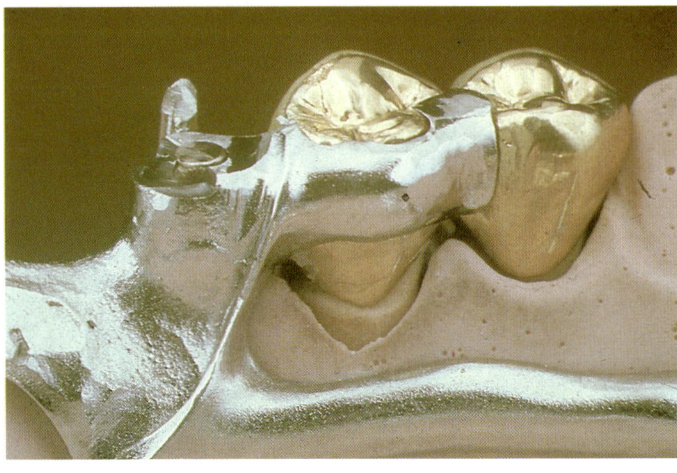

Fig. 365 Chrome framework seated on the master cast.

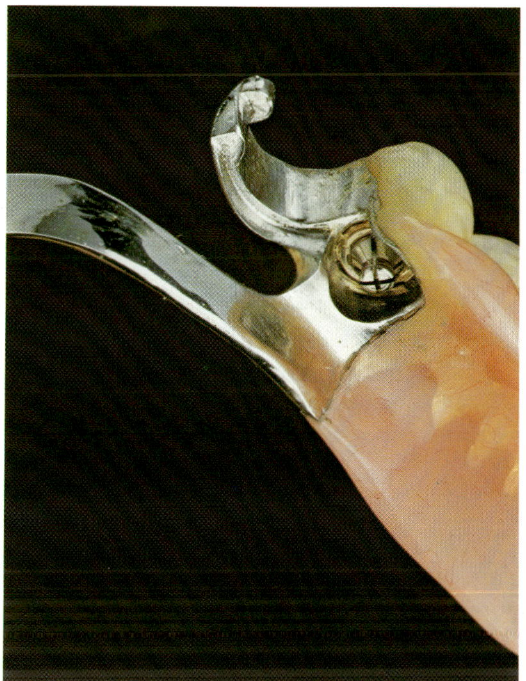

Fig 366   The metal framework surrounds the attachment simplifying plaque control and contributing to the strength of the restoration.

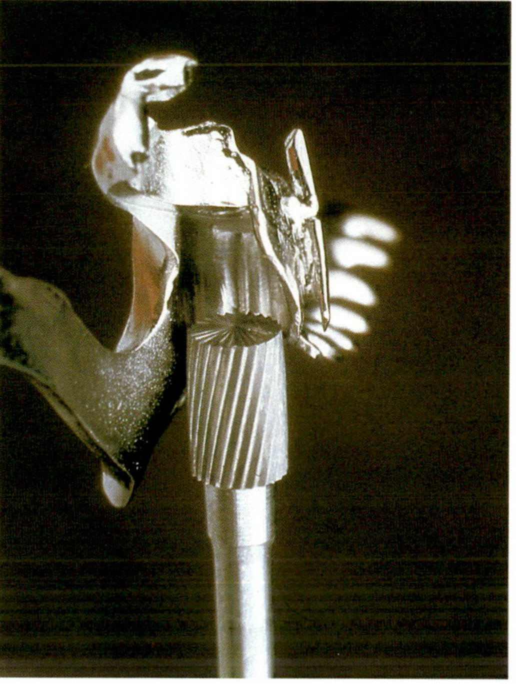

Fig. 367   A special instrument designed for producing a fine finish to the metal surround of the attachment.

hensive kits produced for any attachment (Fig. 370). This kit includes adjusting tools, locating dowels, soldering dowels, finishing instruments, riveting tools and specially modified pliers for holding the attachments. Small wonder that this system is so popular in the laboratory.

Adjustments for retention

The male retaining pin is easily damaged by clumsy or inexperienced attempts at modifying its retention. The manufacturers produce a special adjustment tool for improving the retention, known as the Al instrument. One end of the instrument consists of a wedge-shaped blade (Fig. 371), and the other end incorporates a device for unscrewing the male retaining pins. Since the adjusting tool consists of a wedge, insertion of the wedge between the leaves of the male pin will cause them to separate slightly and it is by judicious use of this taper alone that the retention can be improved (Fig. 372). This blade should never be used for levering the pins apart (Fig. 373). Adjustments of this nature

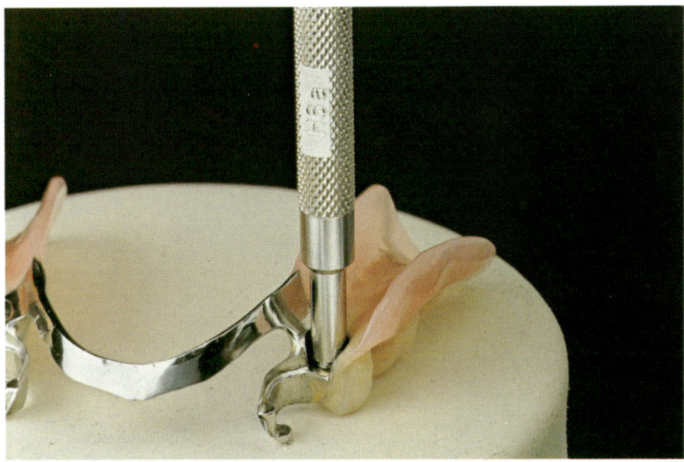

Fig. 368 Using the riveting tool to prevent loosening of the male section.

should be carried out extremely carefully and in stages. No matter how carefully these adjustments are carried out, occasions will arise when it is necessary to slacken retention. Once again inexperience and modifications with longnosed pliers are a certain way of damaging the retention pins.

A special instrument is produced by the manufactures for the purpose of reducing retention. It is known as the H9 unit and is simply placed over the male pin. This procedure can be repeated until the reduction in retention required has been achieved.

When inserting a prosthesis for the first time, the retention of the pins should be slackened as much as possible.

Rebasing

The principles involved in rebasing partial dentures with Ceka attachments are similar to those already described (p. 257). It is a procedure that requires care and attention to detail. Resilient Ceka attachments require the spacer to be inserted over the male pins before the impression is made. It is important that, when the denture is seated, this should be achieved by applying loads to the bracing arm and occlusal rest and never by applying loads distally, as this will introduce a rotational error in the seating of the prosthesis. Where bracing arms and occlusal rest seats have been incorporated, their relationship to their abutment crowns will serve as a guide to ensure that the three-dimensional location of the denture has not been disturbed by the impression procedure. Since the adaptation of the denture base to the proximal surfaces of its abutment is critical, it is recommended that the partial denture, with its reline impression, is

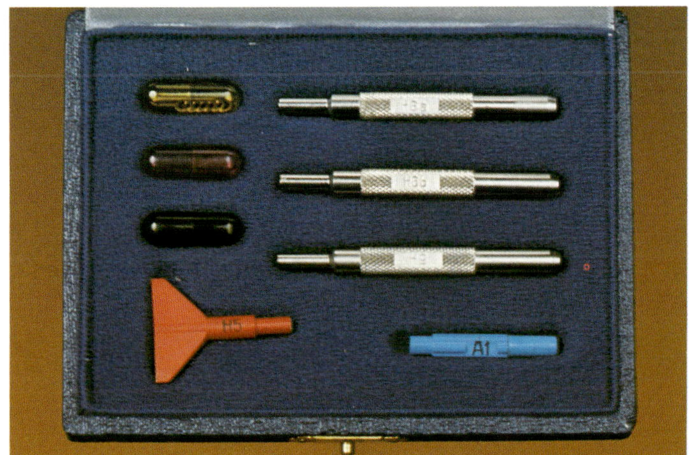

Fig. 369 The Ceka adjustment kit provided for dental surgeons.

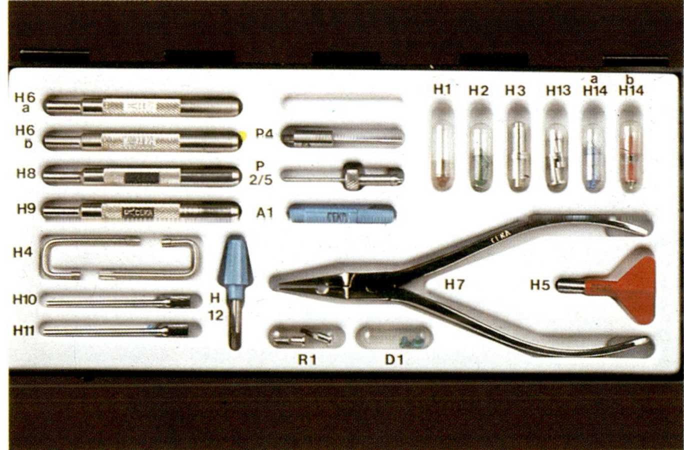

Fig. 370 Possibly the most comprehensive ancillary kit available for any attachment. This Ceka assembly kit for the technician includes devices for adjustments, alignment, riveting, soldering, together with locating dowels for rebasing.

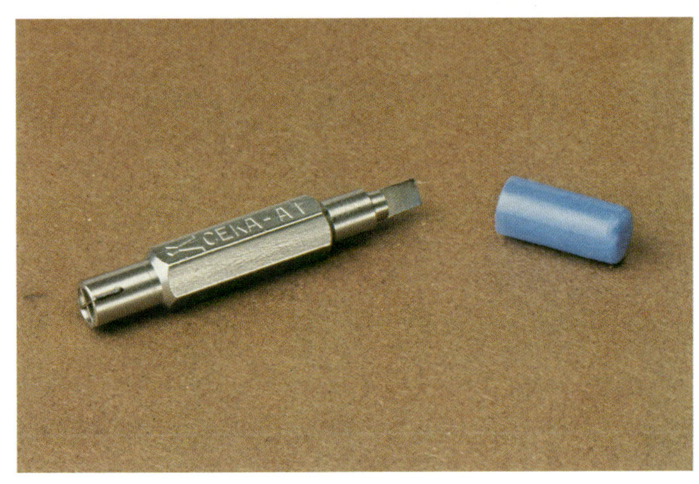

Fig. 371 Wedge-shaped blade for increasing the retention of the Ceka pins. The opposite end is used for replacing retention pins.

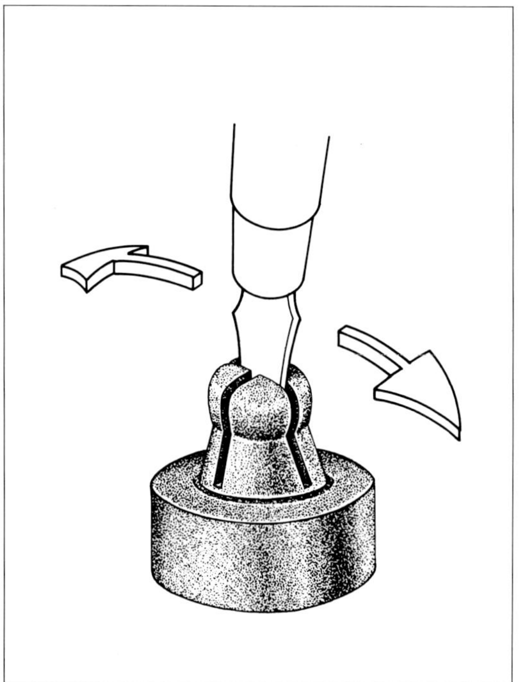

Fig. 372 Retention can be increased by using the taper of the adjusting tool and moving it gently from side-to-side.

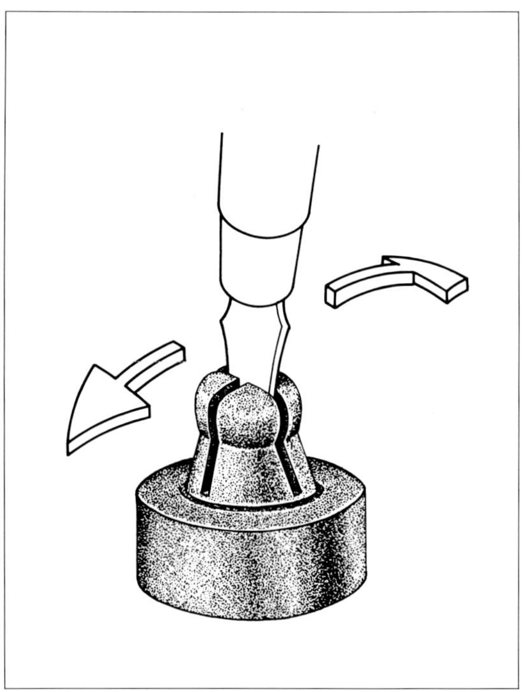

Fig. 373 Never lever apart the leaves of the pins.

removed from the mouth with an overall alginate impression, thereby ensuring that details of the entire arcade of teeth are available.

Before casting the impression, locating dowels known as H13 units are placed over the male pins (Fig. 374). A window in the dowel is provided to ensure that it is correctly seated down over the male pin. The tagging on the dowel incorporates it within the cast of the impression. The dimensions of the dowel surrounding the male pin are identical to those of the female re-

taining ring in the mouth, and ensures that no movement can occur during processing procedures. The male pin is, of course, replaced with a dummy during the processing cycle of the acrylic resin and then replaced prior to reinsertion in the patient's mouth. The riveting procedure must not be overlooked.

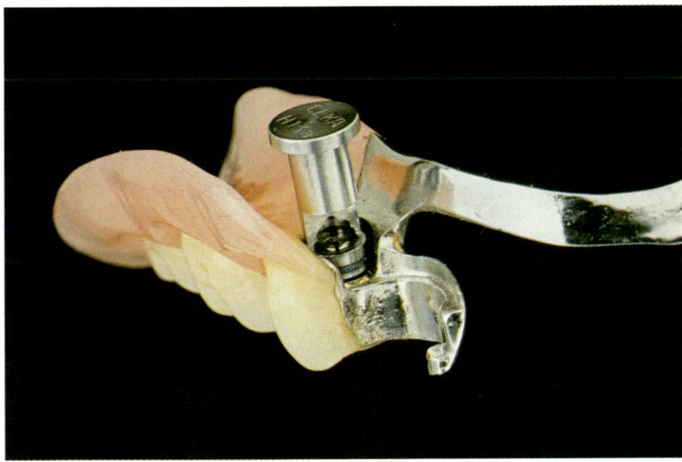

Fig. 374   Ceka locating dowel in place. Its use is essential during rebasing procedures.

Relocation

Following rebasing or relining procedures, the male spring pin may fail to seat completely in its receptacle. The first points to check are the proximal surfaces of the denture in case there is an excess of acrylic resin that is jamming the path of insertion. Once these surfaces have been examined and found to be clear, the problem can often be solved by unscrewing the male pin with the special instrument (H5) and inserting a shim of platinum foil in the screw base before replacing the male pin and tightening it. Nowadays, a special Ceka distance spacer is available that is 0.05 mm thick. More than one shim or spacer can be employed. If the attachment engages, the riveting tool is then employed to prevent accidental loosening of the male pin. This artificial lengthening of the male pin may not solve the problem and suggests that significant movement of one of the attachments has taken place.

This type of movement is most likely to occur with the KS type of attachment that has been buried in acrylic resin and not connected directly to the metal framework of the denture.

The relocating procedure is similar to that described previously (p. 261), but the shape of the Ceka female dictates particularly careful blocking out of the space under and around the attachment. One must not forget to insert the spacer when resilient attachments are employed. Bracing arms and associated occlusal rests ensure correct seating of the denture during the process and contribute to the accuracy with which it can be undertaken. The male spring pin and base is completely separated from the denture and relocated to it in the mouth by means of self-polymerising resin.

It is recommended that this procedure is carried out in two small stages. Once adequate connection has been achieved, the denture is removed with an overall impression of the arcade of teeth, H13 locating dowels placed over the two attachments and the repair completed with heat cured acrylic resin. Dummy spring pins are, of course, substituted during the laboratory stage.

Constructing a duplicate denture

The Ceka system is unique in facilitating what would otherwise be an extremely demanding and time-consuming procedure. A special instrument, known as the H14, is available for this purpose. For practical purpose, the H14 resembles a male spring pin with tagging on it but the spring pin is passive (Fig. 375). The H14 unit is placed within the female receptacle in the mouth and the overall impression subsequently made. The tagging of the H14 unit ensures that it is removed, firmly positioned within the impression and, before casting the impression, the technician places the H13 locating dowels over the H14 unit. These H13 locating dowels are identical to the female circular unit in the mouth so, when the impression is cast, the technician is provided with an accurate duplication of the situation in the mouth with the attachments in their correct relationship to one another. It is then comparatively simple to construct a duplicate denture. This saves the difficult and potentially inaccurate relocation procedures that are necessary with many other units. It can be seen that the versatility provided by this exceptional range of attachments is remarkable and the dental surgeon is strongly recommended to be utterly familiar with the entire system in order to obtain the maximum possible value from it.

Connecting units

These units connect two parts of a removable prosthesis, allowing a certain limited amount of play. They have an apparently similar function to a long and flexible major connector, but act in a more precise and predictable manner.

The Steiger joints are good examples of this type of unit. Changes in clinical techniques have left their production future uncertain, but in their time they were models of careful design and construction. These joints worked extremely well and, since they illustrate the principles involved, a discussion of these units is justified. The Steiger joints were developed between the Wars for joining a denture to its retainers, usually removable sections of the crowns. Steiger recommended his excellent CSP system for the removable crowns, although a simpler telescopic system would nowadays suffice. The joints were also used for joining a denture base to the major connector of a clasp-retained denture.

The female section of the attachment consisted of a vertical sleeve soldered to the removable crowns or the clasp-retained section of the denture. The male unit was a flattened rod, attached to the denture saddle, and fitted within the sleeve. The two parts of the attachment were held together by a small screw passing through the female sleeve and into the male section.

Two basic types of joints were manufactured:

1. *The Axial Rotation joint* (Fig. 376). This connector allowed a limited vertical movement, as a small window was cut out of the female section around the screw. The male section was therefore

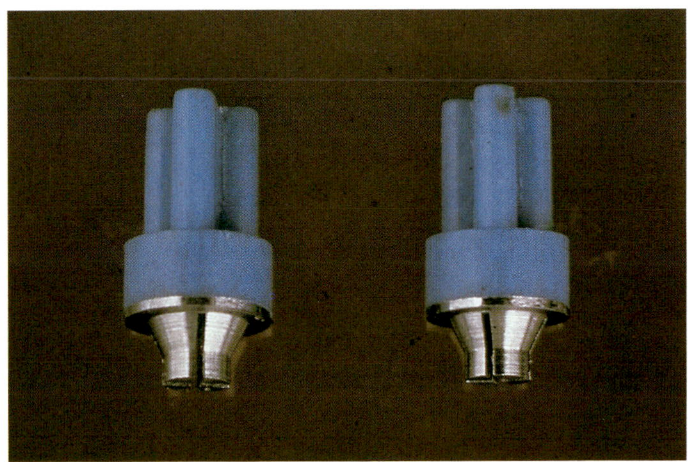

Fig. 375   The H14 instrument resembles a passive male spring pin with tagging. This tagging ensures it is firmly incorporated within the overall impression when a duplicate denture is made.

free to travel up and down within the narrow confine of the window. Rotation and lateral movements was provided by dismantling the attachment and very slightly trimming the male unit. This joint can be incorporated within the Scott attachment.

2. *The Rotation joint* (Fig. 377). This attachment was similar to the axial rotation joint, but there was no window around the screw (Fig. 378). Vertical movements could not therefore take place.

Steiger originally envisaged the axial rotation joints as connectors for distal extension dentures. He felt that the screw should be at the top of the window when the teeth were apart (Fig. 379), and should move downwards as load was applied to the artificial teeth. Since the most favourable distribution of load to the edentulous ridge occurs with a combination of vertical and rotational movements, it was suggested that a small amount of metal be removed from the mesiogingival and disto-occlusal portions by shaving with a hand instrument, and the procedure repeated a week later. In this way, it was felt the degree of movement within the attachment could be adjusted to meet individual requirements. The mesio-occlusal and distogingival portions of the male unit were never adjusted, for they prevented the distal portion of the denture saddle lifting away from the mucosa (Fig. 380).

The Rotation joint was designed for the unilateral distal extension prosthesis, for this type of denture was usually tooth- and mucosal-supported on one side and entirely tooth-supported on the opposite side. Since vertical movement could be damaging to the teeth on the tooth-supported side, *Steiger* designed the Rotation joint to allow only slight rotational and lateral movements in order to minimise torques transmitted from the distal extension base on the opposite side (Fig. 381). A typical unilateral distal extension design would,

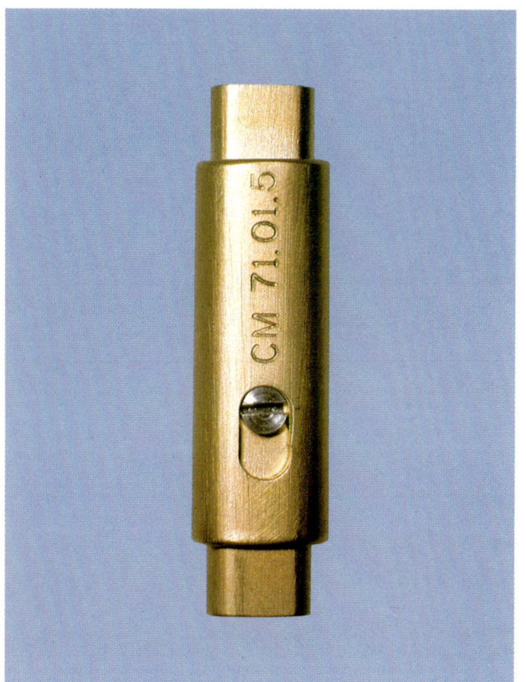

Figure 376

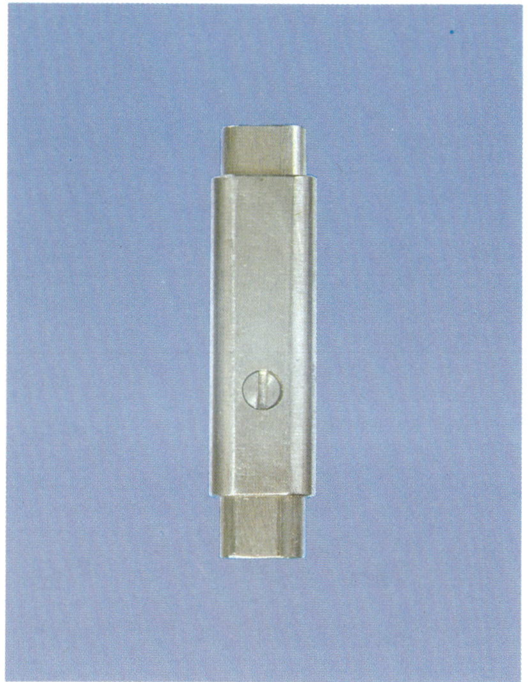

Figure 377

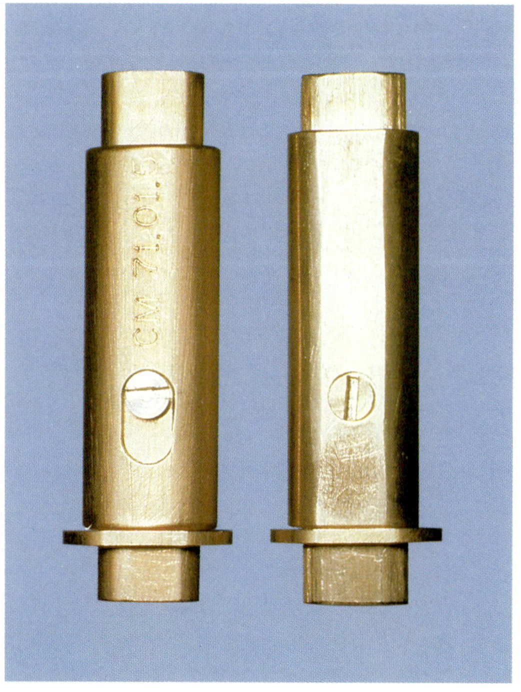

Fig. 376   The Axial Rotation joint. The small window around the screw determines the vertical travel allowed by the joint.

Fig. 377   The Rotation joint allows no vertical play between the two sections of the attachment.

Fig. 378   The Axial Rotation and Rotation joints side-by-side illustrating the soldering rings.

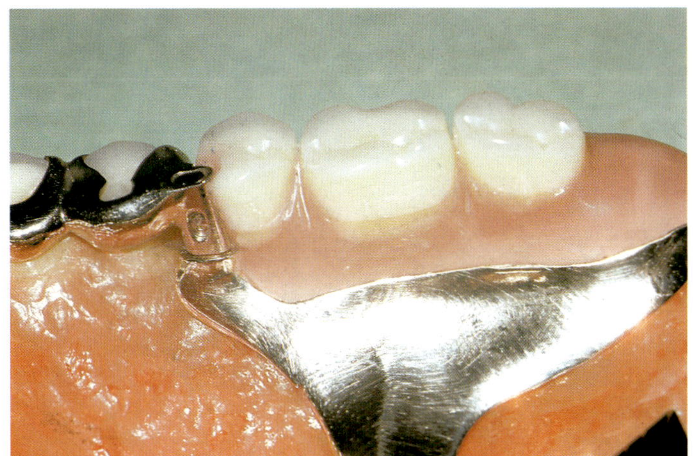

Fig. 379 The Axial Rotation joint is a connector for bilateral distal extension dentures. Steiger felt that the screw should be at the top window with the teeth apart and should move downwards as load was applied to the artificial teeth.

therefore, incorporate an Axial Rotation joint connecting the distal extension base to the retainers and major connector, while the retainers on the opposite, tooth-supported side would be connected through a Rotation joint.

The Steiger joints are one of the few attachments in which the amount and direction of the movement allowance could be determined precisely by the operator. If appreciable wear took place, both parts of the attachment could be removed from the mouth and a replacement soldered on. Many of *Steiger's* original prostheses have stood the test of 20 or 30 years' use. As denture designs and impression techniques improved, it was found that even the slight movement allowance provided by *Steiger's* original design gave too much vertical play and led to possible damage of the distal papilla of the distal abutment tooth. Boitel* found that

better results were obtained by using the Rotation joint for bilateral distal extension base prostheses as well. The window around the screw could be very slightly widened to allow a minute amount of vertical play. Dismantling and shaving the male attachment was unnecessary, for the slight wear taking place between the two units provided the requisite amount of freedom.

It is difficult to calculate the degree and direction of movement that would be allowed by a long flexible major connector. The *Steiger* joints were small and the movement they allowed and the direction in which this movement occurred would be determined with precision. However, we know that a well-designed and constructed denture requires little, if any, movement around the natural teeth.

* personal communication

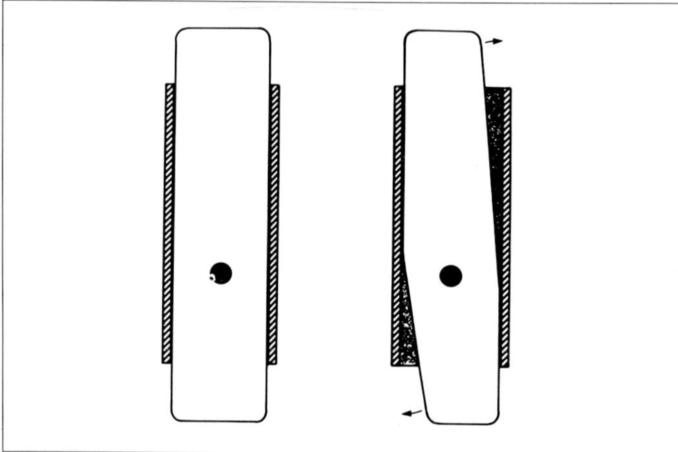

Fig. 380   Exaggeration of the small adjustments necessary to allow slight rotation within the Axial Rotation joint. The metal is shaved only from the mesiogingival and disto-occlusal sections of the male unit. The other surfaces prevent the denture base moving away from the mucosa and should not be touched.

Combined attachments

These units consist of a hinge connector joined to an intracoronal attachment. The hinge unit is buried within the denture so that when it is in position, the attachment closely resembles a rigid intracoronal attachment. Combined attachments usually fit identical female slots to the intracoronal attachments produced by the same manufacturer, so that after tooth loss it may be possible to make a denture substituting a combined attachment for an intracoronal attachment.

The Crismani combined units are typical of this group and have withstood well the tests of time. They require, of course, a box or shoulder preparation within the abutment tooth, while the projecting component requires to be accommodated within the removable prosthesis. Hinge movement is spring-controlled and, in the past, access to the spring chamber was obtained by removing a small screw in the base of the attachment. Since this screw was under continuous load from the spring, accidents were recorded from time to time.

The latest Crismani combined unit features several improvements (Figs. 382 and 383). First of all the intracoronal component has been modified to facilitate insertion and cleansing, and the projecting component features far neater tagging for incorporation in the acrylic resin of the denture. Perhaps the most significant improvement is the fact that the unit can be dismantled by removing the access pin, and that the base of the attachment is one solid component. Retention may be adjusted by the 'U' spring arrangement featured in the larger Crismani intracoronal attachment. The base of the male attachment is then bevelled to facilitate insertion (Fig. 384).

Combined attachments are commonly misused to retain unilateral distal extension prostheses. Following loss of a molar tooth, it is tempting to convert a unilat-

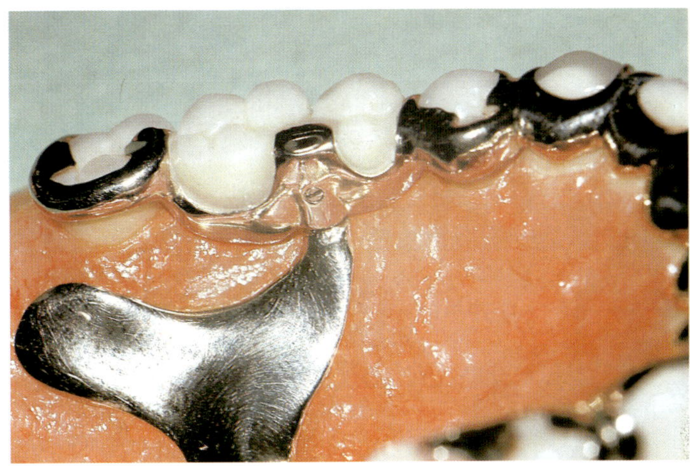

Fig. 381   The Rotation joint in position.

eral posterior 'removable bridge' into a unilateral distal extension denture, merely by substituting a combined attachment for the mesial intracoronal unit. In most cases, however, such a prosthesis nearly always requires support from the other side of the arch.

When the restoration is small, say where a second molar is replaced with an artificial tooth narrower buccolingually and mesiodistally, bilateral support may be considered unnecessary. Provided the abutments are sufficiently rigid, such as a firm second premolar and first molar, a cantilevered fixed prosthesis can be considered. The prognosis of this type of restoration is more favourable when it is opposed by artificial teeth. Whatever the restoration, a 'stress-breaking' attachment should never be used as an excuse for anchoring an unstable denture to a natural tooth.

Combined attachments may be used to retain distal extension prostheses where the strength of the abutment is questionable (Fig. 385). They are more bulky than intracoronal units, and may interfere with the occlusal surface of the first tooth on the denture. Lingual bracing arms are recommended where space allows, and the retention of all these units is adjustable in the same manner as the intracoronal attachments.

Clinical procedures

The importance of healthy supporting structures has been stressed throughout this text. Occasionally, crown lengthening procedures together with orthodontic therapy may be necessary to reposition abutments, ensure periodontal health and to obtain adequate space (Figs. 386 to 388) for the retainers. Ideally, 4 months or so

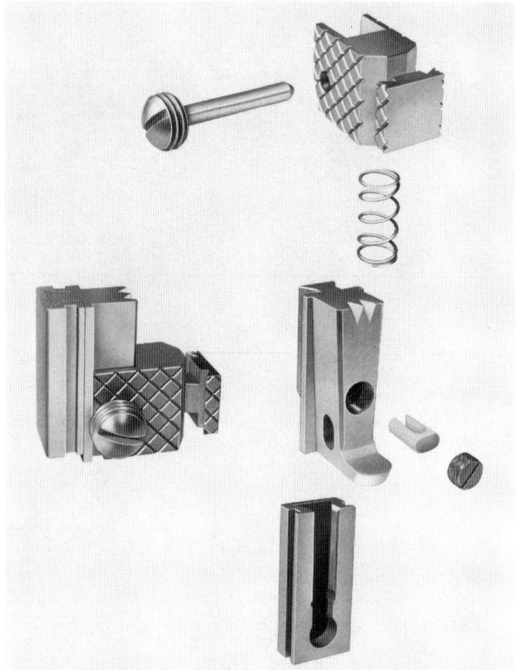

Figure 382

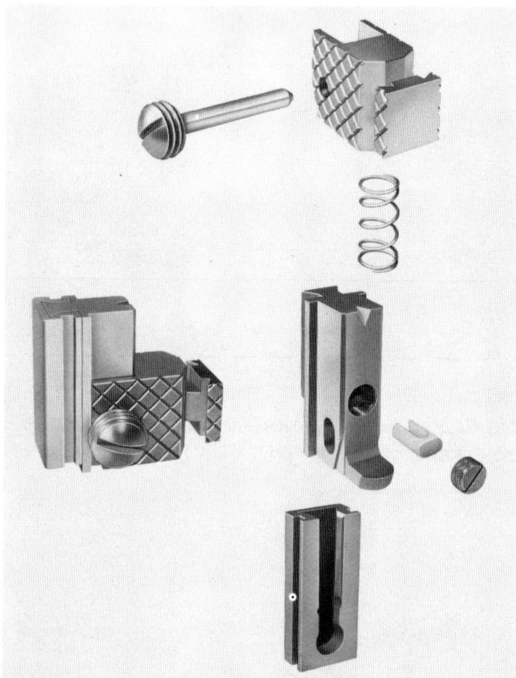

Figure 383

Fig. 382　The new combined Crismani unit. A redesigned access pin strengthens the construction. In the 'bilateral' configuration the lateral walls of the projection are slightly tapered.

Fig. 383　The combined Crismani unit—'unilateral' configuration. The lateral walls of the projection are virtually parallel.

should be allowed from the time of surgery before the definitive crowns are prepared. This allows adequate time for maturation of tissues and for the gingival margin to become established. Where the crown margins can be kept well away from the gingivae, this period can be considerably shortened.

Preparation of the edentulous areas should not be overlooked and is best carried out in conjunction with any muco-gingival surgery. The areas to receive pontics may require minor surgical preparation to allow for subsequent cleansing around the pontic.

Impression techniques

As a distal extension base derives important support from the mucosa, this aspect will be considered in some detail. Since the

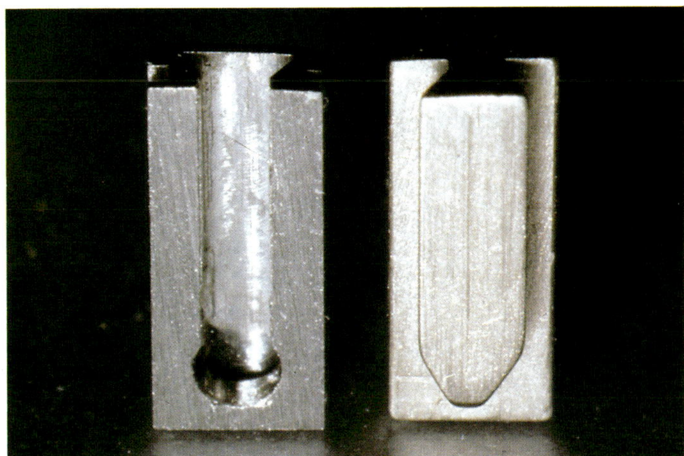

Fig. 384 Male and female of the improved Crismani combined attachment.

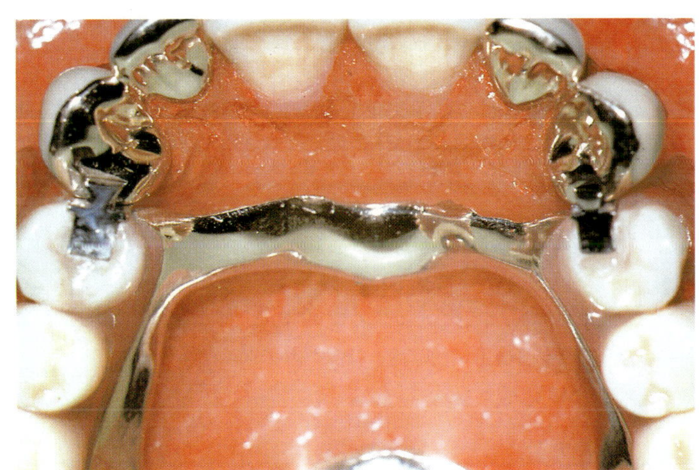

Fig. 385 Bilateral distal extension denture retained by Crismani combined attachments.

mucosa is displaceable, the denture base will tend to sink under occlusal load until an equilibrium is reached between the displacing forces and a combination of mucosal resistance and support from teeth. The mucosa of the denture-bearing area is seldom of even displaceability or thickness, and there can be substantial base movements where the mucosa is poorly supported. The potential base movement can be reduced by using an im-

pression technique that adapts the impression surface of the denture to the shape the mucosa will assume under occlusal load. The base would then have less distance to travel before mucosal resistance developed. On the other hand, it would be undesirable to have the mucosa subjected to a continuous and heavy load from the denture base. The compromise suggested by *Applegate* (1955) was to record mucosal displacement just below the level that produced surface ischaemia, or blanching of the mucosa, with the teeth out of contact.

If it were possible to obtain with one impression details of all the teeth of one jaw, the abutment preparations and a displacement impression of the denture-bearing area, subsequent procedures would be considerably simplified. Improved elastomeric impression materials have made this possible (Fig. 389) and produce excellent impressions of the abutment preparations and their surrounding structures in their correct relationship to one another. This is the method of choice today. Acrylic resin trays are used at one or both stages of the procedure. The limited stiffness of acrylic resin makes it prone to flex under load, and some operators weaken their trays further by incorporating unnecessary retention holes for the impression material. The stiffness of the tray can be ensured by a rib of acrylic resin on the occlusal aspect of the tray. The tray should be spaced 2–3 mm over the abutments and remaining teeth, but closely adapted to the edentulous areas. The importance of accurate borders to the tray has been stressed in Chapter 4.

It is possible to achieve, with one impression, accurate details of the abutments and of the entire edentulous areas. Apart from the difficulty of making the impression, it will be necessary to section the cast to remove the dies of the abutment crowns. It is almost impossible to do this without involvement of the denture-bearing area and for this reason a two stage procedure is recommended.

Stage one
An impression of the abutments and denture-bearing area is made with a polyether material, such as Impregum, or other suitable medium. Reversible hydrocolloid in a water-cooled tray may also be employed for this purpose, provided that the entire denture-bearing area is reproduced. The cast of this impression is sectioned for dies, jaw relation and facebow records made, and the cast then mounted on an adjustable articulator. On this cast the metal work for the abutment crowns is completed, including the incorporation of the aligned attachments.

Stage two
An acrylic resin tray is constructed on the master cast. The tray is spaced 2–3 mm over the natural teeth, the abutment crowns and attachments, but closely adapted over the edentulous areas.

The abutment crowns are tried on their respective teeth and a minute amount of petroleum jelly placed within them before they are seated. Care is taken to ensure they are fully seated. The tray is now tried in the mouth and the border moulding perfected. Large proximal spaces unrelated to the abutments are blocked with soft wax before the impression tray is loaded with Impregum and inserted in the mouth. The castings must be completely dry before inserting the tray. These castings will be removed within the new impression and the first examination is to ensure that no impression material has flowed around the margins of the casting.

The dies are now placed in the castings before the impression is poured. This new

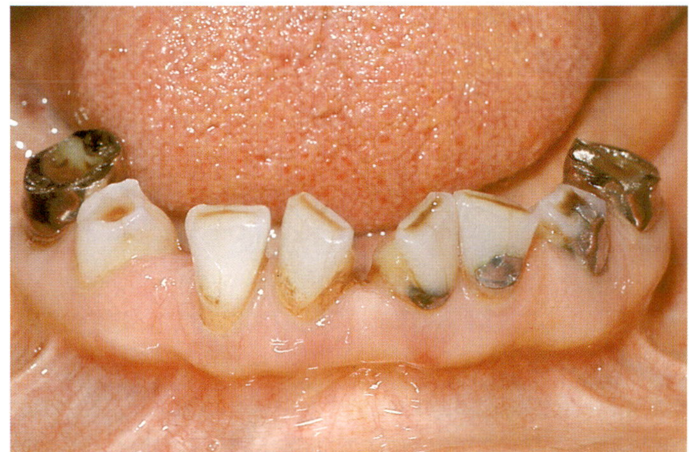

Fig. 386 Malpositioned abutments and inadequate clinical crown height.

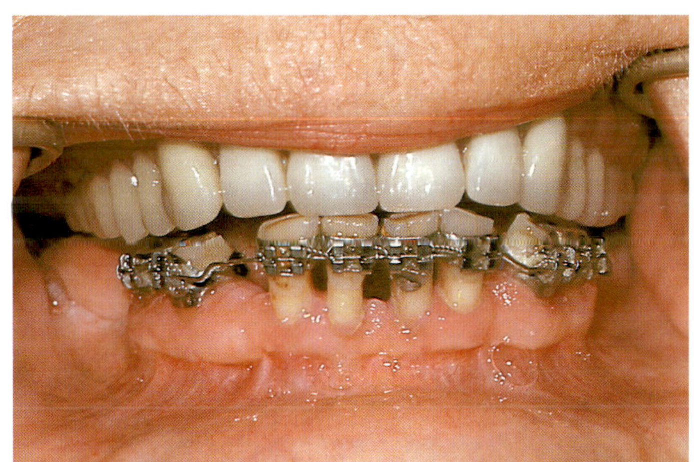

Fig. 387 Preliminary mucogingival surgery followed by orthodontic therapy.

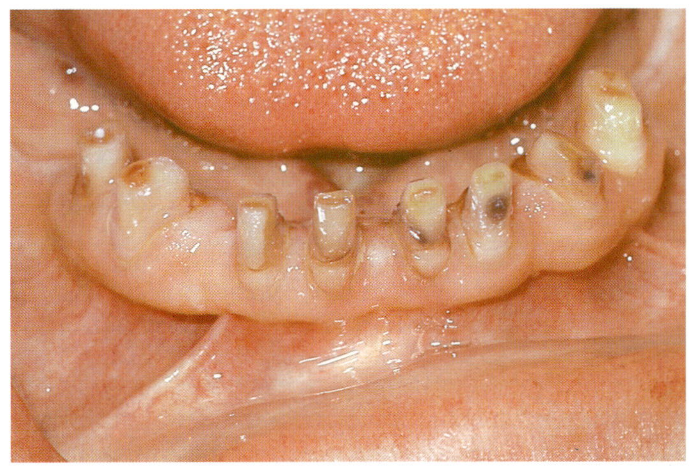

Fig. 388 Outlined preparations.

master cast is employed for the construction of the removable prosthesis.

This technique yields excellent results provided that no movement of the castings has occurred within the impression material.

Other impression techniques

Unlike some aspects of prosthodontics, the operator must be familiar with several techniques to cope with unusual situations. Even more important is to understand the rationale behind the techniques.

Altered cast techniques have been advocated for several decades. Some of the methods allow the impression to be built in stages, thereby allowing the operator some versatility. Furthermore the materials are relatively fast-setting, making it easier to repeat stages.

When at least six, or preferably more, teeth remain in a dental arch with a reasonably prominent curvature, the displacement impression can be made before the metal framework is constructed.

The abutment preparations are completed and impressions of them made in the material of choice.

An acrylic resin tray is constructed on the cast of this impression. The tray consists of a rigid U-shaped strut of acrylic resin fitting over the occlusal surfaces of the teeth. The tray handle is attached to the midpoint of the strut, and the two distal ends of the strut support close-fitting trays covering the mucosa of the denture-bearing area (Fig. 390). This type of tray requires precise location onto the teeth, so that at three widely spaced points occlu-

sal stops are provided between the strut and the teeth. In view of the precise location required, this procedure can be used only where there are widely spaced contacts. It could not be used where there are remaining six anterior teeth in a square arch, for they would be vitually in line.

At the next visit, the temporary crowns are removed and the tray checked in the mouth. The extension of the trays should resemble that of a complete denture, and some relief around the mylohyoid muscle will be required. It is essential that the three occlusal stops make proper contact.

Applegate and co-workers developed a series of impression waxes of known viscosity at mouth temperature.* The hardest of these waxes (No. 1) was designed for use in extending the borders of the denture base, and the softest (No. 4) for use in recording details of the impression surface. The mucosal displacement is obtained when an excess of wax is expelled around the borders of the tray or denture base, rather than by direct pressure applied by the dentist. The amount of mucosal displacement depends upon the viscosity of the wax. Since this has been predetermined, the mucosal displacement is controlled.

The impression wax is best manipulated by softening it in a container surrounded by hot water at approximately 200° F (Fig. 391). Most commercially available thermostatically-controlled water baths can be readily adapted, and it is seldom that more than the two types of wax will be required, although intermediate grades are available. The impression wax can be applied

---

* Korecta Wax, D&R Miner Dental, 14 Lavina Court, Orinda, California 94563, USA.

Fig. 389 Improved elasto-meric materials can provide details of all the teeth of one jaw, the abutment prepara-tions, and a displacement im-pression of the denture-bear-ing areas. In sectioning the cast to make individual dies, the area required for the denture base is likely to be damaged. A later impression made over the uncemented abutment crowns (Fig. 399) will be re-quired for the denture.

Fig. 390 (a) The modified Ap-plegate approach. The acrylic resin tray for making an im-pression of the denture-bear-ing mucosa. The occlusal view of the acrylic resin tray. (b) Im-pression surface of the tray.

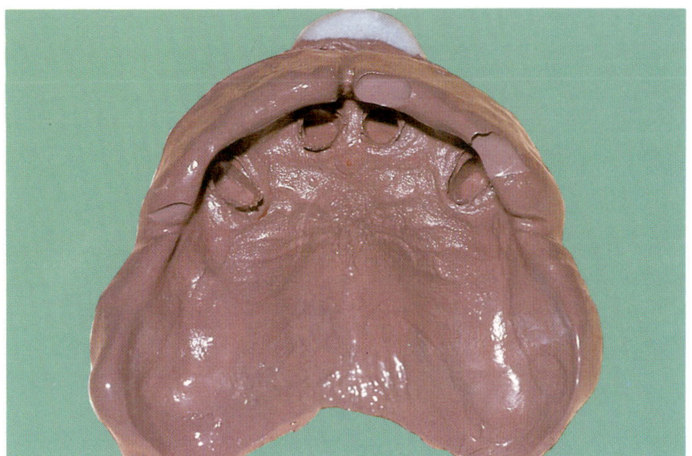

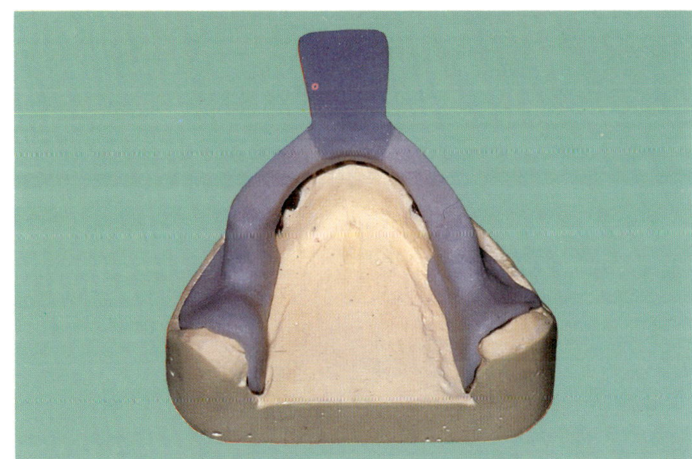

Figure 390 a

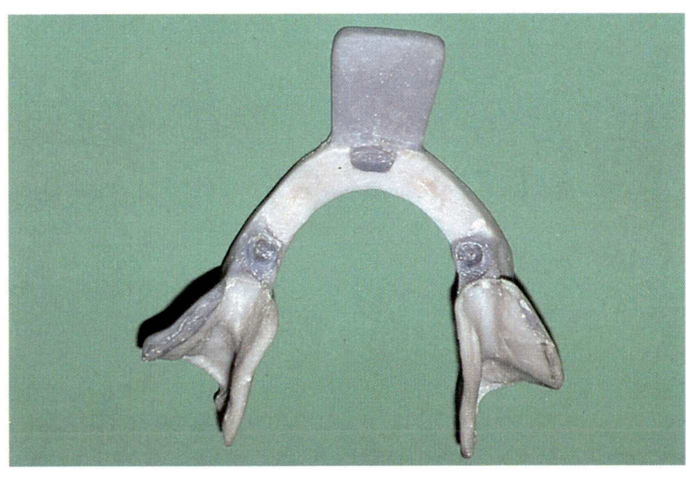

Figure 390 b

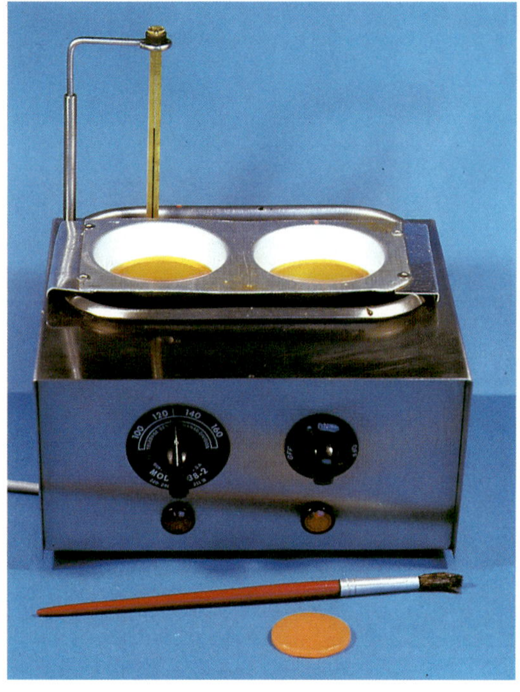

Fig. 391 A thermostatically-controlled water bath suitable for melting impression waxes.

with a small paint brush; a brush with medium stiff bristles 1 cm (3/8") long is suggested by *Applegate*. A separate brush should be used for each wax, as it is important that the waxes should not be contaminated.

A thin layer of wax is painted on the impression surface of the tray, which is then inserted in the mouth. The tray is seated by applying finger pressure over the occlusal stops, never over the denture base area. The bulk of the wax will cause displacement of the mucosa and excess wax will be squeezed out around the periphery of the base. When the area is large, it is helpful to dip the impression tray in hot water just before seating it. While it is true that dipping the tray in water may leach out

some of the constituents of the impression wax, the results appear to be satisfactory and it does overcome the problem of having some parts of the impression warmer than the others when the impression wax first contacts the mucosa. When correctly supported, the impression wax (No. 4) appears glossy. The impression surface should be chilled and dried thoroughly with compressed air before an addition is made, and every care taken to ensure that the occlusal stops of the tray are in contact. The length of time required for the wax to flow varies with the size of the saddle, but at least 4 minutes is usually required.

If the impression has been overbuilt, it may show up by a very high gloss on the im-

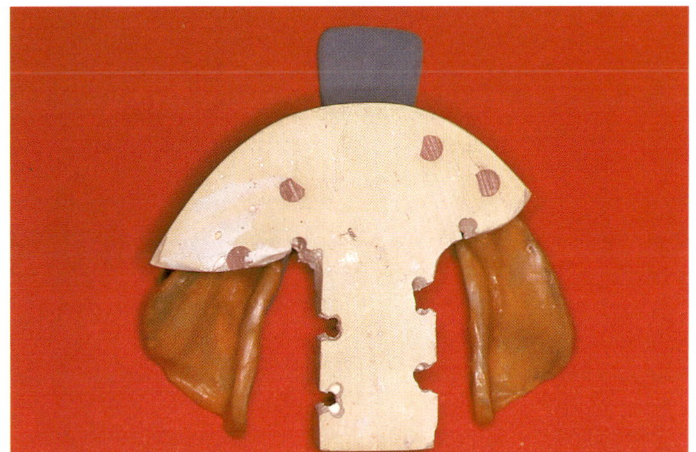

Fig. 392 The edentulous ridges are cut off the cast and the impression tray localised by means of its occlusal stops. Note the dovetails placed in the residual cast.

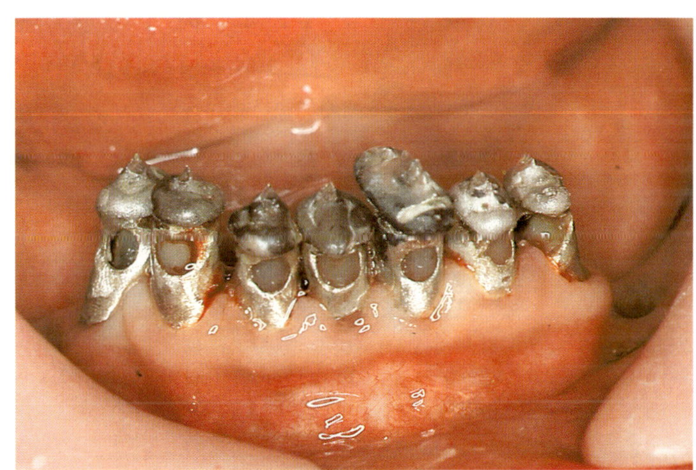

Fig. 393 Metal transfer copings in position. A dated technique, but accurate nevertheless.

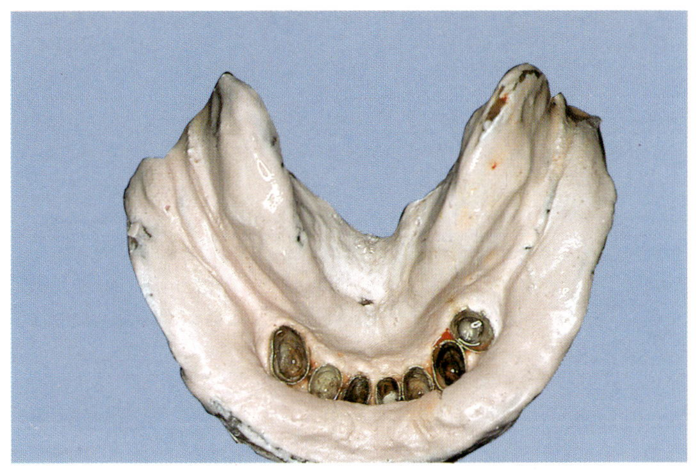

Fig. 394 The plaster locating impression.

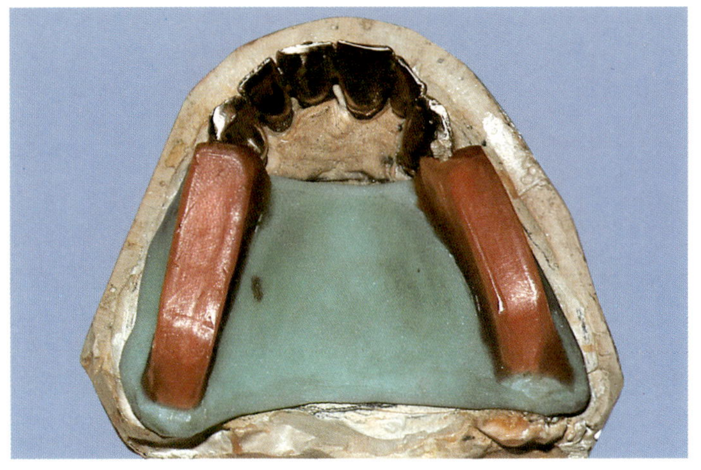

Fig. 395 Upper prosthesis showing close-fitting tray joined to the crowns by means of the attachments.

pression surface and by the occlusal stops which may not seat home. In these circumstances, it is best to scrape out the wax and start again. When a satisfactory impression has been obtained, the impression tray with its recording of the denture-bearing area cannot now be replaced on the cast. Instead, the edentulous ridges are cut off the cast, and the impression tray is reorientated back on the cast by means of the occlusal stops (Fig. 392). The master cast obtained in this manner provides an accurate representation of the residual ridge mucosa under slight load, in its correct relationship to the abutment preparations and to the remainder of the dental arch.

Unfortunately the number or arrangement of the natural teeth frequently fail to provide widely spaced occlusal stops. Another impression procedure is then required.

Rigid extracoronal attachments can be treated like intracoronal units. An impression of the abutment crowns is made with an elastomeric material. Copper tube impressions of individual teeth, transfer copings and a subsequent locating impression may seem dated to some, but are accurate and useful for dealing with awkward problems (Figs. 393 and 394). However it is made, the locating impression must include details of the entire edentulous area.

For upper restorations, a close-fitting tray retained by attachments can be made on the provisional master cast. A wash impression of zinc-oxide eugenol paste is made inside this impression, the jaw relations recorded and both the uncemented abutment retainers and the attached tray removed in an overall alginate impression (Fig. 395). For lower restorations, closely adapted acrylic resin bases are also made on the master cast but are joined to the major connector. Where restorations are to be retained by rigid attachments, the impression procedure is simplified as the

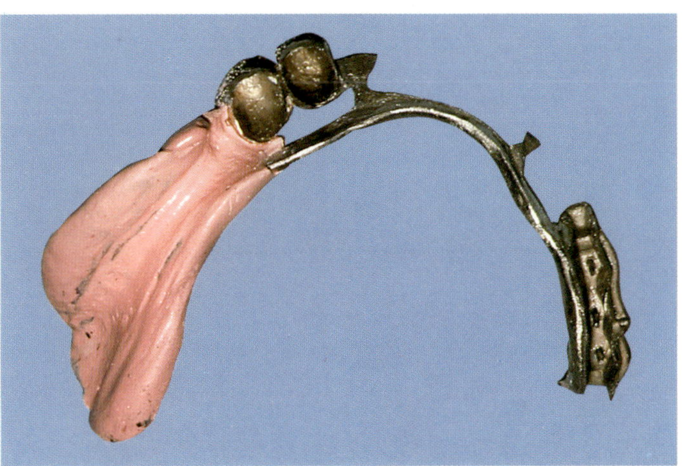

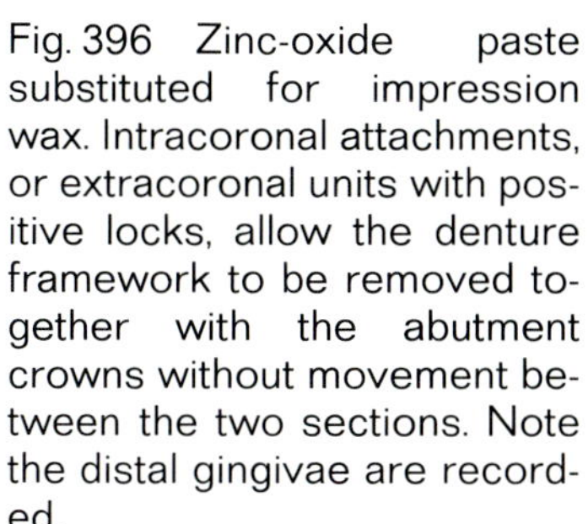

Fig. 396 Zinc-oxide paste substituted for impression wax. Intracoronal attachments, or extracoronal units with positive locks, allow the denture framework to be removed together with the abutment crowns without movement between the two sections. Note the distal gingivae are recorded.

precise path of insertion provided by the attachments is unquestionable.

The abutment crowns can now be placed in the mouth uncemented and the denture slid into place and the bases checked for extension. While an impression in fluid wax can now be produced, virtually indistinguishable results can be obtained with one of the more viscous zinc-oxide eugenol pastes. One practical tip is to remove the abutment crowns attached to the denture in the overall impression, as this ensures that the area representing the distal gingivae is recorded intact (Fig. 396). The master cast is now sectioned, removing the area corresponding with the denture base. This allows the assembled prosthesis to be slid into place on the remains of the cast and stone subsequently poured into the impression areas to reconstitute the master cast.

The advantages of rigid extracoronal attachments with precise paths of insertion and withdrawal become apparent when techniques of this nature are described. But how does one deal with extracoronal attachments with hinge and vertical play? The two stage elastomeric impression has obvious advantages and this is why it is the preferred technique. It is only when an alternative approach is felt necessary that the following is recommended.

The impression of the abutment crown preparations and entire arch is made according to the preferred technique described for rigid intracoronal attachments. Jaw relationships are recorded, the master cast mounted on an adjustable articulator and the metalwork for crowns and denture framework made, including the attachments. Close-fitting resin bases are attached to the major connector (Fig. 397 a).

Once the resin bases have been made, the prosthesis may be tried in the mouth. Apart from movement potential within the attachments, a problem is the small hand-

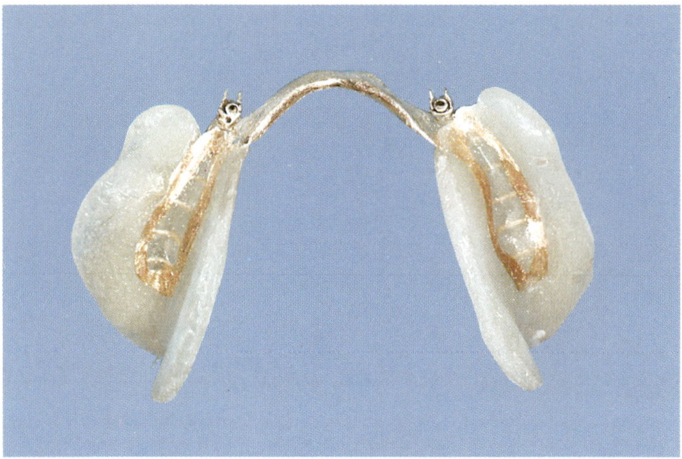

Fig. 397 (a) Dalbo-retained denture base before the wash impression is made. (b) Movement between base and retainers could occur during removal and there is inadequate reproduction of the intervening structures. An overall impression is required to unite the two sections of the prosthesis in their correct relationship, to record the surrounding structures, and to facilitate removal of the impression.

Figure 397 a

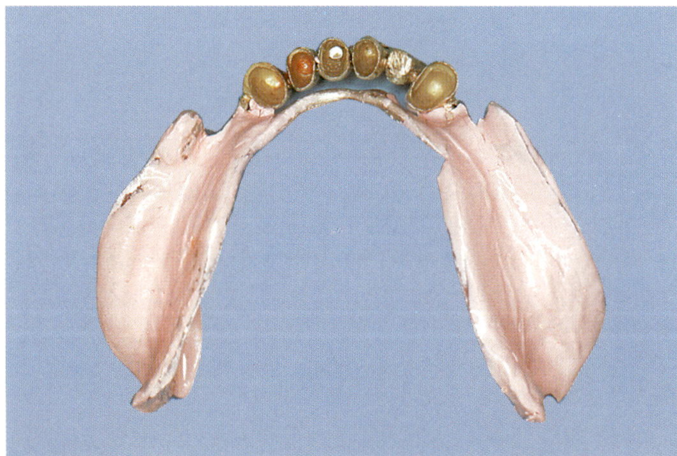

Figure 397 b

ling area available for the operator. The resin should not obscure vision of the attachment in any way and seating load must be applied directly over the attachment. One can then proceed with the impression, provided the location of the attachments is correct. If not, the attachments may be cut from the resin and relocated in the bases. The displacement is then made using fluid wax or zinc-oxide eugenol (Fig. 397b). Excess material is cleaned from the attachments to ensure they are correctly seated and that no tilting has occurred. If all is well, alginate impression material is loaded in a stock tray and inserted over teeth, crowns and base. Both sections of the restoration are removed in this overall impression in their correct relationship to one another (Fig. 398). Apart from removing denture and abutment crowns, the alginate records details of the surrounding tissues. The dies of

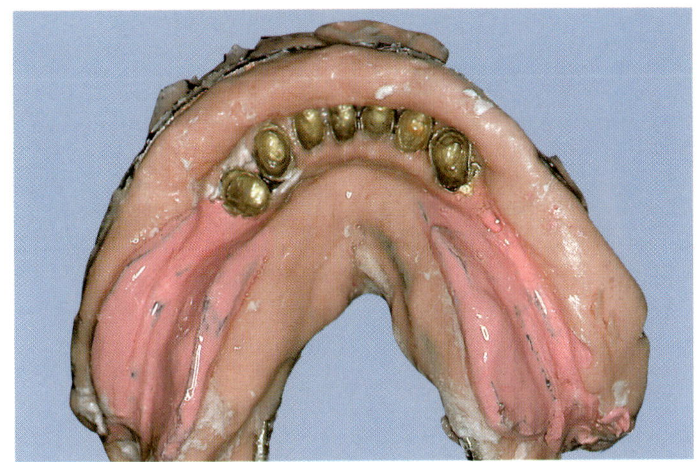

Fig. 398 An overall alginate impression has been employed to remove the two sections of the prosthesis in their correct relationship.

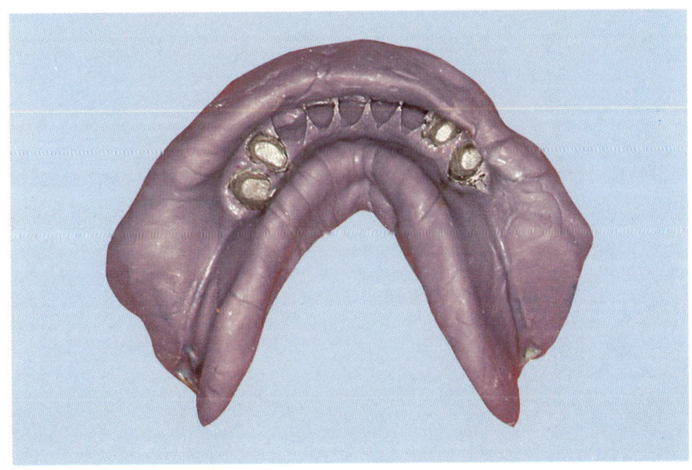

Fig. 399 The most popular technique and one that is normally recommended today. A tray is made closely adapted to the edentulous areas and spaced over the abutments. The uncemented abutment restorations are removed in this impression, the dies placed in their respective crowns and a new master cast produced.

the preparations are inserted into their respective castings and a new master cast produced. Subsequent jaw relations will be necessary to mount this new master cast and for this reason some operators attempt to combine this stage with the impression procedure. This combined result is somewhat easier to achieve with upper impressions than with lower impressions. However, fast-setting artificial stone can be placed on the occlusal surface of the resin tray before the overall impression is made.

In conclusion, it must be stressed that multi-stage impression techniques have a place when exceptional clinical problems manifest themselves. However, the majority of restorations will be made with the two-stage impression techniques. The abutment restorations are made on the cast of the initial elastomeric impression and these uncemented abutment restora-

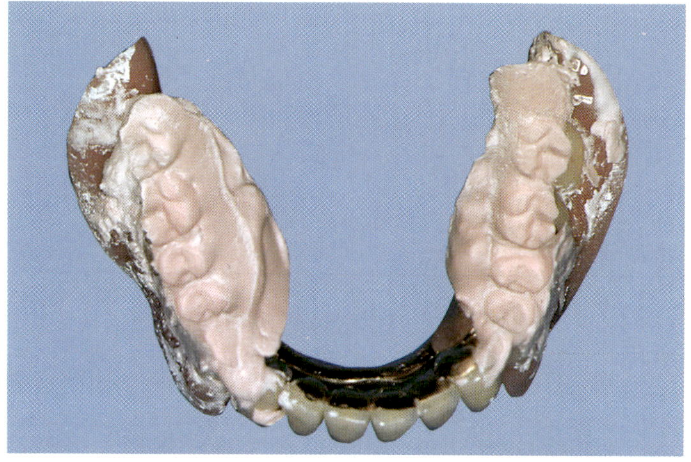

Fig. 400 The check record made when the restoration is inserted in the mouth, but before cementation of the crowns.

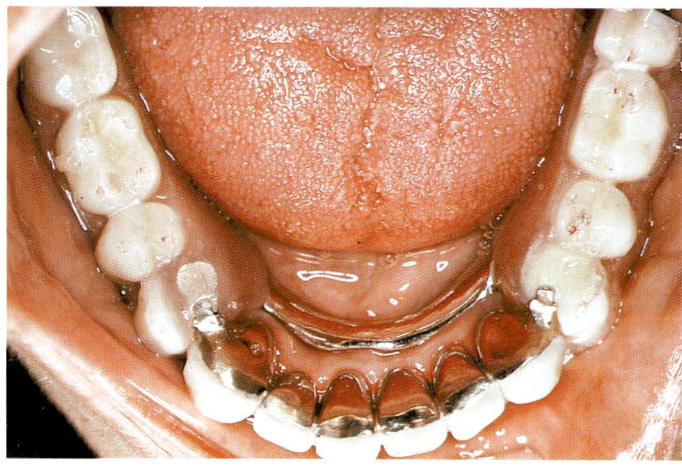

Fig. 401 The completed restoration in the mouth.

tions withdrawn in an overall impression (Fig. 399) upon which the denture is constructed.

Inserting the prosthesis

The adaption of the abutment crowns and that of the denture are rechecked. The attachment positions and their engagement are examined as well. Before the crowns are cemented, further attention should be paid to the jaw relation records. Many of these prostheses oppose complete upper dentures, and it is essential that the jaw relation records be checked with great care if the stability of the upper dentures is not to be impaired. When natural teeth are in opposition, it is equally important to check the jaw relations, in this instance to ensure that undue loads are not placed upon the dentures.

Since mucosal displaceability makes the use of articulating unreliable, a check record procedure is carried out. A centric relation record is made in plaster or fast-setting artifical stone, with the teeth just apart (Fig. 400). The entire prosthesis is now remounted on the articulator, and corrections can be speedily made with the bases mounted on unyielding plaster.

When the crowns have been cemented (Fig. 401), the patient must be shown how to insert and remove the prosthesis. Time should be set aside to demonstrate how the entire prosthesis should be cleaned, while the importance of maintenance needs to be stressed.

Care taken in the construction of the restoration will be rewarded by a long interval before rebasing is required. However, the potential for movement and periodontal breakdown that may be caused by a lapse of plaque control must never be forgotten. Neither must the hazards of springs and other such devices be overlooked, however tempting they may be to use.

Extracoronal attachments have many valuable applications. They are robust, versatile and gaining ever-increasing popularity. Regular inspection and maintenance is essential if they are to provide satisfactory longterm service.

References

Applegate O. C. (1955).
The partial denture base. J. Prosthet. Dent., 5, 5: 636.

Goodman J. J. and Goodman H. W. (1963).
Balance of force in precision free-end restorations. J. Prosthet. Dent., 13, 2: 302.

Heckneby M. (1969).
Distribution of load with the lower free-end partial denture. Acta. Odont. Scand., 27 (Supple. 52), 140.

Kabcenell J. L. (1970).
The resilient partial denture. N.Y. ST. Dent. J., 36: 492.

Lubespere A. and Rotenberg A. (1976).
Attachments et Protheses Combinees. Julien Prelat, Paris.

Marshall W. S. (1938).
Precision attachments and their advantages in respect of underlying tissue. J. Amer. Dent. Ass., 25: 1250.

Mensor M. C. (1968).
The rationale of resilient hinge-action stressbreakers. J. Prosthet. Dent., 20, 3: 204.

Nally J. N. (1961).
The use of prefabricated precision attachments. Int. Dent. J., 11: 192.

Preiskel H. W. (1969).
Precision attachments for free-end saddle prostheses. Brit. Dent. J., 127: 462.

Preiskel H. W. (1971).
Impression techniques for attachment-retained distal extension removable partial dentures. J. Prosthet. Dent., 25, 6: 620.

Rantanen T., Makila E. and Yli-Urpo A. (1972).
Investigations of the therapeutic success with dentures retained by precision attachments. II: Partial dentures. Suom. hammaslaak. toim., 68: 73.

Rushford C. B. (1974).
A technique for precision removable partial denture construction. J. Prosth. Dent., 31, 4: 377.

Schilli G. (1959).
Ein Beitrag zur Versorgung einseitiger Freindlucken mit Hilfe des Dalbo-Gelenkes. Dissertation, University of Freiburg im Breisgau, W. Germany.

Scott J. and Bates J. F. (1972).
The relining of partial dentures involving precision attachments. J. Prosthet. Dent., 28, 3: 325.

Scott W. R. (1968).
A removable telescopic external attachment with an axial-rotation joint. J. Prosthet. Dent., 20, 3: 216.

Steiger A. A. (1951).
Abutment preparation for removable crown and bridgework with a new system of attachment. Dent. Mag. (Lond)., 68: 183.

Steiger A. A. and Boitel R. H. (1959).
Precision Work for Partial Dentures. Stebo, Zurich.

Tabet G. (1961).
Classifications cinematiques des attachments rupteurs des forces. Indication a protheses decolletee. Rev. franc. Odonto-stomat., 8: 6.

Watt D. M. (1972).
Dimple-hinge attachments for partial dentures. Dent. Practit., 22: 12.

Chapter 8

Problems with Attachment Retained Prostheses

Most patients judge the quality of their restoration by its appearance and comfort. According to *John Keats* 'A thing of beauty is a joy for ever, its loveliness increases, it will never pass into nothingness'. Unfortunately his comments do not apply to prosthodontics.

Problems with appearance, comfort and maintenance are frequently traceable to the treatment planning stage and occasionally further back to the history given by the patient. Well-made and good-looking restorations are difficult to produce. It is not just the complications of construction that need consideration, but the wishes of the patient and the eventual appearance. The best way of dealing with prosthodontic problems is still to anticipate them.

A complication of prosthodontics in the past has been the double standards that were accepted in restoring the partially dentate mouth. Competent practitioners would make elaborate and extensive fixed restorations with adequate care and attention to detail; surprisingly these same colleagues appeared perfectly prepared to employ haphazard, slipshod and potentially damaging techniques as soon as a removable prosthesis was required. This was all the more surprising when removable and fixed restorations were made in the same mouth by the same practitioner.

Planning the appearance

The removable restoration provides considerable versatility with the placement of the artificial teeth. It is this versatility that may indicate a removable prosthesis and failure to take advantage of this feature can give rise to disappointment (Fig. 402).

The labial surfaces of the upper anterior teeth provide the red margin of the upper lip with its essential support. Where appreciable bone loss has occurred, there is an understandable tendency to move these teeth back thereby contributing to a thin flaccid upper lip. Newly developed ridge augmentation techniques may have exciting implications in treatment planning once their stability has been assured. However at the present time it is extremely difficult to mask vertical or labio-palatal defects of anterior edentulous areas without the use of artificial mucosa. This artificial mucosa will also allow correct bucco-lingual positioning of the teeth.

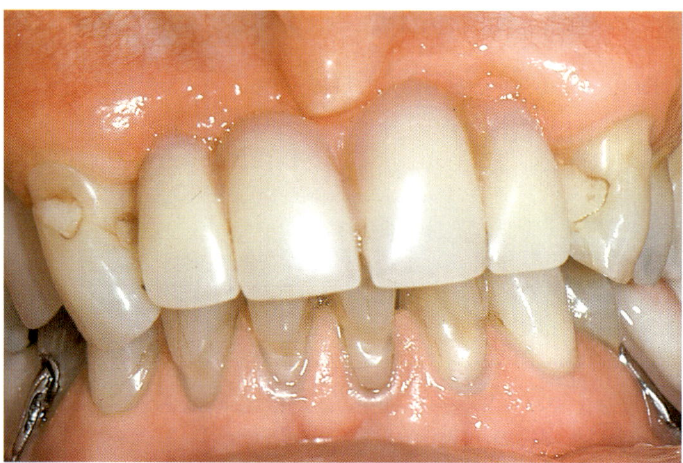

Fig. 402   Poor appearance, inadequate lip support and weakened denture result from this hopeless design.

Other advantages of the removable restoration include the ability to space and rotate teeth at will.

Despite the worthwhile works that are to be found in the literature, a great deal of appearance planning is common sense. It is apparent that prosthodontic replacements should be inconspicuous and blend into the remaining dentition. The teeth must be individual and varied, yet form curves of constantly changing radii. This principle stems from Hogarth's work and has been applied to prosthodontics by several authors.

However, points that seldom receive emphasis are the planning of the denture/abutment interface.

Differing physical properties of materials

Bearing in mind the range of materials that are involved in the denture/abutment interface, one can only express surprise that this area receives scant attention. Between enamel, porcelain, mucosa and acrylic resin the range is enormous.

Colour has three determinants: hue (wavelength), chroma (purity of colour) and value (total reflectance).

McLean (1979) has pointed out that the colour sensation experienced by the observer when viewing a tooth is the result of the amount of absorption of the various colour rays of the tooth dentine and enamel. Porcelain and acrylic resin tooth manufacturers have made advances in producing good-looking teeth arranged in groups of hues. The clinician can help himself in hue selection by staring at a blue background before making his choice. Blue is the complimentary colour to the yellow-brown range.

The chroma of a tooth depends on its colour saturation or strength of hue. The degree of saturation is of considerable importance in its appearance.

Value is sometimes considered the quantivative aspect of colour. *McLean* (1979) illustrates the point by stating that when all spectrum colours are absorbed equally an object appears black. On the other hand, when all the spectral colours from a white light source are reflected with the same intensity as they are received the object appears white.

Objects may therefore have the same hue and chroma, but appear different because of their reflectance properties. With partial denture design the value of a denture tooth may be altered by a metal backing or denture component, such as an attachment within the tooth. A similar problem occurs with the metal of ceramo-metal crowns compared with porcelain crown. Translucency is a function of light reflection and refraction. Regular reflection is in accordance with mirror-like effects. It is often found when smooth and highly polished surfaces reflect light. With diffuse reflection, the incident light is dispersed in many directions. Contoured surfaces will produce this type of reflection. However, to obtain any effects of translucency, light has to pass through the object concerned. Suffice to say that the refractive index between two substances varies as the speed of light through these substances, which in turn depends on their densities.

Yet another problem stems from metamerism, which is the apparent change in colour as the light source is altered. These summaries are set out to give some idea of the problem involved and for further details the reader is referred to the bibliography.

For practical purposes, mixing a variety of restorative materials in the anterior region of the mouth can only have a disappointing result and this must be appreciated when the treatment is planned. For example, attempting to match an acrylic denture tooth, thinly covering a metal attachment, to a porcelain or ceramo-metal crown, is a daunting task. At best it will only look reasonable under certain light conditions and that is assuming it does not break.

Methods of retention

At one time it was only the appearance of the retainers that was considered an aesthetic problem. The need to disguise retaining clasps while placing them inconspicuously in strategic points still applies today, but the methods available have been improved. Where buccal retainers are necessary, they can be placed in such a way that reflected light from them is minimised. Well-designed prostheses will reduce the bulk of any buccal retainers to a minimum. However, with the development of semi-precision and precision retainers, buccal arms can be virtually eliminated. Even so, the contours and method of construction of the crown need to be taken into account to prevent the introduction of aesthetic problems.

The path of insertion

The path of insertion selected for the removable prosthesis is a major element in its design. Apart from the important contacts between metal denture base and abutments, it determines the contours of the artificial mucosa. However, when attachments, overdentures, or telescopic prostheses are to be constructed the contour of these structures are determined by the path of insertion of the removable prosthesis. Unfortunately, these stages of treatment are often planned the wrong way around, with the abutments or copings being constructed before consideration has been given to this path.

Planning the path of insertion highlights the problems of integrating fixed and removable prostheses. Due to compartmentalised undergraduate education, the dental surgeon often prepares teeth for crowns and fixed prosthesis before considering the removable partial denture. Different commercial laboratories may be employed for fixed and removable components so that one might have the extraordinary situation of a technician in one laboratory aligning attachments or guide planes of a crown without any consideration of the design requirements of the partial denture. Unsightly gaps around abutments, together with inadequate base extension, are often found with the result disappointing both patient and practitioner (Fig. 403).

Long before any tooth preparation is made, the selection of the path of insertion should be made and marked on the diagnostic cast. All subsequent preparations can be undertaken with this pathway in mind.

Space

Space is possibly one of the most precious commodities in restorative dentistry. Errors in assessment can produce unsightly and ineffective restorations at best;

at worst the restoration may never reach the mouth.

Adequate vertical space around the abutments is required for the retention of abutment crowns, plaque control, guide planes, attachments, or other retainers, and for the artificial teeth themselves. Insufficient vertical space discovered late in prosthodontic therapy can produce devastating results for there can be few more unsightly restorations than a loose partial denture with its artificial teeth half the height of the abutments.

Buccolingual space measurement is critical where attachments are concerned. Last minute attempts to overcome these problems by means of paper thin facings and bulging contours are not only ugly, but prone to fracture as well.

Manual dexterity

Assessment of a patient's manual dexterity is not always easy. Patients may volunteer a history of accident proneness, or this may become apparent from a few moments conversation. Close observation of the patient during plaque control instruction may provide important clues.

Intracoronal precision attachments are relatively more difficult for a patient to manipulate than some of the extracoronal units. Furthermore, clumsy or careless manipulation of the prosthesis is more likely to damage this type of attachment and the damage can be almost impossible to repair if the female slot is distorted. Replacement of a male unit is possible, but complex, costly and difficult.

No attachment retaining system will with-

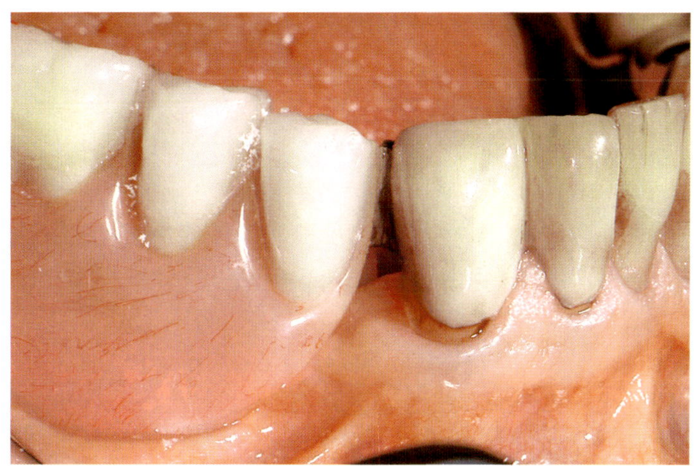

Fig. 403 Unsightly gap produced as a result of an incorrectly selected path of insertion. Elimination of the space will entail remaking the entire restoration.

stand a patient who attempts to bite a removable prosthesis into place; worse still is the individual who attempts to remove a prosthesis by levering it on one side and exerts enormous torque on the other through the major connector. The answer lies in patient education; but, if any lingering doubts remain, the clasp retainer should be considered carefully.

Extracoronal attachments that allow rotational movements also allow the initial insertion of the prosthesis close to the determined pathway before the components guide it into place. This slight freedom can be useful for a wide group of individuals whose manual dexterity may be slightly suspect, despite good intentions.

Rebasing and relining

Rebasing may be considered replacement of the entire impression surface of the denture; relining involves replacement of part of it. Either way, any laboratory procedure that involves curing the denture base introduces potential problems with accuracy and possible alteration of occlusal position or attachment alignment.

Surprisingly, dentures retained by intracoronal attachments are relatively straightforward to rebase or reline. The reasons are that the relationship between the denture base and the abutments are clearly established by the attachments—if the attachments are completely seated the relationship must be correct. Furthermore, intracoronal attachments are generally soldered to the major connector of the denture, thereby eliminating any possible malalignment as a result of processing changes.

It is often claimed that dentures retained by intracoronal attachments require less frequent rebasing than those retained by extracoronal units. Some advocate that the entire impression surface of the denture be metal covered, thereby making it virtually impossible to rebase. It will, however, be easier to maintain plaque free. Jaw relationships, base extension and the care with which the mouth is prepared and the denture constructed are probably the answers to this claim, which is unsupported by scientific evidence. It is true, however, that extracoronal attachments allowing hinge movement are more difficult to rebase. Furthermore, failure to rebase in time could lead to a vicious circle of an unstable base contributing to bone resorption and still more instability.

Fractured dentures

The most common type of damage is fracture of the acrylic resin surrounding an attachment. This is often traced to poor treatment planning with inadequate space provided. Before attempting repair, the cause of the fracture should be ascertained and eliminated as far as possible. With certain extracoronal units, like the Dalbo or Ceka attachments, it may be possible to substitute smaller male units that occupy less vertical space. Metal occlusal and lingual surfaces may be required to provide adequate strength.

Since the proximal surfaces of an attachment retained denture are critical, an overall locating impression will be required. Locating dowels must be placed over any extracoronal unit before casting this impression.

Fracture of a major connector is more serious as it usually represents a design or casting fault. Distortion of the major connector usually requires the operator to section it to allow the two bases to be placed correctly in position. The two ends of the connector should be covered with Duralay, or other hard resin, before the entire denture is removed with an overall impression. A rigid impression material, such as Impregum or plaster, is best for this purpose and the locating dowels should not be overlooked.

Once a master cast has been prepared, a new major connector can be produced. Only rarely will soldering be worthwhile as, in many instances, this would require burning off the entire acrylic work.

Fractures of attachments themselves are remarkably rare. When they do occur, replacement of the removable units will be required according to the methods outlined. It is a tribute to the attachment manufacturers that failure of properly used components forming part of the abutments are almost unknown.

Problems with attachment-retained prostheses simply highlight the complexities of the science and art of prosthodontics. Once the principles of sound prosthodontic treatment are established, attachments have an extremely important and worthwhile part to play in the treatment of the partially dentate mouth.

References and further reading

Frush J. P. and Fischer R. (1959).
Dentogenics: its practical application. J. Prosthet. Dent., 9: 6, 914.

Goldstein R. E. (1976).
Esthetics in dentistry. J. P. Lippincott Co., Philadelphia, Pa.

Grajower R., Revah A. and Sorin S. (1976).
Reflectance spectra of natural and acrylic resin teeth. J. Prosthet. Dent., 36: 5, 570.

Krajicek D. D. (1969).
Dental art in prosthodontics. J. Prosthet. Dent., 21: 2: 122.

Lee J. H. (1962).
Dental Aestetics. John Wright & Sons Ltd., Bristol, England.

Lemire P. A. and Burk B. (1976).
Color in Dentistry. J. M. Ney Co., Bloomfield, New Jersey.

Lombardi R. E. (1973).
The principles of visual perception and their clinical application to denture esthetics. J. Prosthet. Dent., 29: 4, 358.

Lombardi R. E. (1974).
A method for the classification of errors in dental esthetics. J. Prosthet. Dent., 32: 5, 501.

McLean J. W. (1979).
The Science and Art of Dental Ceramics. Volume I Quintessence Publishing, Chicago, Ill.

J. D. Preston (1984).
Dental aesthetics: an objective consideration. In Proceedings of the International Prosthodontic Symposium: 'Restoration of the Partially Dentate Mouth'. (Bates J. F., Neill D. J., Preiskel H. W. eds.) Quintessence Publishing, Berlin.

Sproull R. C. (1973).
Color matching in dentistry: I. The three-dimensional nature of color. J. Prosthet. Dent., 29: 4: 416.

Sproull R. C. (1973).
Color matching in dentistry: II. Practical applications of the organization of color. J. Prosthet. Dent., 29: 5: 556.

Zarb G. A., Bergman B., Clayton J. and MacKay H. F. (1978).
Prosthodontic Treatment for Partially Edentulous Patients. C. V. Mosby Co., St. Louis, Mo.

Appendix

This book concerns the principles of attachment application, employing individual units as examples. The reader should thus be enabled to assess the relative merits of manufactured units and apply them to the restoration of his patient's mouth. Attachment designs change from time to time but the principles are unlikely to vary. The following list may not be complete and is provided solely for the convenience of readers.

Attachment Manufacturers

Ancorvis, Galleria del Oro 3, Bologna, I-40100.

J. Bird Moyer Co. Philadelphia, PA 19132 USA.

Ceka N. V. Maria Henriettalei 6–8, bus 5, B-2000, Antwerpen, Belgium.

Cendres et Métaux SA, Rue de Boujean 122, Biel-Bienne 2501, Switzerland.

Columbia Dentoform Corporation, 49 East 21st Street, New York, NY 10010, USA.

Degussa, Geschäftsbereich Dental, D-6000 Frankfurt (Main), Germany.

J. F. Jelenko & Co. Inc., 170 Petersville Road, New Rochelle, New York 10801, USA.

Cav. G. Lipparini, Piazza Calderini 2/2, Bologna, Italy.

Métaux Précieux SA, Avenue du Vignoble 2, CH-2000 Neuchâtel, Switzerland.

D & R Miner Dental, 14 Lavina Court Orinda, CA 94563 USA.

Precision Attachments Ltd., 1114 Hillside Road, West Vancouver 237, B.C. Canada.

Reliant Dental Mfg. Co. Worth, Illinois, USA.

APM Sterngold, 320 Washington Street, Mt. Vernon, New York, 10553, USA.

The J. M. Ney Co., Maplewood Avenue, Bloomfield, Connecticut, 06002, USA.

Ultratek Attachments and Technology Inc., 1041 Shary, Circle, Concord, California 94518, USA.

Usine Genevoise De Dégroississage d'Or, Place Volontaires 4, CH-1211, Geneva 11, Switzerland.

Attachment Selectors

Whaledent International, 236 Fifth Avenue, New York, NY 10001, USA.

Bell International Inc., 1320 Marston Road, Burlingame, CA 90401, USA.

Index